PHYSICAL FITNESS
The Pathway to Healthful Living

SEVENTH EDITION

ROBERT V. HOCKEY, Ed.D.

Professor
Department of Physical Education and Athletics
Trinity University
San Antonio, Texas

with 255 illustrations

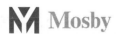 Mosby

St. Louis Baltimore Boston Chicago London Philadelphia Sydney Toronto

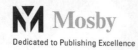

Dedicated to Publishing Excellence

Editor-in-Chief: James M. Smith
Acquisitions Editor: Vicki Malinee
Developmental Editor: Cathy Waller
Project Manager: Karen A. Edwards
Production Editor: Amy Adams Squire Strongheart
Designer: Liz Fett
Manufacturing Supervisor: Theresa Fuchs

SEVENTH EDITION

Printed in the United States of America

Mosby–Year Book, Inc.
11830 Westline Industrial Drive
St. Louis, Missouri 63146

Library of Congress Cataloging-in-Publication Data

Hockey, Robert V.
   Physical fitness : the pathway to healthful living / Robert
V. Hockey. —7th ed.
     p. cm.
   Includes bibliographical references and index.
   ISBN 0-8016-6566-3
   1. Aerobic exercises. 2. Physical fitness. 3. Health.
I. Title.
RA781.15.H63 1993   92-40451
613.7—dc20   CIP

94 95 96 97 GW/DC/DC 9 8 7 6 5 4 3 2

Foreword

Many complex factors contribute to a person's healthful lifestyle and performance. Dr. Robert V. Hockey has magnificently captured the essence of what it takes to become physically fit, splendidly depicting the conceptual way to achieve success.

Nothing is as powerful as the idea whose time has come. The conceptual approach of "coaching a person," using scientifically based exercise and medical programs is the key to success. Dr. Hockey has demonstrated his brilliance in capturing this approach.

Physical Fitness: The Pathway to Healthful Living is a real pearl of knowledge. Its practical approach to making complicated medical and physiological data understandable by graphically displaying the material is unique. The reader is greatly rewarded with the opportunity to structure his or her own personal lifetime wellness program.

Today, more than ever before, each of us needs a guidebook for fitness. Although we have reached astonishing heights through medical research, enabling us to treat diseases that were not treatable just 10 years ago, hypokinetic disease plagues our society because we don't get enough exercise to live a quality life. In addition, approximately 80% of American schoolchildren could not pass the 1991 President's Council on Physical Fitness evaluation. These alarming data indicate that a national health care crisis exists.

The great philosopher, Socrates, believed that all individuals have an obligation to society to take care of their health. Dr. Hockey has provided an ideal source to help you improve your fitness and health. Chapter 6, Nutrition and Fitness, will provide lifelong, valuable information. The chapters on exercise, flexibility, and weight and stress management; Key Terms; and Laboratory Experiences provide you with the key ingredients for a productive fitness program. The book is a must for your personal and professional growth.

LARRY THIRSTRUP, M.D., M.Ed.
Founder of Medical Fitness Centers of America

Preface

Most Americans are now aware that they can greatly influence their state of health with everyday decisions, particularly those relating to exercise and nutrition. However, it is apparent that many of them either do not know how to improve their health or else just lack the motivation to improve it.

"I would like to exercise regularly and eat better, but I just can't get myself to do it." I hear this statement just about every day from students who have a hard time finding time to exercise regularly and who are often fighting to control their body weight. Many of them have been on one diet or another, and yet they have experienced very little success because they lack the discipline necessary to establish consistent habits relative to exercise and nutrition.

One problem is that there is so much conflicting information available that the average person has a hard time knowing what to believe. *Physical Fitness: The Pathway to Healthful Living* contains accurate, scientific information about exercise, nutrition, health, and fitness. This information is presented in the hope that the reader will become more knowledgeable concerning each of these, will evaluate the information objectively, and will then make a wise decision about the importance of each related factor.

With the increased mechanization of modern society, the body does less and less physical work. Therefore everyday tasks must be supplemented with a systematic exercise program. The emphasis throughout this book is on aerobic exercise—activities that stimulate the heart and circulatory system and develop cardiovascular endurance. The added health benefits associated with an optimal level of cardiovascular fitness are clearly identified.

Although the primary emphasis is on cardiovascular fitness, the other health-related physical fitness components of strength, muscular endurance, flexibility, and body composition are also discussed in detail. In addition, the importance of nutrition and stress management is emphasized.

By understanding the material presented in this book, the reader should:
- Become more knowledgeable concerning exercise, nutrition, health, and fitness
- Be able to assess his or her present habits and status relative to each of these
- Learn how to make appropriate changes in his or her lifestyle to promote optimal health and wellness

Physical Fitness: The Pathway to Healthful Living is one of the few physical fitness textbooks currently on the market that has enjoyed the success of six previous editions.

AUDIENCE

Many universities and colleges across the country offer an introductory course emphasizing the scientific approach to exercise and fitness. These classes have titles such as "Concepts of Lifetime Fitness" and often combine lectures and laboratory experience. This book is designed primarily for use in these classes. In addition, it provides useful background information for students interested in exercise physiology and/or sports medicine.

The growing interest in recent years in health and wellness has prompted a tremendous increase in the number of health clubs and exercise facilities. Because of the lack of knowledge by participants, these clubs have been forced to offer classes in weight management and physical fitness. Very few books with accurate scientific information in this field have been written for the general public. Most have been written specifically for college students. The material presented in this book is designed to serve the needs not only of college students but also of all those interested in fitness and nutrition, regardless of their background and experience. What people like most about this book is the simple way in which complex information is presented.

NEW TO THIS EDITION

The seventh edition has been planned carefully, and comments and suggestions from the many instructors who have used this book have been implemented in the revision.

Major changes include the following:
- Self-assessment laboratory information is included at the back of each chapter to ensure greater continuity within each chapter. This includes questionnaires; worksheets; and simple, practical tests that readers can take to see how they rate. There is at least one Laboratory Experience included with each chapter.
- A new chapter—Chapter 8, Weight Management—synthesizes much of the current information into a unique weight management program that can be easily implemented by those who need to lose weight and/or body fat. A new self-evaluation form allows individuals to accurately determine the consistency of their exercise and eating habits.
- The addition of many new line drawings and photographs helps to clarify the text. There are now over 250 illustrations in this edition.
- The chapter on stress management includes relaxation techniques, warning signs of stress, coping strategies, effective ways to deal with stress, and physical and physiological effects of stress on the body.
- A new Food Composition Table and Fast Food Composition Table are listed in the appendixes to provide quick reference on the nutrient value of a variety of foods.
- Objectives included at the beginning of each chapter identify important concepts. These are stated in terms of what each student should be able to do when he or she understands the material contained in the chapter.
- A summary is included at the end of each chapter to help students review the important concepts.

SUPPLEMENTS
Instructor's manual

An Instructor's Manual is available for use with this textbook. It contains a course outline, a proposed schedule of classes, and suggestions for grading. This material should help the instructor to organize a class.

A section is also included on each chapter, including a chapter summary; identification of important topics; proposed class activities; discussion topics; and a series of short answer, essay, and multiple choice questions that can be used to evaluate students.

Physical fitness software package

The Physical Fitness Software Program provides a computerized printout for many of the self-evaluation activities included in the book. It is available free to qualified adopters.

ACKNOWLEDGEMENTS

Over the past 23 years I have become indebted to many people for the development and production of this textbook. Without their help, it would never have materialized, and this revision would not have been possible.

I am particularly indebted to Vicki Malinee, Cathy Waller, and Cheryl Gelfand-Grant at Mosby–Year Book College Publishing. They have been very patient, helpful, and understanding.

I would also like to thank the following reviewers for their valuable input. Each of them will be able to read the book and identify changes and additions that are the direct result of their comments and suggestions:

Dr. Thomas Battinelli
Fitchburg State College
Fitchburg, Massachusetts

Thomas G. Phillips
Saint Leo College
Saint Leo, Florida

Charges H. Manes
Thiel College
Greenville, Pennsylvania

Lori D. Richards
Utah Valley Community College
Orem, Utah

Dr. Gary Oden
Sam Houston State University
Huntsville, Texas

Dr. Jerry Stieger
Valparaiso University
Valparaiso, Indiana

New photographs for this edition were taken by David Garza, and the subjects were Dina Aitken, Jesse Sturgeon, Linda Baker, Marsha Marcus, and Lori Siemen. I am indebted to the Concord Athletic Club in San Antonio, Texas, for permission to use their facilities to take the new photographs. The new line drawings for this addition were rendered by Clate Grunden, a student at Trinity University, and by Betsy Cooper.

I am also grateful to Margaret Boman, Amy Heckathorn, Carol Etzel, and Hugh Lewis for their assistance and to my good friend, Dr. Larry Thirstrup, the founder of Medical Fitness Centers of America, for graciously writing the foreword for this edition.

The following individuals made valuable contributions to previous editions of this book: Dennis Hickey, Jerry Morrow, Betsy Gross, Marilyn Peterson, Rico Zenti, Georgia Horton, Shirley Reucher, Carol Laituri, Martha Shine, Shirley Rushing, Dr. Jesse MacLeay, Jane Blake, Don Pavloski, Susan Wilson, David A. Young, John Rodriguez, and Jeannine Pfluger. I also appreciate the constant help and understanding from my wife Judy and my children Michael and Dianne.

Finally, I owe much to the many students with whom I have come in contact in college classes during the past 28 years and to the people with whom I have worked in adult physical fitness classes, weight management classes, and health and fitness clubs throughout the country. The feedback I have received from these people and the data I have accumulated over the years have been invaluable in the preparation of this book.

ROBERT V. HOCKEY

Contents

Exercise and Physical Fitness

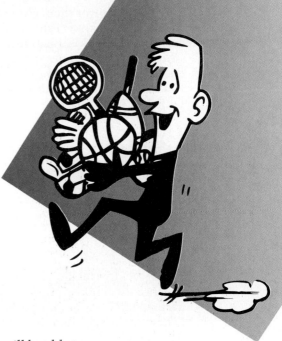

CHAPTER OBJECTIVES

When you understand the material in this chapter, you will be able to:

- Explain why so many Americans are unfit despite the all-time high interest in exercise, physical fitness, and nutrition
- Discuss the importance of exercise in today's world and explain why it is more important today than it was in the past
- Identify the positive changes that take place in the body as a result of regular exercise and explain why an active body is a more efficient body
- Identify the prominent health problems associated with lack of activity that are "lifestyle induced" and know how these can be prevented
- Define physical fitness and identify

and define each of the five health-related components
- Subjectively determine whether you have at least an adequate level of physical fitness and understand fully the benefits of striving to achieve an optimal level
- Determine your present status concerning diet and nutrition, stress, exercise and weight control, smoking, alcohol and drug use, and health and safety so that you know which of these areas need to be improved
- Identify positive changes you can make in your lifestyle that will greatly influence your health and wellness

During the last decade we have discovered that good health is no longer a matter of chance, but rather a matter of choice. If *you* choose to take responsibility for your health by exercising regularly and by consistently adopting other positive lifestyle habits, you can not only promote better health, but also you can decrease your risk of disease, disability, and premature death. Perhaps this is the reason why enthusiasm for exercise and fitness and interest in nutrition is presently at an all-time high in the United States.[16]

Although most Americans recognize the importance of regular exercise and good nutrition, many of them either do not know what to do or else they lack the motivation to do it. "I know I should exercise regularly and eat better, but I just can't get myself to do it." This is a statement that I hear just about every day from college students who seldom find time to exercise and who blame college life for their poor eating habits or from adults enrolled in weight management programs who have not found time to exercise consistently and who have constantly been on one diet or another, with very little success.

> In a recent national survey, 85% of the American adult population agreed with the following statement: "I can do more for my health by what I do and what I eat than anything doctors or medicine can do."[27]

In recent years, because of increased mechanization, the need for regular exercise has increased; however, many of us, because of our busy lifestyle, do not make time available to exercise. Because of this we never achieve an adequate level of physical fitness, and we frequently suffer from diseases associated with inactivity. One of the basic problems is that there is so much conflicting information available, that we have a hard time knowing what to believe, and, in many cases, we just do not know what to do.

Because of this, we wind up doing nothing. Almost 80% of the American adult population admit that they need assistance if they are to make a commitment to change their exercise and eating habits.

By understanding the material in this book, you will become more knowledgeable concerning health, physical fitness, and exercise and nutrition, and you will learn how you can positively influence your health. However, in addition to learning what to do, you must be willing to implement these changes in your lifestyle. This will take motivation and dedication, but the end result will be worthwhile. You will be a winner.

> Unfortunately, many of us spend more time worrying about our health than we spend taking steps to improve it.

CURRENT TRENDS IN EXERCISE AND FITNESS

The present exercise-fitness revolution is now almost 25 years old. It was probably initiated in part in 1968 when Dr. Kenneth Cooper's first book, *Aerobics*, was published. This book helped the American public to understand the importance of aerobic fitness and challenged them to counter the epidemics of heart disease, obesity, and other health-related problems.

Early in the 1970s a national survey indicated that almost 60% of all adults in the United States did not participate in any form of physical activity.[26] From that time on, it would appear as if millions of Americans have taken up the exercise challenge in an attempt to get in shape and to improve their health[1,8] (Fig. 1-1).

The results from surveys such as this, however, tend to be misleading. A closer look at the most recent statistics shows that the average number of days of participation was fewer than 6 per month for each participant. This is insufficient for the development of aerobic fitness and would tend to support the conclusion of Brooks that "most Americans are not knowledgeable about the frequency, duration and intensity recommended for exercise to strengthen the heart and lungs."[5] The results from her survey show that approximately 60% of adults do not exercise regularly, and yet more than 80% of them consider themselves to be active and are "somewhat" or "very" satisfied with their fitness level.

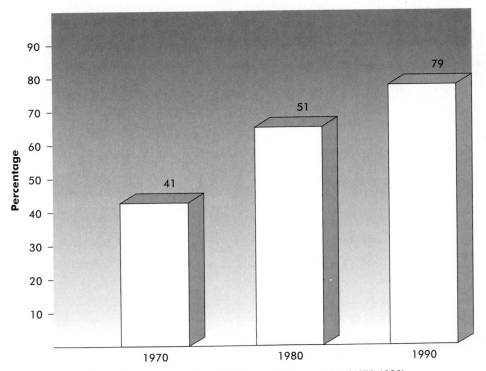

Fig. 1-1 Percentage of adults "involved" in exercise (1970-1990).

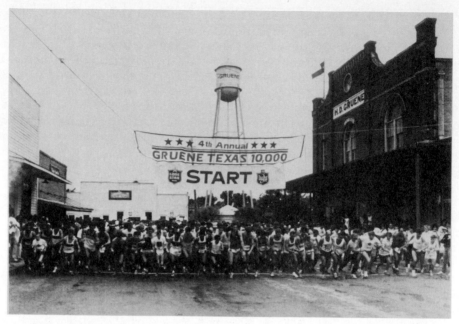

Fig. 1-2 More people than ever before are participating in some form of exercise.

Several other surveys have been completed.[15,16] However, the problem is that many of them lack consistency relative to the procedures involved. Despite this drawback, it would appear that the following summary best depicts the situation that presently exists in the United States relative to participation in various forms of physical activity[24]:

- Of American adults, 35% exercise on a regular basis at the required intensity and duration to result in maximal aerobic development.
- Of American adults, 35% exercise less frequently and at a lower level of intensity, probably not frequently enough and not strenuously enough to develop or maintain desirable levels of aerobic fitness.
- Of American adults, 30% do not participate in any organized physical activity and could be classified as sedentary.

(See Fig. 1-2.)

Despite the widespread fitness boom, far too few Americans get sufficient strenuous exercise, and the average American is far from fit.

Why so many Americans are unfit

Most Americans are aware of the benefits that can be derived from regular exercise, and many of them intend to exercise more, but for one reason or another, they just do not get around to doing this. One problem with changing their current habits is that the present lifestyle of people has little effect on their health now. The absence of any immediate effect is a serious barrier to change. However, individuals must remember that they are building or laying the foundation for what their health will be 20, 30, or 40 years from now.

Excuses for nonexercise. More than half of those who recognize the importance of exercise never actually take the time to exercise on a regular basis. There are many excuses used in an attempt to justify this:

"I don't have the time."
"I work hard all day, and I am too tired."
"It is inconvenient."
"My lifestyle is busy enough; I don't need exercise."
"I am too old."
"I am out of shape."
"I just don't enjoy exercise."
"I don't like to sweat."
"Exercise will mess up my hair."
"When I exercise I get sore muscles."
"It is too late to change the way I live."

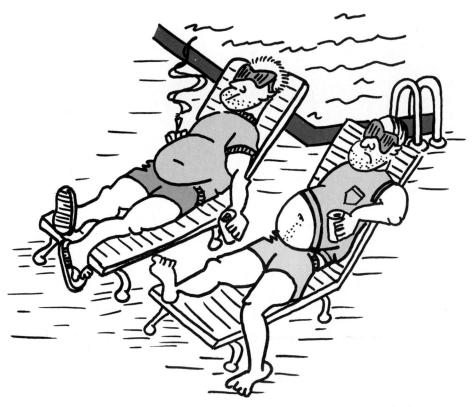

If I knew life was going to be this good, I would have taken better care of my body.

Lack of sufficient time is by far the most common excuse. All it takes is a minimum of 20 minutes of aerobic exercise, every other day to stay in "reasonable shape." If a person believes strongly enough in exercise, he or she will make time available to participate in an activity program on a regular basis. Unfortunately, too few Americans believe strongly enough to do this. Lack of time, obviously, is not as big a problem as lack of desire or lack of self-discipline.

The President's Council on Physical Fitness suggests several ways to persuading people to exercise regularly:

- Show them how to fit exercise into their busy schedules.
- Convince older people that age is not a barrier to exercise.
- Appeal to their concern for health and an attractive appearance.
- Convince them that exercise can be enjoyable.
- Present more information to them on the types of exercise that are best and the amount of exercise necessary to develop and maintain adequate fitness.

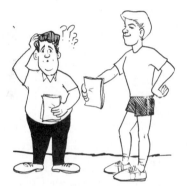

Each of us can program our daily activities to positively influence our health and well-being.

For most people the major problem is "finding time" to exercise. When the schedule gets tight and there are specific things to do at school, at work, or at home, exercise is usually the first thing to go. We rationalize by saying that we will get back to it tomorrow, or the day after when things settle down. Unfortunately, for many of us, this never happens. There is no reason why you cannot schedule exercise each day just like you schedule other activities.

It is now well documented that those who are well informed about exercise and nutrition tend to be more active than those who are not, and they also make more intelligent decisions each day. It should be emphasized at this time, however, that having knowledge is not enough. More than 95% of entering college freshmen "indicate" that exercise is important to them. These students also claim that the attainment of an "adequate" level of physical fitness is a worthwhile objective. However, when these issues are investigated further, the results are rather confusing. Less than 30% of these same students exercise regularly, and even a lower percentage believe that they presently have even an adequate level of physical fitness.

Obviously consistency is important in any exercise program. Those who wait until they "find" time to exercise very seldom develop the consistency that is necessary to be successful.

Finding time to exercise is a problem for many college students. Classes, study, assignments, dating, and other commitments place heavy demands on their time, and, if they work part-time, as many of them do, this makes it even more difficult for them to find time to exercise regularly. In many cases, students who do not exercise regularly find that they have a higher level of stress, they tend to gain weight more readily, and they are frequently sick. These can detract from their success, and college life often becomes a struggle. On the other hand, exercise can contribute to their success by making them more alert and productive and by reducing their level of stress and in general making college life "more enjoyable."[25]

> Whether or not you exercise regularly will be determined by whether or not you believe strongly enough that exercise is important to you. If you do, you will find the time necessary to participate on a regular basis.

THE IMPORTANCE OF EXERCISE

The following are three good reasons why exercise should be important to you:
1. The body functions more efficiently if it is active.
2. Many of our leisure activities are sedentary in nature.
3. Inactivity contributes to many of the prominent health problems that exist today.

Efficiency of an active body

Modern technology has resulted in a substantial decrease in the number of tasks that require a significant expenditure of energy.

- Driving has replaced walking. (Note the number of people who have become so lazy that they will circle the parking lot several times to obtain a parking place close to where they are going.)
- The majority of the working population are now involved in positions requiring mental rather than physical work.
- People use escalators or elevators at airports, stores, and office buildings, rather than walking up or down the stairs or just simply walking.
- Many of the daily household tasks have become mechanized, for example, mowing the yard and washing dishes and clothes.

The result of this is that the tasks of daily life no longer provide sufficient vigorous activity to develop and maintain adequate levels of physical fitness, and we must now go out of our way to "program" exercise back into our lifestyle. This is important because our body was designed and constructed for movement and vigorous activity, not for rest. It functions more efficiently when it is active. Notice what happens when an arm or leg is placed in a cast and not used for an extended period. The muscle mass decreases in size, resulting in loss of strength, endurance, and flexibility. It is obvious that as far as the body is concerned "that which is used becomes stronger and that which is not becomes weaker."

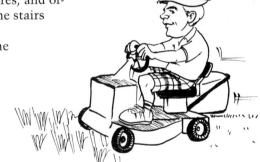

Lack of activity is prevalent in today's society.

Many factors are involved in helping the body to become stronger and more efficient. However, the underlying principle is that the functioning of the body requires

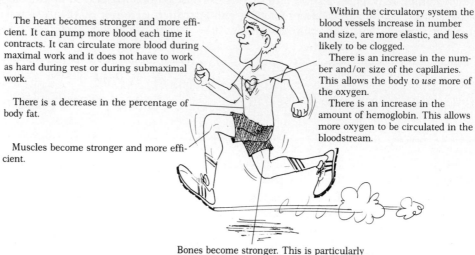

The heart becomes stronger and more efficient. It can pump more blood each time it contracts. It can circulate more blood during maximal work and it does not have to work as hard during rest or during submaximal work.

There is a decrease in the percentage of body fat.

Muscles become stronger and more efficient.

Within the circulatory system the blood vessels increase in number and size, are more elastic, and less likely to be clogged.

There is an increase in the number and/or size of the capillaries. This allows the body to *use* more of the oxygen.

There is an increase in the amount of hemoglobin. This allows more oxygen to be circulated in the bloodstream.

Bones become stronger. This is particularly important for women who face a higher risk of osteoporosis—a degenerative bone disease.

Fig. 1-3 With regular exercise our bodies function more efficiently.

energy, which in turn depends on the ability of the heart, lungs, and blood vessels to process oxygen and deliver it to the muscles, where it becomes the fuel for energy If you exercise regularly, your body is able to process and use greater amounts of oxygen because the intake and supply channels have become more efficient. Some of the changes in the body that result in an increase in efficiency are summarized in Fig. 1-3.

Stated simply, a person who does not exercise regularly may lack sufficient energy to perform simple everyday tasks such as sitting, standing, and walking. This is because the body functions inefficiently and is therefore forced to "overwork" to provide the energy necessary for the performance of these tasks. A person who exercises regularly will have an extra energy reserve because of the increase in effciency

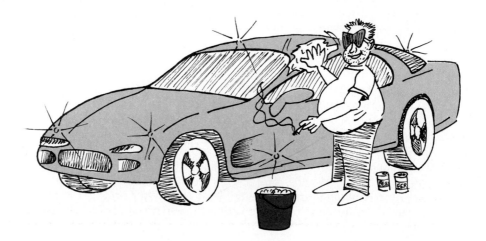

of the functioning of the body. This person will have more drive and increased energy, will feel good, and possibly will be more productive.

Most people take better care of their automobiles than they do of their own bodies. They depend on their cars and they want them to look good, go fast, and last a long time. Yet, unlike the automobile, the human body comes with no guarantees or trade-ins in case it wears out prematurely. There are many people who frequently neglect the preventive maintenance necessary for their body to function efficiently. The old saying "If you don't use it, you lose it" certainly applies to your body in relation to physical fitness.

The sedentary nature of leisure activities

With increased mechanization, many tasks that once required physical work and a considerable amount of time can now be accomplished very quickly by pushing a button or setting a dial. Additional time is therefore available for leisure activities. The problem, however, is that many of our leisure activities are sedentary.

Many of our leisure-time activities
have suddenly become inactive.

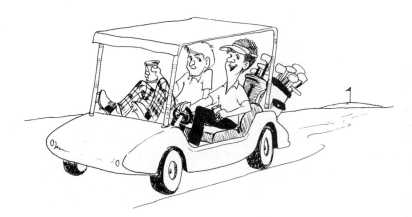

Adults and children spend a considerable amount of leisure time using the home computer or playing video games. Previously, much of this time was spent more actively. Because of increased mechanization and changes in the use of our leisure time, it is now important to program vigorous, sustained physical activity into our daily schedules if we are to achieve and maintain an optimal level of physical fitness.

Consider the following statistics relative to television viewing[10]:

AVERAGE TELEVISION VIEWING	(HOURS PER WEEK)
Older women	37
Older men	33
Younger women	32
Younger men	28
Teens (12 to 17)	23
Children (2 to 11)	25

Prominent health problems associated with inactivity

The sedentary way of life has had a negative effect on the human body and has been associated with many serious health problems. These are often referred to as **hypokinetic diseases**. The following are of specific interest:

- Cardiovascular disease
- Hypertension
- Obesity
- Diabetes
- Low back pain

Cardiovascular disease. The United States still has the highest incidence of cardiovascular disease in the world. The most recent figures released by the American Heart Association indicate that 44% of all deaths in this country can be attributed to cardiovascular diseases (945,000 deaths per year).[18] This is true despite the fact that there are over 200,000 coronary bypass operations per year. Research has clearly shown that regular vigorous physical activity is associated with a reduced overall risk of coronary heart disease and that the rate of sudden cardiac death is lessened in those who exercise regularly compared with those who are inactive. This positive effect of exercise has been shown to be independent of such other risk factors as smoking, obesity, and hypertension.[33]

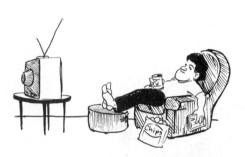

The number one reason for inactivity given by those who recognize that they do not get enough exercise is "insufficient time."

Hypertension. Approximately 60 million Americans have elevated blood pressure, thereby increasing their risk of death and illness. Several research studies have shown that regular physical activity can reduce the risk of developing hypertension and that exercise can be used to control hypertension.

Obesity/Overweight. Sixty-four percent of the adult population can now be considered overweight or obese.[28] This figure has shown an increase every year since 1987. Substantial research shows that physical activity is positively associated with weight control, and it is well established that those who are more active weigh less than those who are sedentary.

Diabetes. Diabetes is one of the most common afflictions of modern society. Approximately 11 million Americans suffer from some form of this disease. Recent research shows that physical activity results in certain metabolic and hormonal changes within the body that might prevent or postpone the development of certain forms of diabetes. Over 80% of adult-onset diabetes occurs in individuals who are obese and/or overweight.[24]

Low back pain. The incidence of low back pain in the United States continues to increase. It has been estimated that 75 million Americans suffer from low back pain, with a resulting cost of over $1 billion in lost productivity and $250 million in worker's compensation each year. It has also been estimated that over 80% of all low back pain problems are caused by improper muscle development.

The basic premise of this book is that exercise is not only good for you but also essential if you are going to function efficiently and achieve an optimal level of **physical fitness**. The information presented in this book will allow you to develop your own individualized exercise program. If exercise is really important to you, you will then participate regularly in this exercise program.

It can clearly be seen that several of today's most serious health problems are the result of our sedentary way of life and that indeed "exercise may be the cheapest preventative medicine in the world."

WHAT IS PHYSICAL FITNESS?

Despite the widespread interest in physical fitness, it is still difficult to define. The average person does not know exactly what physical fitness is, what level of fitness he or she needs to achieve, how to develop that level of physical fitness, or how to evaluate his or her present level of physical fitness.

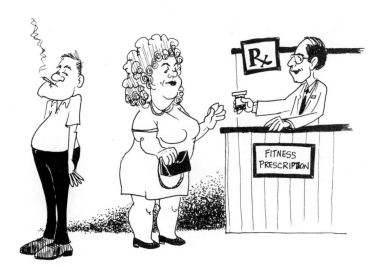

If fitness came in a pill, it would be the most widely prescribed medicine by far.

Physical fitness has frequently been defined as "the ability to carry out everyday tasks with vigor and alertness, without undue fatigue, and with ample energy to enjoy leisure-time pursuits and to meet unforeseen emergencies."[6] The problem with this definition is that our modern way of life has changed. We have seen that many of our everyday tasks now require very little energy expenditure and several of our leisure-time pursuits that once involved a reasonable amount of energy expenditure now require considerably less.

It would appear that a high level of fitness may no longer be needed to work in today's world dominated by technological innovations.[24] Therefore if physical fitness is defined as the level of fitness needed to function in modern society, a large percentage of the American adult population would be considered physically fit. As you will see later in this chapter, this definition can be used to define what would be considered to be an *adequate* level of physical fitness.

Physical fitness means different things to different people. It must be viewed as an individual matter and as such has little meaning unless considered in relation to the specific needs and interests of each individual. Consider what physical fitness means to the following five people.

1. Shirley, a 21-year-old secretary, participates four times each week in an aerobic dance class. She is single, and her major reason for exercise is to maintain a neat trim figure.
2. Jim is a 30-year-old construction worker. He is very strong, has well-developed muscles and appears to have very little body fat. He does not participate in any organized exercise program because he feels that he gets all the physical activity he needs each day at work.
3. Jean is a 40-year-old "avid runner." Her objective is to someday complete a marathon in less than 3 hours. She runs between 40 and 50 miles each week.
4. George is a 45-year-old man who is presently recovering from heart bypass surgery. His exercise program consists of 20 minutes of slow walking, 4 days per week, to improve the functioning of his cardiorespiratory system.
5. Ann is a 20-year-old varsity tennis player who feels that if she is going to reach her potential and compete at the national level, she must practice her skills on the tennis court 2 to 3 hours per day, at least 5 days per week.

To each of these people physical fitness would appear to be important, but it is apparent that each of them views it somewhat differently.

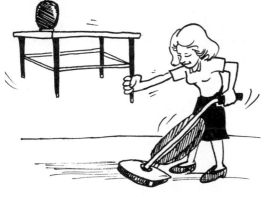

Performance of everyday tasks with vigor and alertness.

They would probably all agree with the statements that "regular exercise is good for you" and that "it is good to be physically fit." It should also be clear that physical fitness is not the same for everyone. It is a desirable quality that can be developed in numerous ways for a variety of reasons.

It may be beneficial to find a way to quantify physical fitness. A logical approach might be to consider physical fitness as existing on a scale, or continuum. A person who is seriously ill and who needs help to function would possess a very minimal level, whereas a highly conditioned person would be close to the maximal level. This concept is suggested by Clarke and Clarke,[6] who state that "physical fitness is a positive and dynamic quality extending on a continuum from 'death' to 'abundant life'." This concept is illustrated in Table 1-1, where physical fitness is represented on a 10-point scale. The table is arbitrarily divided into the following five categories:

1. Maximal
2. High
3. Adequate
4. Minimal
5. Very low

TABLE 1-1 Physical fitness continuum

Criteria	Category/Rating*		Activity criteria
Maximization of your functional capacity	Maximal	10	Able to complete an hour or more of high-intensity aerobic activity and still have energy left at the completion of the activity
Highly conditioned person		9	Excels in all physical fitness components
Energy for vigorous well-rounded life	High	8	Able to complete at least an hour of organized aerobic activity and not feel tired at the end or following the exercise
Increased energy and vitality		7	
Able to make the most of what life has to offer			Exhibits high ratings on physical fitness components
Ability to function normally without undue fatigue	Adequate	6	Able to complete at least 30 minutes of aerobic activity. May be tired or fatigued at the end or following the activity
Some energy left at the end of the day		5	Average ability on all physical fitness components
Barely able to perform everday tasks	Minimal	4	Unable to complete 30 or more of continuous aerobic activity
Little or no energy left at end of day		3	Performs less than average on several of the physical fitness components
Tires easily in completing daily tasks			
Seriously ill	Very low	2	Cannot participate in any form of exercise on a regular basis
Heart problems		1	Cannot complete most of the physical fitness tests
Often needs help to function			
Unfit for work			

*Circle the score that you feel best represents your present level of physical fitness.

Notice that specific criteria are presented relative to each of these categories, and an attempt is made to relate each category to the amount of exercise that is possible.

We have seen that there is an optimal level of efficiency for the functioning of the body and that it is only through regular, sustained physical activity that this can be achieved. To achieve this, it would appear that your level of physical fitness would have to be classified as "high" or "maximal" according to the criteria presented in Table 1-1. These are the levels of fitness for which everyone should strive.

COMPONENTS OF PHYSICAL FITNESS

There has been much confusion in past years as to what the components of physical fitness actually are. To clarify the situation, existing components have been grouped in two categories—health-related and skill-related.

Health-related physical fitness components

It is now generally agreed that only those components that contribute to the development of health and that increase the functional capacity of the body will be classified as health-related physical fitness components. These are identified in Fig. 1-4.

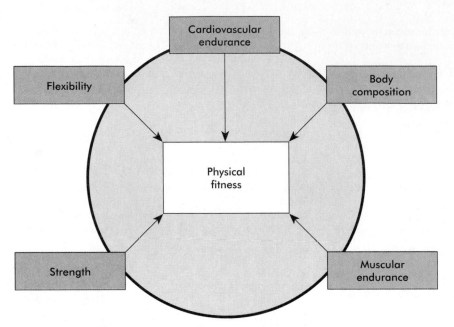

Fig. 1-4 Health-related physical fitness components.

Skill-related physical fitness components

There are several essential components for the successful execution of various sport skills, often referred to as *skill-related*, or *performance-related*:

1. Agility
2. Balance
3. Coordination
4. Speed
5. Power
6. Reaction time

Highly skilled athletes possess an extremely high level of these components. It should be emphasized, though, that a high degree of athletic ability is not essential for the development and maintenance of physical fitness because there are many activities that can be included in your physical fitness program that require minimal amounts of skill. However, for those who thrive on competition and who have a reasonable level of skill, several activities are excellent for development of physical fitness (Fig. 1-5 on p. 15).

a suitcase. Your level of muscular endurance will determine how long you can carry the suitcase. If you are constantly experiencing sore or aching muscles, this is probably an indication that you need to improve your level of muscular endurance.

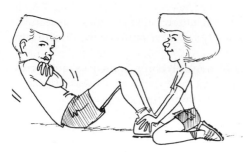

Muscular endurance is the performance of a maximum number of repetitions.

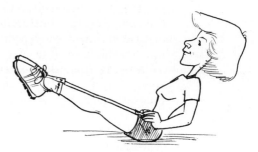

Muscular endurance is sustaining a given contraction.

Body composition

Body composition is also included as one of the health-related physical fitness components. It refers to the relative amounts of fat and **lean body weight** (or fat-free mass) that comprise your body. Your fat-free weight consists of all the tissues of the body other than fat. When you have an excessive amount of fat, you can be classified as obese. An obese person has an increased risk for several serious medical problems such as various cardiovascular diseases and diabetes. In addition, excess fat limits the amount of work that you can perform and may contribute to a decrease in the performance of various sports skills. The percentage of total body weight attributable to body fat is referred to as your **percentage of body fat**.

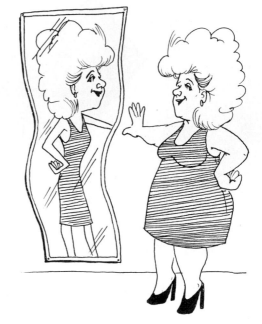

HEALTH AND WELLNESS

It is apparent that to many people the term *health* still means simply the "absence of disease" and that a large percentage of those who have no outward signs of disease or sickness consider themselves to be healthy. A recent survey conducted by Friedman[11] warrants such a conclusion. His study showed that 90% of those surveyed indicated that they considered themselves to be in good health. However, a risk-appraisal survey revealed that 62% of these same people needed to improve their health habits and that 25% of them were in such poor health that they needed to be referred to their physician for treatment. It is unfortunate that many of these people rely on an annual physical examination to determine their level of health. In most cases this examination is not very thorough, and the person is given "a clean bill of health." This then tends to reinforce their existing lifestyle regardless of whether it incorporates healthy or unhealthy practices.

The word "health" should be associated with the term **wellness**, rather than being simply considered the "absence of disease." The relationship between these two terms will be much clearer if we view health as existing on a continuum (Fig. 1-6). In the center of this continuum is a neutral point that reflects a state of no discernible disease or illness. Most people find themselves at this neutral point of the continuum most of the time.

Moving from the center to the left of this neutral point indicates a progressively deteriorating state of health where signs and symptoms of illness appear. If medical treatment is sought, this will usually alleviate the symptoms of the illness, and the person will return to the neutral point. If medical treatment is not sought, the condition will usually get worse and in many cases it will result in premature death.

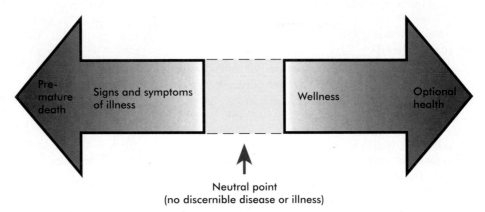

Neutral point
(no discernible disease or illness)

Fig. 1-6 Illness-wellness continuum.

Simply being at the neutral point and being free from disease and illness is not really ideal. One must move beyond the neutral point and be constantly striving for optimal health. This side of the continuum is often referred to as the wellness side, which involves a personal approach to health where each person accepts the responsibility for his or her own lifestyle as he or she tries to prevent illness and disease and strives for optimal wellness.[29]

The balance among all the choices we make each day will determine our position on the continuum. Some of our choices will negatively affect our position while others will move us up on the continuum. By becoming more knowledgeable concerning health-related topics and by developing consistent positive lifestyle behaviors, we can approach our optimal state of health.

It is apparent that in today's world we can do much to influence our state of health. Consider, for example, the following quote from Dr. Richard Winter, Chairman of the Board for National Health Services, which appeared in *Newsweek* magazine in 1987.[38] "Prevention is still the best medicine. Quite simply, if you take care

TABLE 1-2 Leading causes of death in the United States (1989)[18]

Disease	Approximate percentage of deaths
Diseases of the heart and blood vessels	34
Cancer	23
Accidents	4
Chronic obstructive pulmonary disease	4
Pneumonia and influenza	4
Diabetes mellitus	2
Suicide	1

of yourself, most probably someone else won't have to. All that it requires is learning some very basic health and fitness principles, and then applying them—with common sense—to everyday living. It's hardly a high price to pay for our greatest asset . . . good health."

Attainment of a high level of health would appear to be most important in today's world where the most prominent health problems can be considered "lifestyle induced." The six leading causes of death are identified in Table 1-2.

These statistics indicate that approximately 60% of all deaths in the United States are related to cardiovascular disease and cancer. It has been estimated that approximately 80% of these deaths are "lifestyle induced" and could be prevented. The Surgeon General's Report on Health Promotion and Disease Prevention[17] states that "Americans annually lose 15 million years of living from preventable causes." Consider the following facts:

1. High blood pressure (hypertension), a contributing factor to heart attacks and strokes, affects 28% of the American adult population. It is easily identifiable and in most cases can be easily controlled with the right treatment.
2. Cigarette smoking is related to approximately 30% of all cardiovascular heart disease deaths each year, prematurely killing approximately 170,000 Americans.
3. Cigarette smoking is also related to 30% of all cancer deaths each year, accounting for approximately 129,000 premature deaths.
4. Highway accidents account for almost 50,000 deaths annually. The majority of these can be attributed to lack of seat belt use, excessive alcohol consumption, and/or excessive speed.
5. Tobacco use contributes to the majority of the deaths associated with chronic and obstructive pulmonary diseases.
6. The rate of suicide is increasing rapidly in the United States. A high level of stress is the major determining factor in the majority of these cases.
7. Approximately 60% of the American adult population can be considered overweight or obese. This is another risk factor associated with cardiovascular disease, and in most cases it is caused by lack of exercise and/or poor eating habits.
8. The overall risk of heart attack is 40% lower among people who exercise regularly than for those who do not.[2,3]

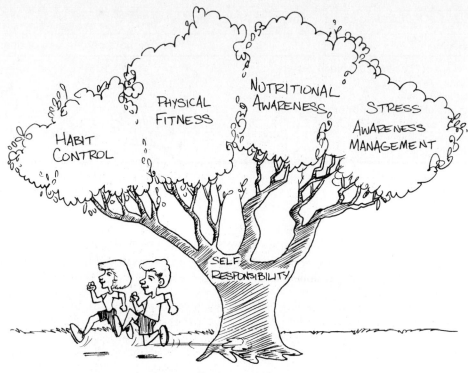

Fig. 1-7 The wellness umbrella.

9. Type II diabetes accounts for approximately 90% of all the cases of diabetes and afflicts approximately 10 million Americans. Eighty-five percent of all those with type II diabetes are obese and/or overweight.[24] (Fig. 1-7).

The following results from a recent national survey indicate that most Americans are now aware of the fact that they can greatly influence their health by the decisions that they make each day, particularly the ones relating to diet and nutrition and to exercise.[28]

	AGREE	DISAGREE
I can do more for my health by what I do and eat than anything doctors or medicine can do.	85%	5%
If I exercise and eat right, I am almost certain to stay healthy.	85%	15%
I would make a commitment to improve my exercise and eating habits if assistance was available.	79%	21%

Notice that almost 80% of the population claims to need assistance if they are to make a commitment to change their exercise and eating habits. There would appear to be three steps involved in this process:

1. Become more knowledgeable concerning exercise and nutrition.
2. Assess your present habits.
3. Learn how to make appropriate changes.

> We have seen an increase in recent years in the number of Americans who have accepted the responsibility for their own health. Perhaps we will be more successful as people become more knowledgeable concerning exercise and nutrition.

EXERCISE AND HEALTH

Research indicates that those who exercise regularly become more health conscious. This is because the number one reason that people gave for "working out" was "their quest for health." It appears that an increase in fitness leads to an increase in self-esteem, and as you feel better about yourself, you are much more likely to have a greater sense of control over the factors that influence your health.

Two different surveys[14,15] showed that those who worked out regularly became more health conscious and were much more likely to implement other health practices. For example, there was a larger percentage of exercisers compared with nonexercisers who were able to quit smoking, to reduce their sugar intake, to reduce their body weight, to increase their fruit and vegetable intake, and to control their level of stress. The differences between the two groups were significant for each of these variables.

Another interesting finding from one of these surveys was that the amount of exercise was very important. It appears that "the more you sweat, the more leverage you have on your habits." The advantages were far greater for those who exercised for 5 hours or more per week, compared with those who exercised for only 1 to 1½ hours per week. Possibly this is due to the discipline one learns from participating in a regular exercise program. The discipline of exercise results in positive feedback and possibly results in a greater sense of control. Remember that "lack of discipline" was one of the top three reasons given for nonparticipation by those who recognized that they do not get sufficient exercise.

It should be emphasized that regular exercise alone does not necessarily ensure better health nor reduce the risk of certain diseases. Consider the following Case Study:

CASE STUDY: DON

Don is a 30-year-old man who exercises very regularly, running 4 or 5 miles at least 5 days each week. He takes great pride in his accomplishments and has no problems maintaining his weight at a desirable level. However, Don smokes two packs of cigarettes a day and has an extremely high level of stress and very poor eating habits. He also figures that because he exercises just about every day that he can reward himself by drinking a six-pack of beer every day. Because of his eating and drinking habits, his cholesterol level is very high.

Despite the fact that Don exercises regularly and maintains a desirable weight, he is still at a high risk for cardiovascular disease because of the other poor habits that influence his health.

MAKING CHOICES

We have seen that how successful a person will be basically depends on the balance that exists between the choices that he or she makes each day.

Prevention magazine[28] has identified 21 key health-promotion questions, which they have used to assess the nation's health. Each of these associated behaviors can be controlled by the individual and has been shown to affect disease or disability. Each question is then "weighted" for its health impact as judged by a group of experts, and a composite score, based on a scale of 1 to 100, is calculated. This is referred to as *The Prevention Index.* A score of zero would therefore mean that nobody had adopted any of these positive behaviors, and a score of 100 would indicate that everyone was carrying out all 21 of them.

Standardized national surveys conducted each year from 1984 to 1992 have shown a gradual increase in The Prevention Index (Fig. 1-8). This indicates that more people than ever before are trying to positively influence their health.

Note that The Prevention Index for 1990 and 1991 remained exactly the same. In 1992 it jumped to 67—the highest score ever. Investigators concluded that if our index score were a grade, we would still barely pass. However, since 1984, we have been moving in the right direction.

> Even though people today know more about healthful living, many of them do not "put into practice" what they know.

You can determine your Personal Prevention Index by completing Laboratory Experience 1-2. This questionnaire includes the 21 questions used by *Prevention* magazine to assess health in the United States.

The important choices that you make each day basically relate to the following:
- Diet and nutrition
- Exercise and weight control
- Stress
- Smoking
- Alcohol and drugs
- Health and safety

By completing the Health and Wellness Questionnaire in Laboratory Experience 1-3, you can determine the area or areas on which you need to concentrate if you are to improve your level of health. Additional information relative to each of these areas is presented in later chapters together with more precise methods of evaluation. This information can be used to help you modify your lifestyle and make better decisions.

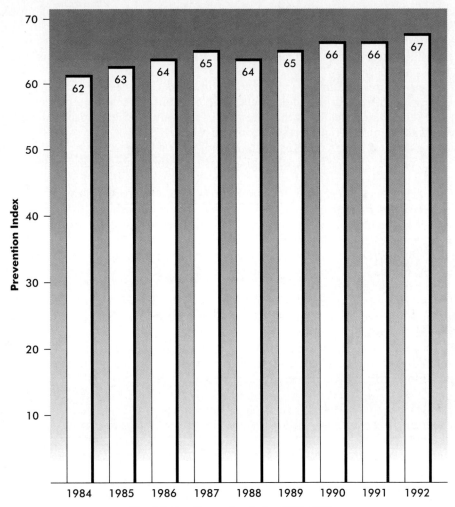

Fig. 1-8 The Prevention Index 1984-1992.

PERSONAL BENEFITS OF EXERCISE

Many advantages result from the development of an optimal level of physical fitness. Several of these are difficult to measure objectively; however, people who exercise regularly report the following:

They feel better and have more energy. Physical fitness promotes a feeling of increased vitality because more energy is available to perform daily tasks. Those who are fit are usually eager to get up in the morning and experience more drive throughout the day. They exhibit a "zest for life."

They look better. Those who are physically fit usually have an improved personal appearance. They are usually stronger and have better muscle tone, decreased weight, and reduced body fat. These factors contribute to better posture and an increased efficiency in the functioning of the body and may result in a delay of the aging process.

They have a reduced level of stress and tension. Those who are fit can usually cope better with daily problems, such as worry, anxiety, pressure, frustration, anger, and fear. They are more able to relax; many work off their tension with some form of exercise.

They are more productive in their everyday tasks. Physically fit people can do more work with less effort and are thus more efficient. Fitness also promotes alertness and self-confidence. Thus they are more successful and less susceptible to mistakes and accidents that often result from fatigue.

They exhibit a better sleeping pattern. Not only do physically fit people require less sleep, but they usually fall asleep sooner, sleep more soundly, and wake up more refreshed.

They experience fewer physical complaints. Those who are physically fit usually have a better resistance to disease. For example, low back pain and the common cold occur less frequently among those who are fit. The benefits are obvious—reduced medical expenses and less time off from work.

They enjoy life more. Those who are physically fit have sufficient energy left at the end of the day to participate in active recreational activities rather than falling asleep in front of the television.

They experience improved psychological benefits. Fitness usually promotes self-confidence and results in enhanced self-esteem and improved body image. The result is an increased feeling of well-being.

Many other specific benefits that result from participation in regular exercise are related to cardiovascular disease and to each of the components of physical fitness. Information on these benefits is presented in later chapters.

SUMMARY

The following summary will help you to identify some of the important concepts covered in this chapter:

- Enthusiasm for exercise and fitness and interest in nutrition is at an all time high in the United States.
- A large percentage of Americans are unfit because they lack motivation and self-discipline.
- Most college students "believe" that exercise is important, but the majority of them just do not "find" the time to exercise regularly.
- The body functions more efficiently if we "take" time to exercise regularly.
- Because of today's "inactive" lifestyle, we must now take time to "program" exercise into our busy schedules.
- Many of the serious health problems that exist in this country are "lifestyle" induced and could be prevented.
- Health-related physical fitness relates to the efficiency with which the body functions, and it is only through regular, sustained exercise that a desirable level can be achieved.
- The components of health-related physical fitness include cardiovascular endurance, flexibility, strength, muscular endurance, and body composition.
- Because of the associated health-related advantages, attainment of an optimal level of cardiovascular endurance is advantageous.

- In today's world, our everyday decisions greatly influence our health.
- Regular exercise does not necessarily ensure good health. We must also be concerned with other health-related practices.
- There are many advantages associated with working hard to build a new lifestyle around exercise, physical fitness, and good nutrition.

KEY TERMS

aerobic activity Any organized activity that is rhythmic in nature and that involves continuous movement using large muscle groups. Examples include walking, jogging, aerobic dance, swimming, cross-country skiing, and a variety of other activities.

aerobic fitness See cardiovascular endurance.

body composition A comparison of the relative amounts of lean body weight and fat tissue in the body.

cardiovascular disease All disease pertaining to the heart and blood vessels, includes hypertension, coronary heart disease, rheumatic heart disease, and stroke.

cardiovascular endurance Extremely high efficiency in the functioning of the heart, lungs, and blood vessels that results in increased efficiency in the performance of continuous work involving large muscle groups. Also referred to as *aerobic fitness* or *cardiorespiratory endurance.*

flexibility The range of motion that is possible at a joint or joints.

health A state of complete physical, mental, and emotional well-being.

hypertension Blood pressure that is consistently higher than normal.

hypokinetic disease A disease related to or resulting from lack of sufficient activity, includes such diseases as cardiovascular disease, osteoporosis, low back pain, hypertension, type II diabetes.

lean body weight The total amount of body weight that is not attributable to fat, includes muscles, ligaments, tendons, bones and fluids.

muscular endurance The ability of a muscle or muscle group to exert a force repeatedly or to sustain a contraction over a period of time.

percentage of body fat The percentage of total body weight attributable to body fat.

physical fitness An optimal level of efficiency in the functioning of the body.

strength The amount of force that can be exerted by a muscle or muscle group against a resistance.

wellness Accepting responsibility for one's lifestyle and making decisions that will result in a high level of physical well-being.

REFERENCES

1. Aldana SG, Stone WJ: Changing physical activity preferences of American adults, *Journal of Physical Education, Recreation and Dance*, pp 67-71 April 1991.
2. Blair SN: Physical activity leads to fitness and pays off, *The Physician and Sports Medicine* 13(3):153-157, 1985.
3. Blair SN, Jawles DR, and Powell KE: *Relationship between exercise or physical activity and other health related behaviors*, Public Health Reports 100, 1985.
4. Brehm BA: Physical activity and wellness, *Fitness Management*, March/April 1987.
5. Brooks CL: Are Americans fit? Survey data conflict, *The Physician and Sports Medicine* 14(11):24, 1986.
6. Clarke HH, Clarke DH: *Application of measurement to physical education*, Englewood Cliffs, NJ, 1987, Prentice Hall.
7. Cohen S: Fitness as in wellness, Health and fitness supplement, *Newsweek*, 1987.
8. Corbin CB, Lindsey RI: *Concepts of physical fitness*, ed 7, Dubuque, Ia, 1991, Wm C Brown.

9. DeWitt PE: Extra years for extra effort, *Time*, p 66, March 17, 1986.

10. *Exercise becomes you—start taking charge*, Bob Hope International Heart Research Institute, Seattle, p 24 1984.

11. Friedman G: *Group health analysis for standard population*, Health Advancement Services, Tempe, Ariz, 1985.

12. Getchell B: *Physical fitness: a way of life*, ed 3, New York, 1983, John Wiley & Sons.

13. Greenberg JS, Pargiman D: *Physical fitness: a wellness approach*, ed 2, Englewood Cliffs, NJ, 1989, Prentice Hall.

14. Harris TG, Gurin J: Look who's getting it all together, *American Heart*, pp 42-47 March 3, 1985.

15. Harris TG, Gurin J: Taking charge: the happy health confidants, *American Health*, pp 53-57, March 1987.

16. *Health: choice or chance?* American Dietetic Association, Chicago, Ill, 1991.

17. *Healthy people: the Surgeon General's report on health promotion and disease prevention*, Public Health Service Pub No 79-55071, Washington, DC, 1979, Department of Health, Education, and Welfare.

18. *Heart facts*—1990, American Heart Association, Dallas, Tex.

19. Hoeger WWK: *Lifetime physical fitness and wellness*, ed 2, Englewood, Colo, 1989, Morton.

20. Kusinetz I, Fine M: Your guide to getting fit, ed 2, Palo Alto, 1991, Mayfield.

21. LaPorte RE et al: Physical activity or cardiovascular fitness: which is more important for health? *The Physician and Sports Medicine* 13(3):145-149, 1985.

22. Lawson BR: The identification and analysis of selected wellness programs in educational institutions in the state of Texas, unpublished dissertation, Stillwater, Oklahoma, 1985, Oklahoma State University.

23. Levine A, Wells S: New rules of exercise, *U.S. News and World Report*, pp. 52-56, August 11, 1986.

24. Nieman DC: *Fitness and sports medicine fitness: an introduction*, ed 2, Palo Alto, 1990, Bull Publishing.

25. Prentice W: *Fitness for college and life*, ed 3, St Louis, 1991, Mosby–Year Book.

26. President's Council on Physical Fitness and Sport: national adult physical fitness survey, Newsletter, pp. 1-27, May 1973,

27. *Prevention index '89*, Emmaus, Penn, 1987, Rodale Press.

28. *Prevention index '91*, Emmaus, Penn, 1991, Rodale Press.

29. Robins G, Powers D, and Burgess S: *A wellness way of life*, Dubuque, Ia, 1991, Wm C Brown.

30. Rosato FD: *Fitness and wellness: the physical connection*, St Paul, Minn, West Publishing.

31. Rosenstein AH: The benefits of health maintenance, *The Physician and Sports Medicine* 15(4): 57-68, 1987.

32. Richter EE, Schneider SH: Diabetes and exercise, *American Journal of Medicine* 70:201-209, 1981.

33. Siscovick DA et al: Habitual vigorous exercise and primary cardiac arrest: effect of other risk factors on the relationships, *Journal of Chronic Disease* 37:625-632, 1984.

34. Siscovick DS, LaPorte RE, and Newman JM: The disease specific benefits and risks of physical activity, Public Health Reports 100, pp 180-188, 1985.

35. Stone WJ: *Adult fitness programs: planning, designing, managing and improving fitness programs*, Glenview, Ill, 1987, Scott, Foresman & Co.

36. Toufeis A: A national obsession, The U.S. turns on to exercise, *Time*, p 77, June 16, 1986.

37. The shape of the nation, despite the exercise boom, Americans are far from fit, *Time*, p 60, October, 1986.

38. Winter RE: A message from the executive health group, *Newsweek*, 1987.

Subjective Evaluation of Present Level of Physical Fitness

How do you know if you have an adequate level of physical fitness? You may be able to subjectively determine this by answering the questions in Laboratory Experience 1-1.

	YES	NO
1. Do you feel tired when you wake up in the morning and often do not really want to get out of bed?	___	___
2. Do you yawn regularly throughout the day?	___	___
3. Do you become fatigued from tasks requiring minimal energy such as climbing several flights of stairs or walking around in a shopping mall?	___	___
4. Do you run out of energy by the middle of the day or the early afternoon and often wish that you had the opportunity to lie down and take a nap?	___	___
5. When you look at yourself do you wish you weighed less and/or had less fat in specific areas of your body?	___	___
6. Do you frequently fall asleep in the evenings while reading or watching television?	___	___
7. Are you often too tired to participate in active leisure activities?	___	___
8. Are you vulnerable to frequent aches and pains?	___	___
9. Do you often drive around a parking lot looking for a parking space close to the entrance?	___	___
10. Do you buy a new pair of exercise shoes every year or so because the old ones are dirty rather than worn out?	___	___

Overall evaluation

Do you generally lack energy and vitality?	___	___

If several of your responses are "Yes," then this may indicate that you have less than an adequate level of physical fitness.

Your Personal Prevention Index

The Prevention Index takes stock of the nation's health, but you can also score your own prevention profile by taking the test below.

Please carefully check "yes" or "no" to each of the following questions:

	YES	NO
1. Do you have a blood pressure reading at least once a year?	___	___
2. Do you go to the dentist at least once a year for treatment or a checkup?	___	___
3. Is your body weight within the recommended range for your sex, height, and bone structure?	___	___

4. Do you exercise strenuously (that is, so you breathe heavily and your heart and pulse rate are accelerated for a period lasting at least 20 minutes) 3 days or more a week?   _____ _____

5. Do you smoke cigarettes now?   _____ _____

6. Do you consciously take steps to control or reduce stress in your life?   _____ _____

7. Do you usually sleep a total of 7 or 8 hours during each 24-hour day? (If you usually sleep either more or less than this, please mark "no.")   _____ _____

8. Do you socialize with close friends, relatives, or neighbors at least once a week?   _____ _____

9. In general, when you drink alcoholic beverages, do you consume less than 14 drinks per week and less than five drinks on any single day? (Mark "yes" only if the answer to both parts of this question is "yes." If you never drink at all, also mark "yes.")   _____ _____

10. Do you wear a seat belt all the time when you are in the front seat of a car?   _____ _____

11. Do you drive at or below the speed limit all the time? (If you don't drive, please mark "yes.")   _____ _____

12. Do you ever drive after drinking? (If you don't drink, please mark "no.")   _____ _____

13. Do you have a smoke detector in your home?   _____ _____

14. Does anyone in your household ever smoke in bed?   _____ _____

15. Do you take any special steps or precautions to avoid accidents in and around your home?   _____ _____

16. Do you try to avoid eating too much salt or sodium?   _____ _____

17. Do you try to avoid eating too much fat?   _____ _____

18. Do you try to eat enough fiber from whole grains, cereals, fruits, and vegetables?   _____ _____

19. Do you try to avoid eating too many high cholesterol foods, such as eggs, dairy products, and fatty meats?   _____ _____

20. Do you try to get enough vitamins and minerals in foods or in supplements?   _____ _____

21. Do you try to avoid eating too much sugar and sweet food?   _____ _____

NOTE:

A drink is defined as a shot of hard liquor, a can or bottle of beer, or a glass of wine.

The correct answer for questions 5, 12, and 14 is "no."

The correct answer for all the other questions is "yes."

Add up your total number of correct responses and then divide that number by 21, which tells you the percentage of the 21 Prevention Index Behaviors that you practice.

Number of Correct Responses = _____

Personal Prevention Index

= Number of Correct Responses /21

= _____ /21

= _____

Health and Wellness Questionnaire

Please answer each question as honestly as possible. When completed, add together the total points for each of your responses.

Diet and nutrition

1. How often do you consciously limit both your salt and sodium intake by not adding salt to prepared foods and by selecting foods that are low in sodium?
   _____ (2) Frequently (almost every day)
   _____ (1) Sometimes (every few days)
   _____ (0) Rarely (once a week or less)
2. How often do you eat a well-balanced nutritious breakfast?
   _____ (4) 7 days each week
   _____ (3) 5 or 6 days each week
   _____ (2) 3 or 4 days each week
   _____ (1) 1 or 2 days each week
   _____ (0) Never
3. During your waking hours, how often do you go longer than 5 hours without eating something nutritious?
   _____ (0) Frequently (almost every day)
   _____ (1) Sometimes (every few days)
   _____ (2) Rarely (once a week or less)
4. How often do you drink at least six 8-oz glasses of water?
   _____ (3) Frequently (almost every day)
   _____ (1) Sometimes (every few days)
   _____ (0) Rarely (once a week or less)
5. How often do you eat at fast-food restaurants?
   _____ (0) Often (three or more times a week)
   _____ (1) Occasionally (one or two times a week)
   _____ (3) Seldom (maybe once a month)
6. Foods that are usually high in fat include cheese, chips, mayonnaise, salad dressings, red meat, Mexican food, fried foods, butter, margarine, and nuts. How would you describe your fat intake?
   _____ (0) High (I usually eat at least two of these foods just about every day.)
   _____ (1) Moderate (I usually eat one of these foods just about every day.)
   _____ (3) Low (Most days I do not eat any of these foods.)
7. Foods that are usually high in simple sugar include candy, cookies, cakes, pastries, ice cream, and sodas. How would you classify your intake of simple sugars?
   _____ (0) High (I usually eat at least one of these types of foods each day.)
   _____ (1) Moderate (I usually eat these types of foods two or three times each week.)
   _____ (3) Low (I hardly ever eat foods that are high in sugar.)
8. Caffeine is contained in coffee, tea, and many soft drinks. How many 8-oz cups of caffeinated beverages do you drink in an average day?
   _____ (4) None

_____ (3) 1 or 2
_____ (2) 3 or 4
_____ (1) 6 to 10
_____ (0) More than 10

9. How many days a week do you eat a well-balanced diet that includes at least two servings from each of the following food groups: milk or dairy products, fruits, vegetables, bread or grains, and meat or meat substitutes?
_____ (3) Every day
_____ (2) 5 or 6 days
_____ (1) 3 or 4 days
_____ (0) Less than 3 days

10. On an average day, how many servings do you get of fruits, vegetables, and grain products? (A serving size is 1 cup of raw vegetables; ½ cup of cooked vegetables, rice, cereal, pasta, or spaghetti; or a medium-sized piece of fruit.)
_____ (3) 8 or more servings
_____ (2) 6 or 7 servings
_____ (1) 4 or 5 servings
_____ (0) Less than 4 servings

Stress

11. How frequently do you experience one or more of the symptoms of excess stress such as tension, migraine headaches, or pain in the neck or shoulders?
_____ (0) Often (three or more times a week)
_____ (1) Occasionally (a few times a week)
_____ (3) Rarely (less than once a week)

12. How frequently do you find it difficult to concentrate on what you are doing because of either deadlines or other tasks that also must be completed?
_____ (0) Often (most working days)
_____ (1) Occasionally (a few times a week)
_____ (3) Rarely (less than once a week)

13. Do you become irritable when you have to wait in a line or at a traffic light?
_____ (0) Yes
_____ (2) No

14. In response to stress and tension, how frequently do you eat, drink, smoke, or take tranquilizers in an attempt to reduce the stress or tension?
_____ (0) Frequently (at least 5 days a week)
_____ (1) Sometimes (every couple of days)
_____ (3) Rarely (once a week or less)

15. How often do you worry about your work and/or other deadlines at night or on at weekends?
_____ (0) Frequently (just about every day)
_____ (1) Sometimes (every couple of days)
_____ (3) Rarely (once a week or less)

16. How often do you wake up in the night thinking about all the things you must do the next day?
_____ (0) Frequently (at least 4 nights a week)

_____ (1) Sometimes (a few times a week)

_____ (3) Rarely (once a week or less)

Exercise and weight control

17. How would you rate your present level of aerobic fitness compared with other people of your age and sex? (If you have completed an aerobic fitness test use your classification from that test.)

_____ (5) Excellent

_____ (4) Good

_____ (3) Average

_____ (2) Fair

_____ (1) Poor

18. How many times per week do you participate continuously for at least 20 minutes in any form of organized aerobic activity such as walking, swimming, bicycling, or jogging?

_____ (0) Rarely (almost never)

_____ (2) Sporadically (one or two times per week)

_____ (4) Regularly (three or more times every week)

19. How often do you spend time warming up and stretching before and/or after participating in your exercise program or sports?

_____ (0) Seldom (hardly ever)

_____ (1) Occasionally (when I have time for it)

_____ (2) Regularly (just about every time I exercise)

20. How would you best describe your present weight?

_____ (5) I am happy with my present weight.

_____ (4) I would like to weigh more than I presently do.

_____ (4) I would like to reduce my weight by less than 10 lb.

_____ (2) I would like to reduce my weight by 10 to 19 lb.

_____ (0) I would like to reduce my weight by more than 19 lb.

Smoking

21. With regard to cigarette and cigar smoking:

_____ (5) I never smoke.

_____ (3) I smoke one to two per day.

_____ (1) I smoke three to twelve per day.

_____ (0) I smoke more than 12 per day.

22. With regard to smoking while lying in bed:

_____ (0) I smoke frequently while lying in bed.

_____ (1) I smoke occasionally while lying in bed.

_____ (3) I never smoke while lying in bed.

Alcohol and drug use

23. What is the average number of alcoholic drinks (beer, wine, or hard liquor) that you consume **per week?**

_____ (5) None
_____ (4) 1 to 5
_____ (2) 6 to 10
_____ (1) 10 to 14
_____ (0) More than 14

24. How often do you take prescription drugs that have been prescribed for someone else?

_____ (3) Never
_____ (1) Occasionally
_____ (0) Frequently

25. How often do you consume drugs other than alcohol, such as marijuana, uppers, or downers?

_____ (3) Never
_____ (1) Occasionally
_____ (0) Frequently

26. How often do you combine alcohol with any other types of drugs or with medications such as sleeping pills, pain pills, or cold pills?

_____ (4) Never
_____ (2) Occasionally
_____ (0) Frequently

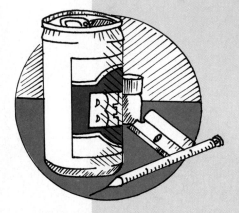

Health and safety

27. How often do you wear a seat belt when driving or when riding in the front seat of an automobile?

_____ (4) Always
_____ (2) Sometimes (about half of the time)
_____ (0) Hardly ever

28. Do you have your blood pressure measured at least once a year?

_____ (3) Yes
_____ (0) No

29. Do you have your cholesterol measured at least once every 2 years?

_____ (3) Yes
_____ (0) No

30. Do you have a complete physical examination at least once every 2 years?

_____ (4) Yes
_____ (0) No

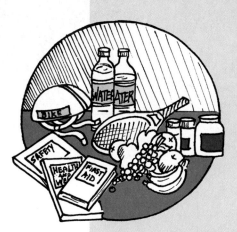

Interpretation of Scores

Excellent	80-100
Good	60-79
Average	40-59
Fair	20-39
Poor	<20

Cardiovascular Endurance

CHAPTER OBJECTIVES

When you understand the material in this chapter, you will be able to:

- Explain why cardiovascular endurance is the most important component of physical fitness
- Differentiate clearly between aerobic and anaerobic work
- Define each of the terms associated with the cardiovascular system and be able to discuss their importance in relation to cardiovascular endurance
- Describe the relationship between oxygen consumption and energy expenditure
- Define maximal oxygen consumption and discuss the changes that take place in the body as a result of regular aerobic exercise, which positively influence this variable
- Design and evaluate an exercise program specifically planned to develop your level of aerobic fitness
- Calculate your target-zone heart rate and your critical heart rate and understand their importance in the development of cardiovascular endurance
- Evaluate your level of cardiovascular fitness using different methods of assessment
- Define each of the key terms

Cardiovascular endurance, which is also referred to as physical work capacity or aerobic fitness, is the most important component of physical fitness. Attaining a high level of cardiovascular endurance helps to reduce your risk of cardiovascular disease and will result in an increase in the efficiency with which your body functions. You will be able to exercise at a higher level of intensity, and you will be able to sustain this level for a longer period.

Cardiovascular endurance depends on how efficiently the lungs, the heart, and the blood vessels can provide the necessary oxygen to the working muscles and how efficiently these muscles can use this oxygen. Cardiovascular endurance can therefore be defined as the efficiency with which you can perform heavy, continuous physical work, involving large muscle groups and lasting for an extended period. The more oxygen that can be supplied and used, the higher the level of work that can be sustained (Fig. 2-1).

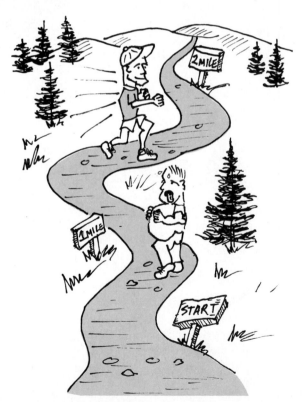

Fig. 2-1 A fit person's body functions more efficiently, and a fit person can run further than an unfit person in the same amount of time.

How much continuous work you can perform before you become fatigued and exhausted, and at what level you can work, will reflect your level of cardiovascular endurance.

EFFICIENCY OF PERFORMANCE

The intensity of effort required for an activity can be measured by your heart rate response. This will reflect the efficiency with which you perform the task. A person with a low level of cardiovascular endurance will have a higher heart rate response to a submaximal standardized task compared with a fit person and will fatigue much faster (Fig. 2-2).

Efficiency of performance is reflected by a fit person's ability to:

- Work at a higher intensity level than an unfit person without fatigue
- Perform more work than an unfit person before reaching exhaustion
- Recover faster than an unfit person following exercise; the heart rate will return to its resting rate much faster

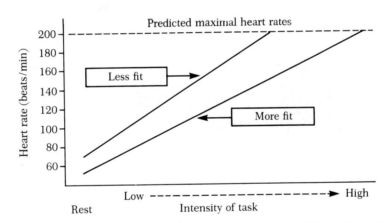

Fig. 2-2 Comparison of heart rate patterns for individuals with different fitness levels.

ANAEROBIC AND AEROBIC WORK

Within the body there are two systems that can supply energy—the anaerobic system and the aerobic system. The type of task you perform determines which system will make the major contribution.

Anaerobic system

This provides energy for tasks requiring a high rate of energy expenditure for a short period. The 100-yard dash is an example. With this system a large amount of energy is released to supply the immediate needs of the body. The amount of work you can perform anaerobically is limited, and you will usually be able to perform this type of exercise only for up to 2 minutes. Lactic acid is produced with this process, and an accumulation of lactic acid in the body contributes to muscle fatigue.

Aerobic system

This provides energy for **submaximal tasks** requiring a lower rate of energy expenditure over a longer period. Walking and jogging are examples of aerobic activities. Tasks such as these are dependent on a constant amount of oxygen being available for use by the muscles performing the work. The amount of oxygen taken in and used by the body must be sufficient to provide the energy required for the task.

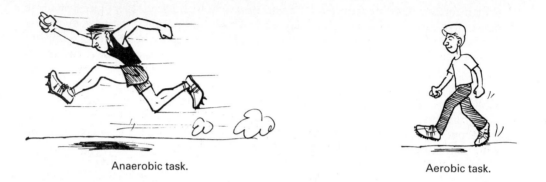

Anaerobic task.   Aerobic task.

The length of time and intensity of the exercise will determine the relative contribution of each of these energy systems. This relationship is summarized in Fig. 2-3. This graph shows that during a 1-minute run, a high percentage of work is performed anaerobically (greater than 60%). It can be seen that when the time of the task exceeds 10 minutes, the anaerobic system becomes less important and accounts for no more than 5% of the oxygen required.

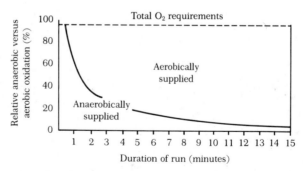

Fig. 2-3 Relative roles of anaerobic and aerobic processes for supplying oxygen.

BASIC PHYSIOLOGICAL INFORMATION

Knowledge of the heart and circulatory system is necessary to understand cardiovascular endurance and the changes that occur in your body that will allow you to function more efficiently.

The heart as a muscular pump

The **heart** is simply a muscular pump that provides the force to keep blood circulating throughout the network of arteries. This hollow, muscular organ is located between the lungs and the diaphragm in what is known as the *medial sternal space.* It is mostly to the left of the midline of the body with its apex pointing down.

The heart actually consists of two pumps. A thick muscular wall, known as the *septum,* divides the heart cavity down the middle into the right side and the left side. On each side is an upper chamber known as the **atrium** and a lower chamber called the **ventricle.** Each atrium is separated from the ventricle by a valve that regulates the flow of blood. These are atrioventricular valves.

The right side of the heart receives blood that has completed its cycle through the body. This blood collects in the right atrium of the heart. This used blood reaches the heart by way of two large veins—the superior and inferior venae cavae. The superior vena cava returns blood from the head and arms, while the inferior vena cava drains blood from the trunk and legs. A third opening into the right atrium is the coronary sinus. This returns blood that is used by the heart muscle itself. From the right atrium blood enters the right ventricle through the tricuspid valve. Blood is pumped from the right ventricle through the pulmonary arteries to the lungs, where it picks up fresh oxygen and gives up carbon dioxide. The function of the right side of the heart, then, is to pump blood to the lungs, where oxygen is picked up and carbon dioxide is eliminated. The blood flow associated with the right side of the heart is illustrated in Fig. 2-4, *A.*

The left side of the heart receives reoxygenated blood, which is returned through the pulmonary veins. This blood collects in the left atrium and passes from this upper chamber to the lower through the mitral, or bicuspid, valve. It is this left ventricle that pumps blood out of the heart. Blood passes through the aorta—the largest artery

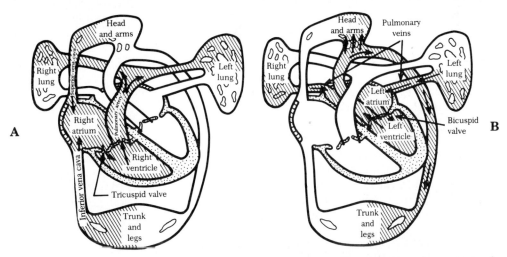

Fig. 2-4 **A,** Blood flow associated with the right side of the heart. Note that the major purpose of the right side of the heart is to pump blood to the lungs where oxygen is picked up and carbon dioxide is eliminated. **B,** Blood, associated with the left side of the heart. Blood is pumped to all parts of the body by way of the aorta.

in the body—to all parts of the body. Fig. 2-4, *B*, illustrates blood flow associated with the left side of the heart.

Valves of the heart

The valves play an important role in regulating the flow of blood. Besides the two atrioventricular valves that have been explained previously, two other valves are located where the pulmonary artery and aorta join the ventricles. These valves, as well as the two atrioventricular valves, allow blood to flow in only one direction. These prevent the backward flow of blood during diastole, when the heart is relaxed. The heart sounds that may be heard with a stethoscope are caused by the closing of the valves of the heart. The sounds that are heard are *lubb-dupp*. The first of these sounds, *lubb,* is caused by the atrioventricular valves as they close when the contraction of the ventricles takes place. At this time the other two valves, the aortic and pulmonary valves, are open as blood is being ejected from the heart. The *dupp* sound is made by the closing of the valves in the aorta and pulmonary arteries as the heart again is filling with blood. If heart valves do not function properly, increased turbulence occurs, and abnormal sounds may be heard. These are referred to as *heart murmurs.*

Blood vessels

A clear distinction is necessary between arteries and veins. Any vessel taking blood away from the heart is an **artery,** whereas any vessel returning blood to the heart is a **vein.** The muscular wall of the normal artery is much thicker than that of the vein. This allows the arteries to be elastic so that when blood is ejected from the heart, they can expand to receive the blood. During the relaxation phase of the cardiac cycle, the muscular walls of the arteries contract to keep blood moving through the arterial system. As fatty deposits accumulate on the inner arterial walls, they tend to lose their elasticity and become smaller. This decreases the circulatory system's ability to function efficiently and increases the possibility of cardiovascular problems. This is discussed in detail in Chapter 10.

Arterial branches become smaller and smaller as they are distributed throughout the body. The smallest branches are known as **capillaries.** It is here that oxygen and nutrients leave the blood to enter body cells and carbon dioxide and metabolic wastes leave the cells to be picked up by the bloodstream.

Blood is returned to the heart through the network of veins. As indicated, veins do not have the thick, muscular walls that most arteries have. For this reason there is less pressure in veins. This does not create a problem for blood returning from the upper parts of the body, since gravity will assist in the return of blood to the heart. However, blood in the arms and legs must rely on the squeezing action of the muscles to be returned to the heart. There is a system of valves in veins that allows blood to flow only toward the heart. These veins are located between skeletal muscles, and when these muscles contract, veins are "squeezed," and blood flows toward the heart. If too much time is spent standing in one place, it is not uncommon for a person to experience fatigue and pass out. Blood is not returned from the lower parts of the body to the heart, and it "pools" in these lower areas. Varicose veins may result from failure of used blood to be returned to the heart fast enough. The accumulated blood causes the veins to swell. Varicose veins often occur in individuals whose jobs require them to stand still or to remain seated for extended periods.

TERMS ASSOCIATED WITH THE CARDIOVASCULAR SYSTEM

There are four basic terms associated with the cardiovascular system that you will need to know to understand the changes that occur in your body as a result of a good aerobic exercise program. These are (1) heart rate, (2) stroke volume, (3) cardiac output, and (4) blood pressure.

Heart rate

For an average person at rest who does not exercise regularly, the heart will beat about 70 to 75 times per minute. This is the **heart rate,** or pulse. It is caused by the impact of blood on the arteries as the heart contracts. It is determined by counting the number of times your heart contracts in a certain period and then converting this number to the standard measure in beats per minute (beats/min).

Measuring your heart rate. Your heart rate can be determined by placing your finger or fingers on your lower arm at the base of the thumb or on one of the arteries in the front of the neck. (See the accompanying box.) Make sure that you press just firmly enough to feel the pulse. Pressing too hard may interfere with the rhythm.

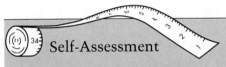 Self-Assessment

MEASURING YOUR HEART RATE

Your heart rate can be determined by counting the number of times your heart contracts in a given period and converting this to beats per minute. Make sure that you press just firmly enough to feel the pulse. Pressing too hard may interfere with the rhythm.

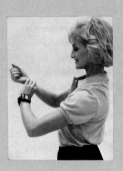 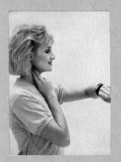

Your pulse can be detected by placing a finger or fingers on your lower arm near the base of the thumb.

Your pulse can also be easily detected over the carotid artery in the front of the neck.

The procedures for determining your resting heart rate and for interpreting your scores are presented in Laboratory Experience 2-1.

Changes with regular exercise. With regular aerobic exercise, your heart becomes stronger and more efficient, which should result in a reduction in your resting heart rate.

Stroke volume

Each time the heart contracts, blood is ejected. This is referred to as the **stroke volume.** For an average person at rest, the stroke volume is about 70 ml. A physically trained person, with a stronger heart, can pump as much as 100 ml with each contraction.

Cardiac output

Cardiac output is the amount of blood the heart circulates each minute. It is determined by how many times the heart contracts each minute (heart rate) and the amount of blood ejected with each contraction (stroke volume). The resting cardiac output for most people will range from 5 to 6 liters and is not dependent on fitness level. The following example clearly shows the relationship between cardiac output, stroke volume, and heart rate.

EXAMPLE:

For an untrained person who has a resting heart rate of 72 beats/min and a stroke volume of 70 ml, the resting cardiac output is calculated as follows:

$$\text{Cardiac output} = \text{Heart rate} \times \text{stroke volume}$$
$$= 72 \times 70$$
$$= 5040 \text{ ml/min}$$
$$= 5.04 \text{ L/min}$$

(NOTE: 1000 ml = 1 liter)

As the heart becomes stronger with regular exercise, it can pump more blood each time it contracts, and it therefore does not have to beat as frequently to circulate the same amount of blood. The example on p. 41 will clarify this relationship.

Blood pressure

Blood pressure is the amount of force that blood exerts against the artery walls. It is generated by the heart as it contracts and is maintained by the elasticity of the arterial walls.

Blood pressure changes constantly during each cardiac cycle. Each time the heart contracts, blood pressure goes up as more blood is forced from the heart into the arterial system. The contraction phase of the cardiac cycle is called **systole,** which creates the systolic blood pressure. The relaxation phase of the cardiac cycle is called **diastole** and creates the diastolic blood pressure.

EXAMPLE:

If the person in the previous example, through regular exercise, is able to change the resting stroke volume from 70 ml to 90 ml, the anticipated change in resting heart rate would be calculated as follows:

$$\text{Cardiac output} = \text{Heart rate} \times \text{stroke volume}$$
$$5.04 \text{ liters} = \text{Heart rate} \times 90$$
$$\text{Heart rate} = 5.04/90$$
$$= 5040 \text{ ml}/90$$
$$= 56 \text{ beats/min}$$

Conclusion: The resting heart rate should drop from 72 to 56 beats/min, with the cardiac output remaining steady at 5.04 L/min.

Blood pressure is measured in millimeters of mercury (mm Hg) and is written as systolic/diastolic. For example, 120/80 indicates that the systolic blood pressure is 120 mm Hg and the diastolic blood pressure is 80 mm Hg. It is difficult to define "normal" blood pressure. However, a score of 140/90 is usually considered to be the highest pressure that could be classified as normal. Blood pressure that is consistently higher than it should be is called **hypertension.** This condition is discussed in Chapter 10 as one of the risk factors associated with cardiovascular disease. Suggestions are given in that section for control of blood pressure.

The procedures for measuring your blood pressure and for interpreting your scores are presented in Laboratory Experience 2-2.

ENERGY AND PERFORMANCE

The major function of the cardiovascular system during exercise is to deliver oxygen to the working muscles. Because aerobic processes account for most of the energy produced in the body, the amount of oxygen that can be supplied directly determines the amount of work that can be performed. Cardiovascular endurance depends on how efficiently the lungs, heart, and blood vessels take oxygen from the air you breathe in, process it, and deliver it to the muscles where it is used. Efficient performance depends on:

- Availability of sufficient oxygen in the inspired air
- Ability of oxygen and carbon dioxide to diffuse across the pulmonary membrane into and out of the blood
- Chemical binding of oxygen with **hemoglobin** in the blood
- A blood flow through the lungs geared to pick up and carry the amount of oxygen required by the body
- Ability of the cells to pick up oxygen from the capillaries in exchange for carbon dioxide and other waste products

> The heart is obviously the key to the entire system. It must constantly beat to keep blood circulating.

The relationship between oxygen consumption and energy expenditure can be summarized as follows:

- Each activity requires energy. Even simple activities, such as sitting and sleeping, require energy.
- To produce energy, oxygen is necessary. Energy is produced by burning foodstuffs, but oxygen is the necessary fueling agent.
- The body can store food, but it cannot store oxygen. A person must breathe to live. If the oxygen supply is discontinued, the body will die quickly, since the oxygen supply in the body will last for only a short time.

When demands for oxygen increase within the body, such as during strenuous exercise, the ability to take in and deliver oxygen to the working musculature will be important in determining how much work can be performed and how efficiently it can be performed. The more oxygen the circulatory and respiratory systems are able to deliver, the longer the person will be able to exercise before becoming fatigued or exhausted. The reason a person becomes fatigued is that he or she reaches the point at which the body cannot process enough oxygen to supply the energy needed.

MAXIMAL OXYGEN CONSUMPTION

The rate at which oxygen is delivered and used by the body is referred to as *oxygen consumption.* It is expressed as a volume of gas per unit of time and is abbreviated as $\dot{V}O_2$.

$$V = \text{Volume (usually expressed in liters or milliliters)}$$
$$O_2 = \text{Oxygen gas}$$
$$\cdot = \text{Per unit of time (usually expressed in minutes)}$$

The more oxygen your body is able to process and use, the more work you should be able to perform before becoming fatigued. The maximal rate at which oxygen can be used by your body is therefore important and is considered by most experts to be the best indicator of cardiovascular (or aerobic) fitness. It is called **maximal oxygen consumption** and is abbreviated $\dot{V}O_2$ max.

Your rate of oxygen consumption is measured in liters per minute, but because those who weigh more will have a higher total score because of their larger size, this score must be adjusted to account for individual differences in size. Comparisons can then be made between individuals of different body weights. Table 2-1 should help you understand this concept.

Note that by dividing the total oxygen consumption (milliliters) by the body weight (kg), the amount of oxygen available for each unit of body weight can be determined. This is expressed as milliliters of oxygen per kilogram of body weight per minute and is abbreviated ml/kgbw/min. The higher this value, the more oxygen that is available for each unit of body weight and thus the more work that you can perform before exhaustion.

TABLE 2-1 **Comparison of maximal oxygen consumption for individuals of different body weights**

Variable	Subject 1	Subject 2
$\dot{V}O_2$ max. (L/min)	4.2 L/min = 4200 ml/min	3.9 L/min = 3900 ml/min
Body weight	185 lb = 84.1 kg	160 lb = 72.7 kg
$\dot{V}O_2$ max. (ml/kgbw/min)	4200/84.1 49.94	3900/72.7 53.65

The sample data in Table 2-1 clearly shows that subject 2 can provide more oxygen for each kilogram of body weight (53.65) than subject 1 (49.94) even though the total oxygen consumption is less.

With regular participation in a good aerobic exercise program, a person can increase his or her maximal oxygen consumption by as much as 30% over a 12-week period, depending on his or her initial level of fitness. The following changes in the body possibly contribute to this:

- An increase in the amount of hemoglobin in the blood, which results in an increase in the amount of oxygen that can be transported in the blood
- An increase in the maximal cardiac output as the heart becomes stronger and more efficient. This means that you can circulate more blood to the working muscles
- An increase in the amount and/or size of the capillaries, allowing for a more efficient exchange of gases, which in turn allows the muscles to use more of the oxygen circulated

DEVELOPMENT OF CARDIOVASCULAR ENDURANCE

A high level of aerobic fitness is an important objective of most exercise programs. Your body was designed to be active, and if you achieve a high level of aerobic fitness and maintain this level, your body will function more efficiently, and you can reduce your risk of cardiovascular disease. To achieve this it is important to determine if your program is too hard, too easy, or just right.

In designing an aerobic fitness program, you must be able to answer the following questions:

- How hard must I exercise? (intensity)
- How long must each exercise session last? (duration)
- How often do I need to exercise? (frequency)
- Which activities are best for me? (mode of exercise)

Intensity of exercise

Intensity of exercise refers to how vigorous an exercise must be in order to contribute toward the development of aerobic fitness. Many people do not understand this concept and exercise at a level that is too high or too low. When you exercise, your heart rate will increase in proportion to the energy required for the performance of the task (Fig. 2-5). As the task increases in intensity, there will be a corresponding increase in your heart rate. Your exercise heart rate can therefore be used to determine the amount of physiological stress placed on the body. It is easy to measure and has become universally accepted as the standard way to determine exercise intensity. Your heart rate response to exercise is obviously an individual matter and will depend

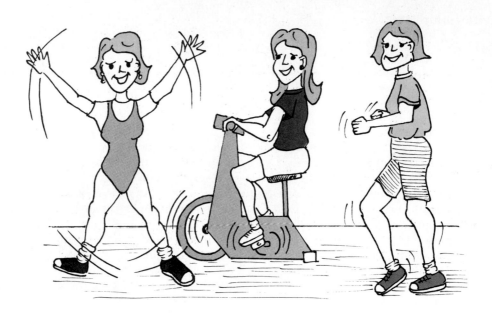

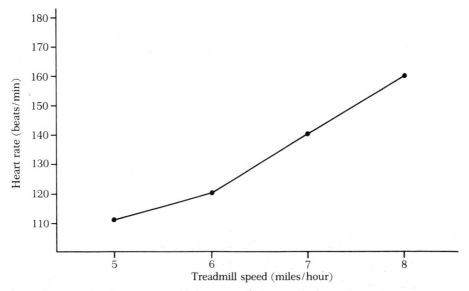

Fig. 2-5 Heart rate response of a 21-year-old subject running on the treadmill at 5, 6, 7, and 8 mph.

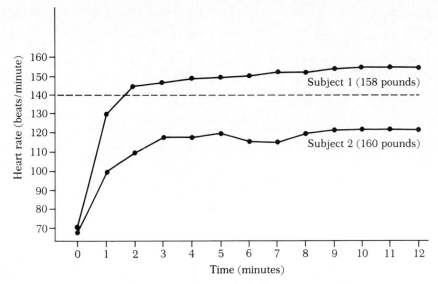

Fig. 2-6 Comparison of heart rate responses for 20-year-old subjects running on a treadmill at 6 mph for 12 minutes.

on the efficiency of your heart and circulatory system. Fig. 2-6 compares the heart rate responses for two people of about the same age and body weight running at the same speed.

With regular aerobic exercise, your cardiovascular system will function more efficiently, and you will have a lower heart rate response for the same task. It is apparent in Fig. 2-6 that subject 2 has a higher aerobic fitness level than subject 1.

For a 20-year-old person, the minimum intensity of exercise needed for an increase in aerobic fitness is a level of work that will produce a heart rate of about 140 beats/min. For subject 1, running at a speed of 6 mph would be sufficient, but subject 2 would have to run faster to obtain the desired results.

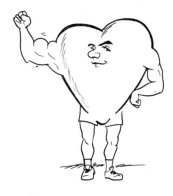

Since the heart is a muscle, like any other muscle, stress is necessary for it to function more efficiently. Unless sufficient stress is used, the changes will be minimal. If a person exercises too intensely, it may be dangerous, and he or she probably will not be able to continue long enough to produce desired results. High levels of exertion often result in muscular injuries.

Target-zone heart rate. For a safe and effective workout, the intensity of the activity must be regulated so that your heart rate is elevated to a predetermined level.[25] This is called your *training heart rate,* or, more commonly, **the target-zone heart rate.** Your target-zone heart rate is 70% to 85% of your **maximal heart rate.** Maintaining your heart rate within this range for an extended time will result in optimal development of aerobic fitness. Procedures for calculating target-zone heart rate follow.

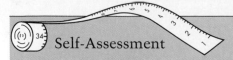

Self-Assessment

DETERMINATION OF YOUR TARGET-ZONE HEART RATE

To determine your target-zone heart rate, you must first estimate your maximal heart rate. This is not influenced by sex or level of fitness. It is almost entirely related to age.

For practical purposes your maximal heart rate can be estimated by subtracting your age (in years) from 220. This will usually be accurate within 10 beats/min.

$$\text{Maximal heart rate} = 220 - \text{age (years)}$$
$$\text{(estimated)} = 220 - \underline{\qquad}$$
$$= \underline{\qquad} \text{ beats/min}$$

Calculate your target-zone heart rate

$$\text{Lower level} = 0.70 \times \text{Maximal heart rate}$$
$$(70\% \text{ maximal heart rate}) = 0.70 \times \underline{\qquad}$$
$$= \underline{\qquad} \text{ beats/min}$$

$$\text{Upper level} = 0.85 \times \text{Maximal heart rate}$$
$$(85\% \text{ maximal heart rate}) = 0.85 \times \underline{\qquad}$$
$$= \underline{\qquad} \text{ beats/min}$$

Target-zone heart rate \underline{\qquad} to \underline{\qquad} beats/min

People who are extremely unfit and/or overweight may have difficulty in working at an intensity where their heart rate exceeds the lower level of their target zone. They may be able to work at a lower intensity and still achieve beneficial results. The appropriate level for these people might be 60% to 70% of their maximal heart rate.

Predicted maximal heart rates and target-zone heart rates for different age-groups are summarized in Fig. 2-7. The heart rates corresponding to 60% of the maximal heart rate are also included for those who need to work at this intensity.

When you are exercising and not using a heart rate monitor and you want to determine your heart rate, you usually stop and count your pulse for 10 seconds. Procedures for this are given in Laboratory Experience 2-3. Table 2-2 allows you to quickly equate your 10-second pulse count to that necessary to reach the required target zone.

Critical or threshold heart rate. An alternate method to evaluate the intensity of an exercise is to determine the critical, or threshold, heart rate that must be exceeded if maximum development of cardiovascular fitness is to result.[12] With this method you obtain a value that you must exceed rather than the range of values you get with the target-zone heart rate method.

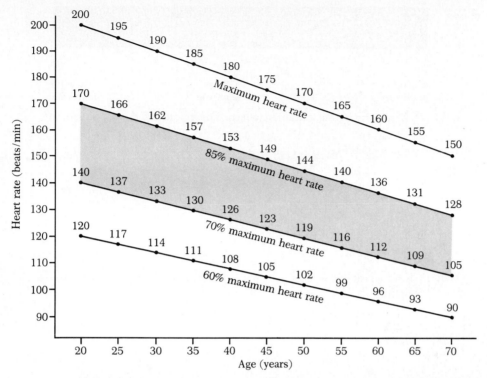

Fig. 2-7 Maximal heart rate and target-zone heart rate in relation to age. Also included is the corresponding 60% level of maximal heart rate.

Your critical, or threshold, heart rate represents the minimal heart rate needed for the development of cardiovascular endurance. It is determined by calculating 60% of the difference between your maximal and **resting heart rates** and then adding this value to your resting heart rate (Fig. 2-8 on p. 48).

TABLE 2-2 Determination of the target-zone heart rate for specified age-groups

Age range	Target-zone heart rate		Number of beats/ 10 seconds
	Lower limit (beats/min)	Upper limit (beats/min)	
20-29	140	162	23-27
30-39	133	154	22-26
40-49	126	145	21-24
50-59	119	137	20-23
60-69	112	128	19-21

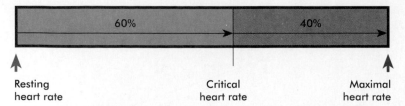

Fig. 2-8 Critical heart rate in relation to resting heart rate and maximal heart rate.

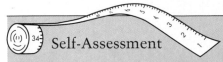

CALCULATION OF YOUR CRITICAL HEART RATE

Your critical heart rate may be calculated as follows:

Critical heart rate = Resting heart rate + 0.60(Max heart rate − Resting heart rate)

EXAMPLE: If a subject has a resting heart rate of 70 beats/min and a maximal heart rate of 190 beats/min:

$$Critical\ heart\ rate = 70 + 0.60\ (190 - 70)$$
$$= 70 + 0.60\ (120)$$
$$= 70 + 72$$
$$= 142$$

To calculate your critical heart rate you must know your resting heart rate and either know or estimate your maximal heart rate. Procedures for obtaining these scores have previously been identified.

Your resting heart rate _____ beats/min
Your maximal heart rate _____ beats/min
Critical heart rate = Resting heart rate + 0.60 (Max heart rate − Resting heart rate)
= _____ + 0.60 (_____ − _____)
= _____ + 0.60 − (_____)
= _____ + _____
= _____ beats/min

You must consistently keep your heart rate above this value while exercising if you want maximum development of cardiovascular fitness.

Use of a heart rate monitor. Various heart rate monitors can be used to determine your heart rate while you are exercising. An advantage of these is that you do not have to stop exercising to determine your heart rate. By knowing your heart rate while exercising, you can adjust the intensity of your workout to sustain your heart rate at the desired level. Most monitors provide a continuous digital readout of the heart rate.

The Polar Vantage Heart Watch (Fig. 2-9) allows you to store heart rates into memory so that you can play them back and record them later. With this monitor, after you have finished your workout, you can see exactly what your heart rate was at any time during your exercise session. In addition, the monitor will alert you if you are exercising at a level that is too low or too high. This takes the guesswork out of exercise.

Computer programs are available to analyze scores from heart rate monitors. These can be used to compare heart rate responses for different activities and to measure aerobic fitness improvement. The Fitness Profile Software, developed for use with this textbook, contains a heart rate monitoring program. Fig. 2-10 on p. 50 contains a sample printout.

Rate of perceived exertion. Despite the fact that the heart rate is used most often for evaluating intensity of exercise, it does have the following limitations:

- Some people have difficulty finding their pulse and/or counting it accurately.
- Errors in estimation of maximal heart rate result in calculation errors of the desired heart rate.
- Several factors can change your heart rate, including room temperature, level of stress, medication, altitude, and smoking.

Because of these limitations, an alternate method has become popular. This is the Rate of Perceived Exertion (RPE), developed in the 1960s by Borg. It uses a scale of numbers from 6 to 20, and each odd number is related to a subjective evaluation of exercise intensity (Table 2-3).

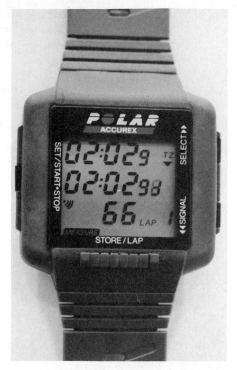

Fig. 2-9 A Polar heart rate monitor. Using a monitor such as this takes the guesswork out of exercise.

TABLE 2-3 **Rate of perceived exertion scale**

Number	Perceived exertion
6	
7	Very, very light
8	
9	Very light
10	
11	Fairly light
12	
13	Somewhat hard
14	
15	Hard
16	
17	Very hard
18	
19	Very, very hard
20	

This technique is based on the premise that you have the ability to determine how hard your body is working during exercise. To use this method you need to see the scale while exercising. Rate your exercise intensity based on how it feels. For college-aged students, adding a zero to the selected number should give an indication of the anticipated heart rate response for that level of work.

Change in exercise heart rate. Your exercise heart rate must be checked regularly because regular participation in a good aerobic exercise program will cause a gradual

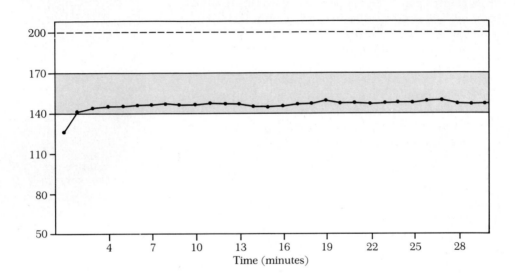

Name: *Freddie Fitness*   *Date:* **6/2/94**
Mode: *Regular running time:* **30 min**   *Total miles:* **3.00**

Exercise Heart Rate Summary

Name	Freddie Fitness
Date	6/2/94
Age (years)	21
Body Weight (lb)	165
Predicted maximal heart rate	199
70% maximal heart rate	139
85% maximal heart rate	169
Mode of exercise	Regular running
Time of exercise (minutes)	30
Total miles	3.00
Aerobic minutes of exercise	29
Average heart rate (beats/min)	144.27
Starting minute	1
Finishing minute	30
Standard deviation	3.71

Fig. 2-10 Sample printout from Fitness Profile Software for the Heart Rate Monitoring Program.

reduction in the exercise heart rate for a standardized task as your heart becomes more efficient. It is necessary to increase the intensity of the task from time to time to maintain your heart rate at the desired level. This is why progression must be built into an exercise program.

Frequency

Research indicates that maximal development of cardiovascular endurance can be attained if you exercise regularly, between 3 and 5 days per week, with the days of rest interspersed with exercise days.[24] Rest periods are essential and need to be built into any exercise program. They result in both physical and mental relaxation. Those who are starting an exercise program are advised against exercising more frequently than this. Exercising 6 or 7 days each week actually produces very minimal additional benefits and may in fact result in poor adaptation by the muscles in the body. The incidence of injury is much higher in those who exercise this frequently compared with those who exercise three to five times each week. It is better to start gradually and take more time in reaching your objectives than to start out at a high level and drop out because of injuries.

Duration of exercise sessions

The length of each exercise session may vary according to the objectives. The plan proposed by the American Heart Association for development of cardiovascular endurance is adequate for most people. This association suggests that each exercise session be divided into three segments[25]:

1. A 5- to 10-minute warm-up and stretching session so that the heart and circulatory system are not suddenly taxed

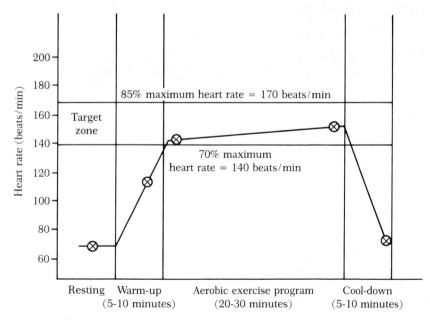

Fig. 2-11 Suggested exercise training pattern for a 20-year-old.

2. A sustained 20- to 30-minute exercise session in which the heart rate remains in the target zone
3. A 5- to 10-minute cool-down session in which the intensity of the task is lessened before the exercise is completely stopped

This plan is summarized in Fig. 2-11 on p. 51.

If you are training to compete in a marathon, or if your objective is to lose weight quickly, this plan would be inadequate. This is simply an exercise plan for optimal development of cardiovascular fitness.

The warm-up and cool-down phases of the program are important. A good warm-up gradually stretches the muscles and therefore reduces the chance of injury. In addition, it allows the heart to adjust to the increase in work. It can significantly reduce muscle soreness, which often results from a poorly planned exercise program.

The cool-down period is of equal importance. Blood relies on contraction of skeletal muscles to be returned to the heart from the lower extremities. If activity ceases abruptly and there is no contraction of these muscles, blood tends to pool in the legs, and there may be insufficient blood returned to the heart for circulation. Any body movement involving your legs will assist in the return of blood and will be beneficial.

Many people who initiate a running program for development of fitness feel that they must run a certain distance each week. However, the distance covered is not as important as making sure you continue long enough at an intensity that is high enough to produce the desired results. Most beginning joggers who are 20 to 30 years of age should be able to cover between 2 and 3 miles in 30 minutes of continuous work. If they exercise 5 days per week, which is the maximum that is recommended, they will cover 10 to 15 miles per week. Cooper[3] suggests that anyone who runs more than 15 miles per week is running for something other than fitness. The program previously described is consistent with his conclusion.

A question often asked is "If 30 minutes of sustained exercise will result in a significant improvement in cardiovascular fitness, will exercising longer result in even greater improvement?" Exercising longer will result only in minimal additional changes. Stone, for example, presents information showing that 15 minutes of exercise resulted in an 8.5% increase in aerobic fitness and with 30 minutes the increase was 16.1%. When the duration was increased to 45 minutes the corresponding change was 16.8%. In this study the intensity of the work remained constant with subjects working within their target zone.[23]

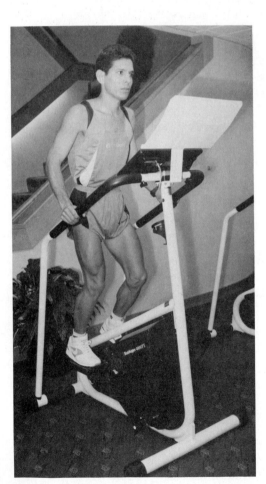

Fig. 2-12 Stair climbing is an excellent form of exercise.

You will not attain a high level of cardiovascular fitness without consistent effort. However, it should be realized that excessive effort is wasted. The old saying "no pain, no gain" simply is not true. You must learn how to exercise for maximum development of aerobic fitness without pain or discomfort. The amount of exercise you need will depend on your present level of fitness and what your objectives are for exercise. Your exercise program should be fun.

Mode of activity

If the criteria for intensity, duration, and frequency are met, it makes no difference what aerobic exercise you use. Any activity that can be maintained continuously and uses large muscle groups will be beneficial. Bicycling, swimming, walking, jogging, aerobics (aerobic dance), cross-country skiing, jumping rope, racquetball, basketball, and stair climbing (Fig. 2-12) are examples of good cardiovascular activities.

With activities such as walking, jogging, and bicycling, the intensity is simply determined by how fast you move and your skill level is of little significance. If your heart rate response is too low, you simply increase your speed until you reach the desired heart rate level (Fig. 2-7 on p. 47). With activities such as cross-country skiing and swimming, your skill level is very important. To a large extent this will determine how continuous the activity will be and how fast you will need to move to maintain your desired heart rate.

With racquetball and squash, not only is your skill level important but also the skill level of your opponent. If you have at least a minimal amount of skill and you play an opponent who is at least at your skill level, you can get a good aerobic workout playing racquetball or squash. The following case study will show how good an activity racquetball can be:

CASE STUDY: ROBERT

Robert is a 54-year-old who enjoys running and playing racquetball. He has participated regularly in these two activities for the last 10 years, not competitively, but simply to develop his level of aerobic fitness.

When running, because of his fitness level, Robert must run at about an $8\frac{1}{2}$-min mile pace, or 7 mph, to sustain his heart rate at the desired level (Fig. 2-13). When playing racquetball, he does not feel that he gets as good an aerobic workout, but despite the stop and start nature of the activity, his heart rate usually averages 10 to 20 beats/min higher for each minute of racquetball than it does when he is running. These scores are compared in Fig. 2-13 on p. 54.

Most racquetball and squash players who have at least a minimal amount of skill are able to achieve and maintain their desired target-zone heart rate. For them, these activities provide a good aerobic workout. Tennis, however, is not nearly as good as racquetball or squash. In tennis the heart rate goes up and down, not remaining in the target-zone long enough to bring about significant training effects. Even those who have an extremely high level of skill in tennis are rarely able to maintain their heart rate in the target zone. However, in racquetball even beginners can usually achieve and maintain the desired heart rate.

It is clear that not all activities are beneficial for development of aerobic fitness. Remember that the activity must be continuous, involve a large amount of musculature, and result in a heart rate consistently high enough to produce a cardiovascular training effect. Activities that usually meet these criteria are considered to be good aerobic activities.

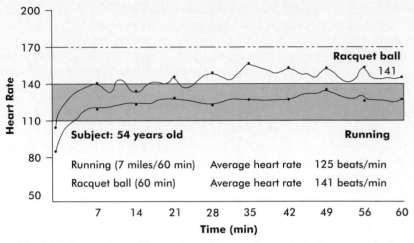

Fig. 2-13 Comparison of heart rates while running and playing racquetball.

Good aerobic activities

Aerobics (aerobic dance)	Rowing
Basketball	Running
Bicycling	Skating (ice and roller)
Cross-country skiing	Soccer
Handball	Squash
Jogging	Stair climbing
Racquetball	Stationary bicycling
Rebound running (mini trampoline)	Swimming
Rope jumping	Walking

Activities that do not meet these criteria are considered to be poor aerobic activities.

Poor aerobic activities

Archery	Gymnastics
Baseball	Softball
Bowling	Tennis
Football	Volleyball
Golf	Weight training

We have seen that your heart rate response to an activity will vary according to your aerobic fitness level (Fig. 2-6 on p. 45). What might be a good aerobic activity for one person may not be a good one for another. The best way to be sure that the activities you select are beneficial is to determine their intensity by measuring your heart rate response. Procedures for this have been identified previously in this chapter. Remember that this must be done regularly because a good aerobic program will change your heart rate response to a given activity. Laboratory Experience 2-3 outlines the procedures you can use to evaluate several of the activities you participate in.

MAINTENANCE OF CARDIOVASCULAR ENDURANCE

When you have reached a desirable level of cardiovascular endurance, you must make a lifetime commitment to exercise to sustain it. If you stop exercising, your fitness level deteriorates quickly, with all gains lost within 5 to 10 weeks.[5] However, you may not have to exercise as often to sustain your fitness level as you do to develop it. One study shows that exercising just 2 days per week is sufficient.

CHANGES IN THE BODY RESULTING FROM REGULAR AEROBIC EXERCISE

The human body was designed to be active, and when you exercise regularly, it will function more efficiently. There are a number of physiological adaptations occurring in the body that contribute to this increase in efficiency. These include the following:

CHANGE	RESULT
An increase in the strength of the heart muscle	An increased resting stroke volume, which means that the heart beats less frequently in circulating the same amount of blood. This also results in an increased maximal stroke volume, which means that your body is capable of circulating more blood when oxygen is needed by the muscles at a higher rate.
An increase in the number and/or size of the capillaries	A greater exchange of oxygen at the cellular level between the blood and cells. Your body is able to use more of the oxygen that you circulate.
An increase in the amount of hemoglobin	Your body can carry more oxygen in the blood to the working muscles.
An increase in the amount of oxygen that your body is capable of using ($\dot{V}O_2$ max.)	You can exercise longer and at a higher level before you become fatigued.

MEASUREMENT OF CARDIOVASCULAR ENDURANCE

The best method to determine cardiovascular endurance is to measure $\dot{V}O_2$ max. This involves the use of a treadmill or bicycle ergometer, and the heart rate, oxygen consumption, and other metabolic variables are monitored continuously during the test. The task is made progressively more difficult until a rate is reached where there is no further increase in oxygen consumption, even though the intensity of the task is increased. When this occurs, a person is said to have reached his or her maximal intake for that task. This relationship is illustrated in Fig. 2-14 on p. 56.

The measurement of $\dot{V}O_2$ max is a difficult procedure that can only be conducted in a well-equipped laboratory. It is not practical with large groups or for class use. An

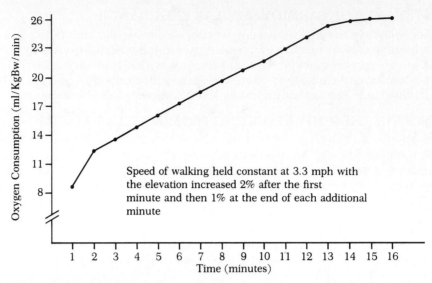

Fig. 2-14 Comparison of minute-by-minute oxygen consumption scores for a female on the Modified Balke Treadmill Test. Note the linear relationship in oxygen consumption until the thirteenth minute and then the leveling off, which occurs at this time.

alternate approach is to estimate **aerobic capacity** by measuring the maximal amount of work that can be performed over a period of time. The most commonly used tests involving this concept are the 12-minute run test and the timed 1.5 mile run.

Valid results can be obtained from these tests if you learn how to pace yourself and you give a maximal performance. If you do not run regularly, you will have a better chance of meeting these criteria if you take several days before the test and practice pacing yourself. Procedures to follow for the 12-minute run test are presented in Laboratory Experience 2-4 and for the 1½ mile run test in Laboratory Experience 2-5.

You can also estimate your aerobic capacity by evaluating the efficiency of your heart and circulatory system. You can measure your heart rate response to a standardized task such as the step test. Laboratory Experience 2-6 presents the information you need to use this evaluation.

SUMMARY

The following summary will help you identify some of the important concepts covered in this chapter:

- Cardiovascular endurance is the most important physical fitness component.
- Your level of aerobic fitness will be reflected by how much work you can perform and by what level you can work at.
- Anaerobic work is high-intensity work, which lasts for only a few minutes.
- Aerobic work is performed at a lower intensity than anaerobic work and can be sustained for a longer period.

- The heart and circulatory system must function efficiently if you are to attain a high level of aerobic fitness.
- The ability of your body to process and use oxygen will determine your level of cardiovascular endurance.
- To increase your aerobic capacity, you must exercise at the right intensity continuously for 20 to 30 minutes at least 3 days each week.

KEY TERMS

aerobic capacity The maximal rate at which work can be performed with the body supplying energy aerobically.

aerobic work Activities using large muscle groups at an intensity that can be sustained for a long period in which the body is able to provide sufficient energy aerobically.

anaerobic work A high intensity activity that can be sustained for only a short period in which energy demands are greater than the capacity of the heart and circulatory system to supply the energy.

artery A blood vessel that transports blood away from the heart.

atrium An upper chamber of the heart (blood being returned to the heart first enters the right or left atrium).

blood pressure The force exerted by blood against the walls of blood vessels.

capillary The smallest blood vessel in which exchange of gases takes place between blood and tissues.

cardiac output The amount of blood circulated by the heart each minute.

critical, or threshold, heart rate The minimal heart rate necessary for the development of cardiovascular endurance.

diastole The relaxation phase of the cardiac cycle when the heart is not contracting.

duration The time that an activity must be continued with the heart rate at a specified level to result in improvement of cardiovascular fitness.

frequency The number of times you must exercise each week to experience improvement in cardiovascular endurance.

heart The muscular pump responsible for the circulation of blood through the circulatory system.

heart rate The number of times the heart contracts per minute.

hemoglobin The iron-containing protein found in blood that is responsible for the transportation of oxygen.

hypertension Blood pressure that is consistently higher than it should be.

intensity Stress placed on the body by an activity. It can usually be measured by the heart rate response to the work involved.

maximal heart rate The maximal heart rate the body is capable of attaining. It can be estimated by subtracting your age from 220.

maximal oxygen consumption The maximum amount of oxygen the body is capable of processing and using. It is considered to be the best measure of cardiovascular endurance. It is also referred to as maximal oxygen uptake, aerobic capacity, and physical work capacity.

resting heart rate The number of times your heart contracts each minute while the body is at rest.

stroke volume The amount of blood pumped from the left ventricle each time the heart contracts.

systole   The contraction phase of the cardiac cycle, occurring when the ventricles contract and force blood out of the heart.

submaximal task   A task performed aerobically at an intensity where the body can supply the necessary energy aerobically.

target-zone heart rate   The heart rate necessary for maximum development of cardiovascular endurance. It is 70% to 85% of the maximal heart rate.

vein   A blood vessel that returns blood to the heart.

ventricle   The lower chamber of the heart. It is responsible for pumping blood away from the heart.

REFERENCES

1. Brehm BA: Understanding energy expenditure, *Fitness Management* 4:1 1988.
2. Consolazio F, Johnson R, Pecora L: *Physiological measurement of metabolic function in man,* New York, 1963, McGraw-Hill.
3. Cooper KH: *The aerobics program for total well-being,* New York, 1982, M Evans & Co.
4. Gibson SB, Gerberich SG, Leon AS: Writing the exercise prescription: an individualized approach, *The Physician and Sports Medicine* 11(7):87-110, 1983.
5. Greer N, Katch F: Validity of palpation recovery pulse to estimate heart rate following four intensities of bench step exercise, *Research Quarterly for Exercise and Sport* 53:340, 1982.
6. Hales D, Hales RE: How much is enough? *Amercian Health: Fitness of Body and Mind* 5:14-17, 1986.
7. Health Information Library: *Aerobic exercise,* Daly City, Calif, 1985, Krames Communications.
8. Hickson RC, Rosenkoetter MA: Reduced training frequencies and maintenance of increased aerobic power, *Medicine and Science in Sports and Exercise* 13(1):13-16, 1981.
9. Hoeger WWK: *Principles and labs for physical fitness and wellness,* ed 2, Englewood, Colo, 1991, Morton Publishing.
10. Jerome J: Getting it all back, *American Health: Fitness of Body and Mind* pp 62-67, June 1982.
11. Johannessen S et al: High frequency, moderate intensity training in sedentary middle-aged women, *The Physician and Sports Medicine* 14(5):99-102, 1986.
12. Karvonen MJ: Effects of vigorous activity on the heart. In Rosenbaum MJ FF, Belknap EL, editors: *Work and the heart,* New York, 1959, Paul B Hoeber.
13. Katch V, Katch F: *Inside exercise, Shape,* November 11, 1984.
14. McArdle WW, Katch F, Katch V: *Exercise physiology: exercise, nutrition and human performance,* ed 3, Philadelphia, 1991, Lea & Febiger.
15. Mirkin G, Shangold M: Getting back in shape, *Nation's Business* 71:36, 1983.
16. Monohan T: Is activity as good as exercise? *Physician Sportsmed* 15(10):181-186, 1987.
17. Ong TC, Sothy SP: Exercise and cardiorespiratory fitness, *Ergonomics* 29(2):273-280, 1986.
18. Phillips G: How does your exercise rate? *Dance Exercise Today* pp 55-58, June/July 1986.
19. Rogers CC: Of magic, miracles and exercise myths, *The Physician and Sports Medicine* 13(5):156-166, 1985.
20. Sheehan G: Beyond fitness, *Physician Sportsmed* 15(10):67, 1987.
21. Stamford B: Predicting your aerobic fitness, *The Physician and Sports Medicine* 13:3, 1985.
22. Stamford B: What is exercise capacity? *The Physician and Sports Medicine* 15:4, 1987.
23. Stone WJ: *Adult fitness programs: planning, designing, managing and improving fitness programs,* Glenview, Ill, 1987, Scott, Foresman & Co.
24. Wenger HA, Bell GJ: The interactions of intensity, frequency and duration of exercise training in altering cardiorespiratory fitness, *Sports Medicine* 3:346-356, 1986.
25. Zohman LR: *Exercise your way to fitness and heart health,* 1974, American Heart Association.

Measuring Your Heart Rate

Your heart rate can be determined by counting how frequently your heart contracts during a given period and converting this number to the standard measure in beats/min. Make sure that you press just firmly enough to feel the pulse. If you press too hard it may interfere with the rhythm.

Determination of Your Resting Heart Rate

There are many factors that influence your resting heart rate. These include stress, food, excitement, room temperature, and previous physical exertion.

Your resting heart rate should be taken while sitting quietly and not after participating in vigorous activity. If possible you should sit quietly for at least 30 minutes before measuring it. Take it several times to make sure it is stable.

Your resting heart rate should not be changing as rapidly as it does following exercise, so you can count for either 10 seconds and multiply by 6, 30 seconds and multiply by 2, or count for the full minute.

RESTING HEART RATE

Trial 1	_____	beats/min
Trial 2	_____	beats/min
Trial 3	_____	beats/min
Trial 4	_____	beats/min
Trial 5	_____	beats/min
Typical score	_____	beats/min

Most highly-trained endurance athletes have low resting heart rates. Most untrained subjects who participate regularly in a good aerobic fitness program will experience a decrease in their resting heart rates. Your score can be evaluated as follows:

RATING	RESTING HEART RATE (BEATS/MIN)
Excellent	<60
Good	60-69
Average	70-79
Fair	80-89
Poor	>89

Measuring Your Blood Pressure

A sphygmomanometer is used to measure blood pressure (Fig. 2-15 on p. 60). An airtight cuff is wrapped around the arm just above the elbow. The cuff is connected to a glass tube filled with mercury. Air is pumped into the cuff by squeezing a bulb. As the cuff becomes tighter, it compresses a large artery in the arm—the brachial artery. This temporarily cuts off the flow of blood to the forearm, and no heart sounds can be heard when a stethoscope is placed on the compressed artery just below the cuff. As the air pressure in the cuff is released, the mercury level drops. Eventually a point will be reached at which the blood pressure in the artery is just greater than the air pressure in the cuff. Blood will now begin to flow through the artery, and the heart sound may be heard through the stethoscope. This is the systolic, or upper, pressure; it is the maximum pressure that can be produced by the heart. As air continues to be let out of the cuff, the sounds heard through the stethoscope will become louder as more blood flows through the artery. Finally, a point will be reached at which the distinct heart sounds disappear as the blood is flowing steadily through the artery. At this point the height of the mercury shows the diastolic, or lower, pressure representing the least amount of pressure in the artery.

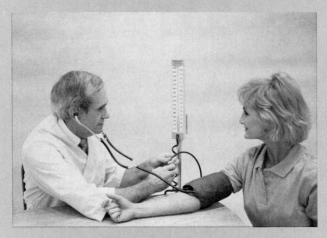

Fig. 2-15 Measurement of blood pressure with a sphygmomanometer.

Record your blood pressure figures in the space provided below.

Blood pressure _____ / _____
Classification _____

Interpretation: *Your blood pressure scores can be evaluated by consulting Table 2-4.*

TABLE 2-4 **Classification of blood pressure scores**

Score	Classification	Values (mm Hg)
Systolic	Good	<116
	Average	116-140
	Poor	>140
Diastolic	Good	<80
	Average	80-90
	Poor	>90

Determination of Exercise Heart Rate without a Monitor

If you do not use a heart rate monitor, it is usually not possible to count your heart rate accurately while participating in most activities. However, an accurate estimate of your exercise heart rate can be obtained if your heart rate is counted immediately after exercising. If you do not start counting within 10 seconds after stopping, the score is likely to be inaccurate.

Count the number of beats in 10 seconds and multiply this value by 6 to convert it to beats/min. Do not count for a longer time because your heart rate begins to slow down as soon as you stop exercising. The more fit you are, the quicker you heart rate will decrease following exercise.

Select several activities that you enjoy. Perform each for 5 minutes, working at a constant level or speed. Record heart rates for each of these activities.

ACTIVITY	BEATS/10 SECONDS × 6 = BEATS/MIN
_____	_____ × 6 = _____
_____	_____ × 6 = _____
_____	_____ × 6 = _____
_____	_____ × 6 = _____
_____	_____ × 6 = _____
_____	_____ × 6 = _____
_____	_____ × 6 = _____

Measurement of Cardiovascular Endurance: 12-Minute Run Test

Description

For 12 minutes run as far as possible and try to maintain a steady pace until the last few minutes, when you should try to speed up slightly depending on how much energy you have left. The number of laps completed during this time is counted and recorded, and the distance covered is calculated.

Results

Record the results in the spaces provided.

Number of laps completed: _____

Distance of 1 lap   _____ feet

Distance covered = laps × distance

= _____ × _____ feet

= _____ feet

To convert to miles, divide by 5280

Distance covered = distance covered (feet)/5280

= _____ /5280

= _____ miles

(calculate to two decimal places)

Interpretation

The results for the 12-minute run test can be evaluated by consulting Table 2-5 (men) or Table 2-6 (women).

TABLE 2-5 **Classification of scores for 12-minute run test** *(men)* **distance (miles)**

Category	Percentile rank	Age (years)					
		<20	**20-29**	**30-39**	**40-49**	**50-59**	**>59**
Excellent	95	2.04	1.91	1.79	1.70	1.58	1.49
	90	1.95	1.82	1.70	1.61	1.49	1.40
Good	80	1.85	1.72	1.60	1.51	1.39	1.30
	70	1.78	1.65	1.53	1.44	1.32	1.23
Average	60	1.72	1.59	1.47	1.38	1.26	1.17
	50	1.66	1.53	1.41	1.32	1.20	1.11
	40	1.60	1.47	1.35	1.26	1.14	1.05
Fair	30	1.54	1.41	1.29	1.20	1.08	0.99
	20	1.47	1.34	1.22	1.13	1.01	0.92
Poor	10	1.37	1.24	1.12	1.03	0.91	0.82
	5	1.28	1.15	1.03	0.94	0.82	0.73
Mean		1.66	1.53	1.41	1.32	1.20	1.11
Standard deviation		0.23	0.23	0.23	0.23	0.23	0.23

TABLE 2-6 Classification of scores for 12-minute run test *(women)* distance (miles)

Category	Percentile rank	Age (years)					
		<20	20-29	30-39	40-49	50-59	>59
Excellent	95	1.70	1.62	1.54	1.44	1.37	1.28
	90	1.61	1.53	1.45	1.35	1.28	1.19
Good	80	1.51	1.43	1.35	1.25	1.18	1.09
	70	1.44	1.36	1.28	1.18	1.11	1.02
Average	60	1.38	1.30	1.22	1.12	1.05	0.96
	50	1.32	1.24	1.16	1.06	0.99	0.90
	40	1.26	1.18	1.10	1.00	0.93	0.84
Fair	30	1.20	1.12	1.04	0.94	0.87	0.78
	20	1.13	1.05	0.97	0.87	0.80	0.71
Poor	10	1.03	0.95	0.87	0.77	0.70	0.61
	5	0.94	0.86	0.78	0.68	0.61	0.52
Mean		1.32	1.24	1.16	1.06	0.99	0.90
Standard deviation		0.23	0.23	0.23	0.23	0.23	0.23

LABORATORY EXPERIENCE 2–5

Measurement of Cardiovascular Endurance: 1¹/₂-Mile Run

Description

The 1¹/₂-mile run test may be preferred to the 12-minute run test because it is easier to administer. You should try to cover 1¹/₂ miles in the shortest time possible. Elapsed time is recorded in minutes and seconds.

Results

Record the results of the 1¹/₂-mile run test in the spaces provided.

Time for 1¹/₂-mile run _____ minutes _____ seconds.

Interpretation

The results for the 1¹/₂-mile run test can be evaluated by consulting Table 2-7 (men) or Table 2-8 (women).

TABLE 2-7 Classification of scores for 1½-mile run test *(men)* time (min:sec)

Category	Percentile rank	Age (years)					
		<20	20-29	30-39	40-49	50-59	>59
Excellent	95	8:50	9:21	10:02	10:30	11:20	11:56
	90	9:17	9:53	10:39	11:11	12:10	12:52
Good	80	9:50	10:32	11:25	12:02	13:11	14:01
	70	10:15	11:00	11:58	12:38	13:56	14:51
Averaage	60	10:35	11:24	12:26	13:09	14:33	15:34
	50	10:54	11:46	12:52	13:38	15:08	16:13
	40	11:13	12:08	13:18	14:07	15:43	16:52
Fair	30	11:33	12:32	13:46	14:38	16:20	17:35
	20	11:58	13:00	14:19	15:14	17:05	18:25
Poor	10	12:31	13:39	15:05	16:05	18:06	19:34
	5	12:58	14:11	15:42	16:46	18:56	20:30
Mean		10:54	11:46	12:52	13:38	15:08	16:13
Standard deviation		1:16	1:28	1:44	1:55	2:19	2:37

TABLE 2-8 Classification of scores for 1½-mile run test *(women)* time (min:sec)

Category	Percentile rank	Age (years)					
		<20	20-29	30-39	40-49	50-59	>59
Excellent	95	10:39	11:00	11:36	12:16	12:46	13:45
	90	11:16	11:46	12:30	13:14	14:00	15:07
Good	80	12:01	12:43	13:35	14:28	15:30	16:48
	70	12:34	13:24	14:22	15:22	16:36	18:01
Average	60	13:02	13:59	15:01	16:07	17:31	19:03
	50	13:28	14:37	15:39	16:49	18:22	20:00
	40	13:54	15:03	16:16	17:31	19:13	20:57
Fair	30	14:22	15:38	16:56	18:16	20:08	21:59
	20	14:55	16:19	17:43	19:10	21:14	23:12
Poor	10	15:40	17:16	18:48	20:24	22:44	24:53
	5	16:17	18:02	19:41	21:25	23:58	26:15
Mean		13:28	14:37	15:39	16:49	18:22	20:00
Standard deviation		1:43	2:09	2:28	2:48	3:25	3:49

Estimation of $\dot{V}O_2$ max from Running Tests

The results of the 12-minute run test or the $1\frac{1}{2}$-mile run test can be used to estimate your maximal oxygen consumption. Knowing the distance covered and/or the time, you can easily determine your average running speed.

EXAMPLE 1

A person who runs 1.6 miles in 12 minutes has an average running speed of 1.6 × 5, or 8 mph. (Multiply by 5 because there are 5 periods of 12 minutes in 1 hour.)

EXAMPLE 2

A person who completes the $1\frac{1}{2}$-mile run test in 10 minutes has an average running speed of $1\frac{1}{2}$ × 6, or 9 mph. (Multiply by 6 because 6 periods of 10 minutes make up 1 hour.)

The approximate $\dot{V}O_2$ values for selected speeds of walking and running are given in Table 2-9.

TABLE 2-9 Approximate $\dot{V}O_2$ values for selected speeds of walking and running

Activity	Speed (mph)	Estimated $\dot{V}O_2$ consumption (ml/kg body weight/min)
Walking	2.5	11.6
	3.0	13.9
	3.5	16.2
	4.0	18.5
Running	5.0	30.1
	6.0	35.7
	7.0	40.9
	8.0	46.6
	9.0	51.8
	10.0	57.1

To estimate your $\dot{V}O_2$ max, simply find your distance covered for the 12-minute run test, and/or your time for the $1\frac{1}{2}$ mile run test in Table 2-10, and your estimated value will be given in the first column corresponding to your score.

Your score can be evaluated by consulting Table 2-11 (men) or Table 2-12 (women).

TABLE 2-10 Estimated maximal $\dot{V}O_2$ based on 12-minute run and $1\frac{1}{2}$-mile run tests

Estimated maximal $\dot{V}O_2$ (ml/kg body weight/min)	12-Minute run distance (miles)	$1\frac{1}{2}$-Mile run time (min:sec)
56	2.07	8:42
55	2.02	8:54
54	1.99	9:03
53	1.94	9:17
52	1.91	9:25
51	1.87	9:38
50	1.83	9:50
49	1.79	10:03
48	1.75	10:17
47	1.71	10:32
46	1.66	10:50
45	1.62	11:06
44	1.58	11:24
43	1.54	11:41
42	1.50	12:00
41	1.45	12:25
40	1.41	12:46
39	1.37	13:08
38	1.33	13:32
37	1.29	13:57
36	1.24	14:31
35	1.20	15:00
34	1.16	15:31
33	1.12	16:04
32	1.08	16:40
31	1.03	17:28
30	0.99	18:10
29	0.95	18:57
28	0.91	19:46
27	0.87	20:41
26	0.83	21:41
25	0.78	23:05

TABLE 2-11 Classification of scores for maximal oxygen consumption *(men)* (ml/kg body weight/min)

Category	Percentile rank	Age (years)					
		<20	20-29	30-39	40-49	50-59	>59
Excellent	95	55	52	49	47	44	42
	90	53	50	47	45	42	40
Good	80	51	48	45	43	40	38
	70	49	46	43	41	38	36
Average	60	47	44	41	39	36	34
	50	46	43	40	38	35	33
	40	45	42	39	37	34	32
Fair	30	43	40	37	35	32	30
	20	41	38	35	33	30	28
Poor	10	39	36	33	31	28	26
	5	37	34	31	29	26	24
Mean		46	43	40	38	35	33
Standard deviation		5.5	5.5	5.5	5.5	5.5	5.5

NOTE: All scores are rounded to the nearest whole number.

TABLE 2-12 Classification of scores for maximal oxygen consumption *(women)* (ml/kg body weight/min)

Category	Percentile rank	Age (years)					
		<20	20-29	30-39	40-49	50-59	>59
Excellent	95	47	45	43	41	39	37
	90	45	43	41	39	37	35
Good	80	43	41	39	37	35	33
	70	41	39	37	35	33	31
Average	60	39	37	35	33	31	29
	50	38	36	34	32	30	28
	40	37	35	33	31	29	27
Fair	30	35	33	31	29	27	25
	20	33	31	29	27	25	23
Poor	10	31	29	27	25	23	21
	5	29	27	25	23	21	19
Mean		38	36	34	32	30	28
Standard deviation		5.5	5.5	5.5	5.5	5.5	5.5

NOTE: All scores are rounded to the nearest whole number.

Measurement of Cardiovascular Endurance: The Step Test

Many versions of the step test are available. Probably the most common is the original 5-minute step test. This test and its variations are not as good as the 12-minute run test or the $1\frac{1}{2}$-mile run test, but because of practical considerations, it is often used, particularly with large groups of students.

An accurate measurement of the heart rate is necessary if the results from this test are to be meaningful. If you have trouble counting your heart rate, the results will not be accurate. For this evaluation the pulse will be counted for $\frac{1}{2}$-minute periods and then converted to beats per minute by multiplying the obtained value by 2. Practice counting your heart rate by taking four $\frac{1}{2}$-minute counts while remaining seated. Refrain from talking and unnecessary movement during periods when heart rates are being counted; these activities can influence your results.

Results should be recorded in the space below.

TRIAL	BEATS/$\frac{1}{2}$ MIN		BEATS/MIN
1	_____	× 2 =	_____
2	_____	× 2 =	_____
3	_____	× 2 =	_____
4	_____	× 2 =	_____

The step test is based on the premise that for a submaximal work task the person with a higher level of cardiovascular fitness not only will have a smaller increase in heart rate but also will have a heart rate that returns to normal much faster following the task than it would in a person with a lower level.

Purpose

The purpose of this test is to obtain immediate knowledge of the level of cardiovascular efficiency.

Method

Do not perform any activity before this test; no warm-up is allowed. A 20-inch bench should be used for men, and a 16-inch bench for women. Step up to and down from this bench at the rate of 30 steps per minute. The same foot must start the "step-up" each time, and an erect posture must be assumed. Continue the activity for a maximum of 5 minutes or until you are unable to maintain the set rate. The heart rate is determined for a $\frac{1}{2}$-minute period, starting exactly 1 minute after completion of the last step (that is, from 1 to $1\frac{1}{2}$ minutes after completion of the task).

Results

Record the results in the spaces provided.

Time of stepping _____ seconds

Heart rate _____ beats/$\frac{1}{2}$ min (1 to $1\frac{1}{2}$ minutes of recovery)

The physical efficiency index (PEI) may be estimated by consulting Table 2-13, or it may be calculated using the following procedure.

CALCULATION OF PEI

$$PEI = \frac{\text{Time of stepping (sec)} \times 100}{5.5 \times \text{heart rate for } \frac{1}{2} \text{ minute}}$$

$$= \frac{\underline{\hspace{1cm}} \times 100}{5.5 \times \underline{\hspace{1cm}}}$$

$$= \underline{\hspace{1cm}}$$

$$= \underline{\hspace{1cm}}$$

$$= \frac{\underline{\hspace{1cm}} \times 100}{5.5 \underline{\hspace{1cm}}}$$

$$= \underline{\hspace{1cm}}$$

Interpretation

The results are interpreted in Table 2-14.

TABLE 2-13 Scoring for the Harvard step test*

Duration of effort (minute) 99	Total heart beats 1-1½ minutes into recovery (score—arbitrary units)											
	40-44	45-49	50-54	55-59	60-64	65-69	70-74	75-79	80-84	85-89	90-94	95-
0-½	6	6	5	5	4	4	4	4	3	3	3	3
½-1	19	17	16	14	13	12	11	11	10	9	9	8
1-1½	32	29	26	24	22	20	19	18	17	16	15	14
1½-2	45	41	38	34	31	29	27	25	23	22	21	20
2-2½	58	52	47	43	40	36	34	32	30	28	27	25
2½-3	71	64	58	53	48	45	42	39	37	34	33	31
3-3½	84	75	68	62	57	53	49	46	43	41	39	37
3½-4	97	87	79	72	66	61	57	53	50	47	45	42
4-4½	110	98	89	82	75	70	65	61	57	54	51	48
4½-5	123	110	100	91	84	77	72	68	63	60	57	54
5	129	116	105	96	88	82	76	71	67	63	60	56

From Consolazio F, Johnson R, Pecora L: *Physiological measurement of metabolic functions in man,* New York, 1963, McGraw-Hill.
*INSTRUCTIONS:
1. Find the appropriate line for the time stepping was continued.
2. Find the appropriate column for the pulse count for the 30-second period; do *not* multiply this by 2—it is a 30-second count that is used.
3. Read the score where this line and column intersect.

TABLE 2-14 **Classification of Harvard step test scores**

Score	Cardiovascular classification
55 or below	Very poor
56-64	Poor
65-79	Average
80-89	Good
90 or above	Excellent

Development of Cardiovascular Endurance

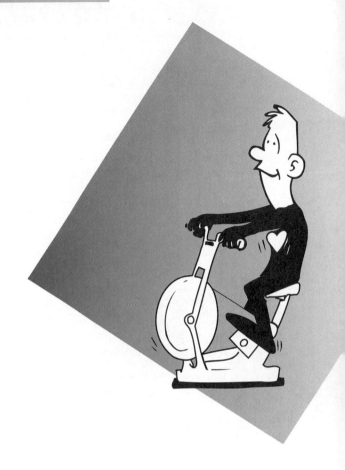

CHAPTER OBJECTIVES

When you understand the material in this chapter, you will be able to:

- Identify the activities that can be used for the development of aerobic fitness and know how to incorporate these activities into a good aerobic fitness program
- Determine the level at which you need to exercise for each of the aerobic activities
- Evaluate and compare the advantages and disadvantages of the various activities and programs
- Discuss the advantages of circuit training as compared with a regular exercise program involving calisthenics
- Design a program using weight training activities that can contribute to the development of cardiovascular endurance

O ne of the most frequently asked questions pertaining to aerobic exercise is "How much exercise do I really need?" The answer to this question basically depends on who is exercising, what his or her fitness level is, and what his or her objectives are. The reasons why most people participate in some form of aerobic exercise can be grouped into three major categories:

Fitness: The overall objective for many people who exercise regularly is to increase their level of cardiovascular fitness so that their bodies function more efficiently.

Weight/body composition: Many people use aerobic exercise to reduce their body weight and/or their percentage of body fat to a desirable level and then to maintain that level.

Health: There are many health benefits associated with regular aerobic exercise. You can add years to your life by reducing your risk for developing cardiovascular disease, diabetes, hypertension, and osteoporosis.

The amount of exercise necessary for attaining each of these objectives will vary. This chapter will provide information concerning several different aerobic activities or programs. By applying the scientific principles presented in other parts of this book, you will be able to achieve an optimal level of aerobic fitness together with the associated health benefits, and you will know how to achieve and maintain a desirable body weight and/or percentage of body fat.

> The secret is to exercise enough so that you will be successful at achieving your goals yet not so much that it becomes an obsession or that you are constantly tired or frequently in pain or injured.

AEROBIC ACTIVITIES

Any activity that is continuous and involves large muscle groups can be classified as an aerobic activity. Aerobic activities that meet these criteria are listed in the accompanying box.

CONTINUOUS AEROBIC ACTIVITIES

Aerobic dance (aerobics)	Bicycling
Cross-country skiing	Jogging/Running
Rebound running	Rope jumping
Ice skating	Roller skating
Stair-stepping	Stationary bicycling
Swimming	Walking

Because of the continuous nature of these activities, all you need to do is to determine at what **intensity level** you need to participate in order to maintain your heart rate at the desired level.

The following Case Study may help you to understand this concept and will help you to get started:

CASE STUDY: JIM

Jim is a 20-year-old college student who wants to start an exercise program for the specific purpose of developing his level of aerobic fitness. He knows how to measure his heart rate, and he knows that if he is to be successful, he must exercise at such an intensity that his heart rate gets to and stays between 140 and 170 beats/min (see Chapter 2). However, he does not know what he needs to do to achieve this. He decides to start out by walking. All he needs for this is a good pair of walking or jogging shoes and a watch.

He measures a distance that is exactly 1 mile and decides to walk this distance at a brisk pace. He finds that it takes him 15 min-

utes. Upon stopping, he immediately counts his pulse for 10 seconds and finds that his heart rate is 120 beats/min (20 beats in 10 seconds). He now knows that by walking a mile in 15 minutes he is not exercising at a fast enough pace to maintain his heart rate in his target zone.

Jim decides to cover the same 1-mile distance again only this time he decides to jog at a very slow pace. He finds that this time it takes him 12 minutes, and his heart rate at the end of the mile is 150 beats/min. Jim has now discovered the pace that he needs to maintain to achieve the right intensity for this type of workout.

When participating in any of the aerobic activities previously listed (see the box on p. 74), it is important to follow the same procedures as identified in the Case Study so that you can determine the correct level at which you should exercise. This will depend on your level of aerobic fitness, which basically reflects how efficiently your heart and circulatory system function. You must also keep in mind that over time your heart rate response to a specific task will change if you develop good, consistent exercise habits. For this reason, you need to periodically check your heart rate response to make sure that you are exercising at the right intensity.

There are also other aerobic activities that are not as continuous as those previously listed. Although these activities involve stop and start motion, because of the nature of the movements involved, many participants in these activities are able to sustain their heart rate in their target zone. These activities can therefore be classified as aerobic activities and include basketball, handball, racquetball, soccer, and squash. Information on several of these activities is presented later in this chapter.

STARTING YOUR PROGRAM

When initiating a program, it is important to start out at a low level and progress slowly. Many problems are caused by doing too much too soon. If you intend to become involved in a running program, most likely you will have to start out by walking and gradually build up your endurance and efficiency until you can run slowly.

Time must be taken in each session to **warm up** and **cool down.** If the correct procedures are followed, muscle soreness can be reduced, and many injuries associated with exercise programs can be avoided. People who have had exercise-related injuries quickly learn to warm up and stretch the muscle groups they intend to use. Information pertaining to warming up and cooling down is presented in Chapter 5.

WALKING

Walking is fast becoming one of the most popular aerobic fitness activities. The results from two recent national surveys are summarized below[25,26]:

- In 1991, over 73% of the adults surveyed indicated that "during the past month" they had done some "walking for exercise." This is significantly higher than a previous survey in 1986 (69%).
- Americans are now walking longer distances when they walk.
- Walking attracts a solid core of long-term enthusiasts. More than 40% of adults who walk for exercise have been walking for "more than 5 years."
- The percentage of walkers increases with age.
- Older adults also walk more frequently. Over 54% of those over 65 years of age walk "several times each week."

One possible reason why walking has become so popular is that walking is a natural activity. Even a sedentary American worker will average 2 to 3 miles/day performing everyday tasks. Unfortunately, the walking that most people get as part of their everyday tasks is not continuous enough to contribute to the development of aerobic fitness.

For a walking program all you need is a good pair of shoes. You need little or no instruction, and you can walk almost anywhere either alone or with someone. Walking can be an enjoyable exercise, and although it is not as intense as jogging or running, it can be used by many people to develop cardiovascular fitness. Sustaining a steady brisk pace will maximize aerobic benefits.

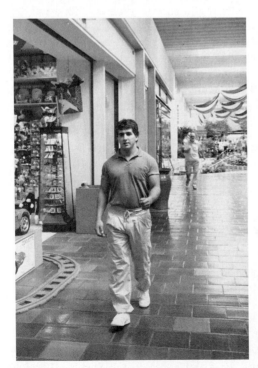 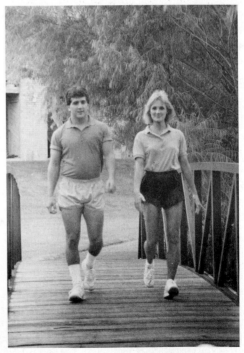

When the weather is inclement, walkers often use shopping malls for their aerobic workout. Many malls promote walking programs *(left)*. Walking is a form of movement in which at least one foot is in contact with the ground at all times *(right)*.

If you use walking to develop your aerobic fitness level, it is important to learn how fast you must walk to sustain the desired heart rate. The normal pace for most people is 3 to 4 mph. You must walk fast enough to keep your heart rate in your target zone but not so fast that you cannot carry on a conversation or so fast that you are constantly fatigued. You should never walk so hard that you are unable to perform the same workout the next day. The procedures for initiating a walking program are included in Laboratory Experience 3-1.

If you use walking in your training program, it may be necessary to spend more than the 20 to 30 minutes per exercise session as suggested previously. This is particularly true if you wish to lose weight as well as develop cardiovascular endurance.

Your heart rate response to walking will depend on your aerobic fitness level. Heart rate responses for two 20-year-old women walking at 4 mph are compared in Fig. 3-1. This speed is equivalent to walking a mile in 15 minutes. Even though each subject's weight is about the same, there is a significant difference in their heart rate responses to the same task. Subject 1 obviously has a higher level of cardiovascular fitness. Her heart is more efficient and therefore does not have to beat as frequently. This task is not of sufficient intensity for her heart rate to reach the target zone. However, for subject 2, walking at the rate of 15 minutes per mile is sufficient to produce the training effect.

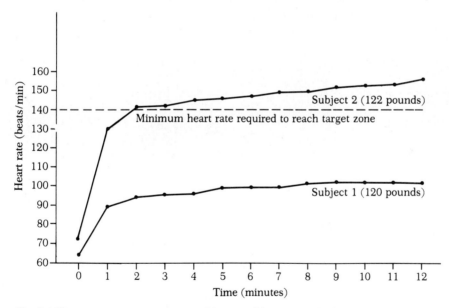

Fig. 3-1 Heart rate response of two subjects walking at 4 mph. *Subject 2* could use walking as her aerobic activity, whereas *subject 1* would need a running program to obtain the same results.

To initiate a good walking program you will need to:
- Know your current level of fitness
- Have a good pair of walking or jogging shoes
- Be able to calculate your target-zone heart rate
- Be able to determine your pulse accurately

You also need to walk correctly. You should always walk with the heel-to-toe method (Fig. 3-2). The heel of the leading foot should always touch the ground before the ball of the foot and the toes. You should land as softly as possible to absorb the shock. When pushing off, the knee is bent so that the heel is raised and the weight is shifted forward. The toes push off, and the leg is accelerated forward to get in front of the body.

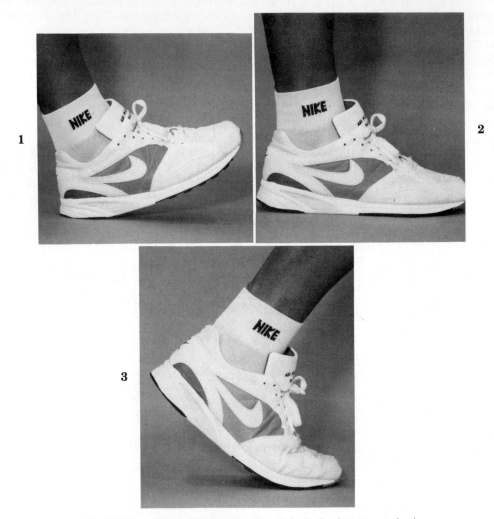

Fig. 3-2 The correct way to run and walk is the heel-to-toe method.

Fast walking and aerobic training

A question often asked is "Is fast walking intense enough to sustain your heart rate within your target zone?" Several studies of fast walking have shown that it can be an effective exercise for most people for the development of aerobic fitness.[24] In one study, for example, which involved 343 subjects, 91% of women and 83% of men were able to reach their target-zone heart rate while walking. In a second study, even young men with a high level of aerobic fitness were able to achieve and maintain this target-zone heart rate during a 30-minute walk. For most adults, it would appear that fast walking can be used as an adequate aerobic training stimulus.

Use of hand weights while walking

In recent years the use of light hand-held weights while walking has become popular. Usually, weights ranging from 1 to 5 lb are held in each hand. The use of such weights while walking can produce a significant increase in both heart rate and caloric expenditure. However, this happens only if the arm movements are accentuated and are more vigorous than they would normally be during regular walking. Simply carrying the weights with little or no arm movement will result in only small increases of energy expenditure. Proper use of hand weights while walking will provide the necessary stimulus for the development of aerobic fitness without the high impact forces associated with running, which often result in injuries to the lower extremities.

Walking on a treadmill

Many people prefer walking on the treadmill to walking elsewhere. It certainly has some advantages:

- There are no hills or wind to cope with and neighborhood dogs will not attack you. Since the surface is flat and even, you will be less likely to twist your ankle.

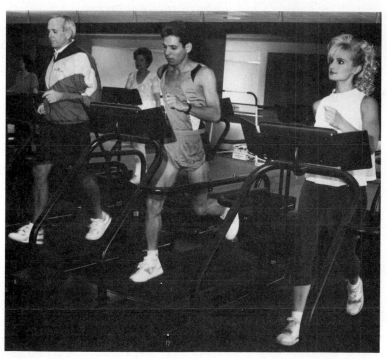

Fig. 3-3 You can either run or walk on a treadmill and still be exercising with a friend and at the right intensity.

- It is easier to maintain a constant pace. You simply set the treadmill at a specific speed and maintain your position on the treadmill.
- You can watch television or read a book while you walk. This helps the time pass more quickly.
- You can control the temperature, and it never rains indoors.
- You can walk with a friend (if two or more treadmills are available) and be walking at different speeds so that you are both exercising at the right intensity (Fig. 3-3).
- If you are walking as fast as you can, and your heart rate is still not up to the desired level, you can continue to walk and increase the elevation until you reach your target-zone heart rate.

JOGGING AND RUNNING

It is not important to set arbitrary standards to distinguish between jogging and running. Jogging is simply a slow form of running that is done at a comfortable pace that can be maintained for a long time. Jogging and running are two of the most widely used methods of developing aerobic fitness, particularly for those who are less than 30 years of age. Possibly, this is because they require a low level of skill compared with other activities, and they give maximum benefits for a minimal investment of time (Fig. 3-4).

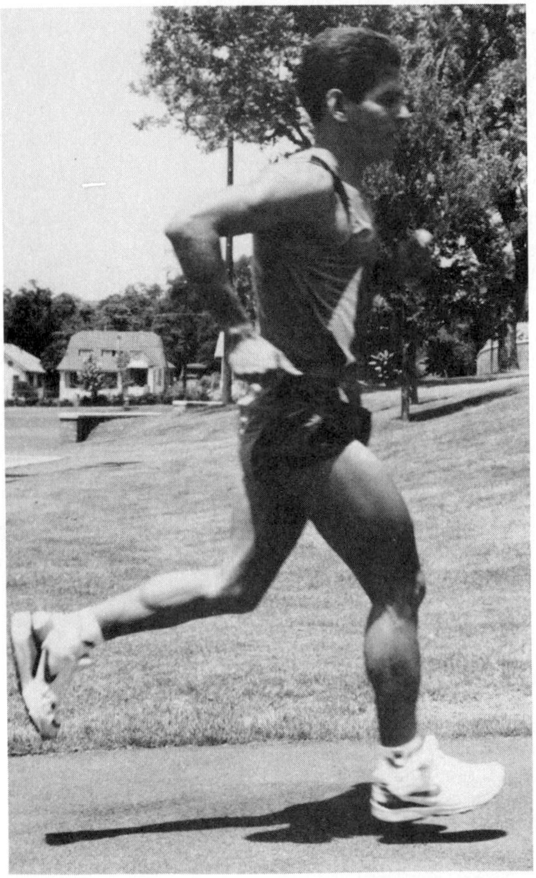

The correct way to run

Although there is not *one* correct way to run, there are procedures that, if followed, can contribute to greater efficiency and possibly result in fewer muscular problems. Possibly the most important aspect is correct foot action. The recommended procedure is the same as described for walking—the heel-to-toe movement (Fig. 3-2 on p. 78). The heel should touch the surface first as softly as possible. The jogger then rocks forward onto the ball of the foot and pushes off with the toes in preparation for the next stride. This procedure can reduce the stress placed on muscles in the leg and can significantly reduce the incidence of shin splints and other muscular problems.

When a person lands on the balls of the feet or runs flat-footed, there is a constant jarring of the muscles. By wearing jogging shoes with padded heels and by landing softly on the heels and rocking onto the toes, this jarring can be reduced significantly.

If you have experienced shin splints in the past, or if you jog or run a lot, particularly on

Fig. 3-4 Jogging is a very popular form of aerobic exercise.

hard surfaces, you need to include an exercise in your program for strengthening the muscles in the front of your lower leg. This will also help to prevent shin splints. Probably the best exercise for this is to sit with your legs straight and in front of you and the bottom of your feet as close to the ground as possible. You now try to bring the top of your feet as close to your upper body while a partner resists this movement by continuously pushing down on the top of your feet (Fig. 3-5). Even though no movement takes place, the muscles in the front of your lower legs will contract. Hold this contraction for at least 30 seconds. If this exercise becomes part of your regular exercise routine, over time this muscle group will become stronger.

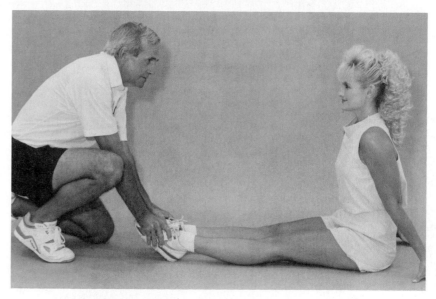

Fig. 3-5 Strengthening the muscles in the front of your lower leg may help you to avoid shin splints.

Jogging should be a natural movement, not one that creates tension and stress. It is important to learn to relax while running and to eliminate extraneous movements that do not contribute to the forward momentum of your body. The length of the stride varies according to speed, and the knees should be lifted only high enough to obtain the desired stride length. The arms should be as relaxed as possible with the forearms about parallel to the ground. Arm action should be minimal and certainly should not be of such intensity that either hand crosses the midline of the body. The key to successful running, regardless of speed, is relaxation.

Jogging shoes

By far the most important piece of equipment for the jogger is shoes. In fact, shoes are the only equipment that make a difference in the type of jogging program suggested. Many beginners make the mistake of starting a serious jogging program with shoes designed for basketball, tennis, or racquetball. These may be expensive shoes, but they are not adequate for the serious jogger.

Running shoes usually have greater arch support than regular tennis shoes and a well cushioned, padded sole raised slightly in the heel. This is particularly important because the heel must absorb most of the shock as the initial contact is made with the running surface. Jogging shoes should not fit quite as tightly as regular shoes, and a thick pair of socks can protect against blisters and sore feet (Fig. 3-6).

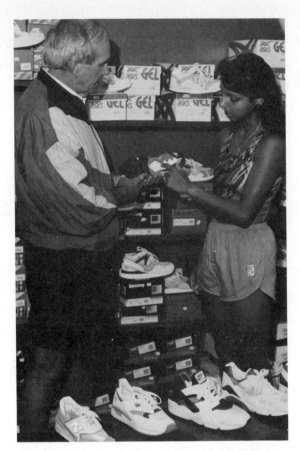

Fig. 3-6 If you are going to walk or jog regularly, you need to purchase a good pair of walking or jogging shoes.

Initiating a jogging program

Before starting a jogging program, it is important to make sure that your fitness level is such that when walking as fast as you can, your heart rate is below your desired target-zone level (see Laboratory Experience 3-1). Your starting speed will be influenced greatly by your initial level of aerobic fitness. The following suggestions are offered for those who have not participated regularly in a jogging program:

Step 1. Select a realistic distance to start your program. Recommended distances based on your aerobic fitness classification from either the 12-minute run test or the 1.5-mile run test are listed below. (NOTE: If your aerobic fitness classification is either "very poor" or "poor," you will probably need to start out with a walking program.)

Aerobic fitness classification	Suggested distance for step 1 (miles)
Very poor	1
Poor	1
Average	2
Good	2
Excellent	3

Your initial objective is to jog continuously and cover the selected distance. If the initial distance selected is too easy or too difficult, make another selection so that you have a realistic objective. If you are unable to jog continuously and cover the entire distance, alternate periods of jogging and walking. You should gradually strive to reduce your walking time until you can run continuously at a constant speed and cover the entire distance. Exercise only 3 days per week at first, and progress slowly. This is the time when you are susceptible to muscular problems. Make sure that you warm up and cool down before and after each exercise session.

Step 2. After you have achieved the objective in step 1, check your heart rate to see if the intensity is correct. If your heart rate is within your specified target zone, your pace is good, and you should continue at that speed. If it is below the target zone, you must increase your speed slightly until it reaches the required level. If it is above the target zone, the intensity should be reduced slightly.

Step 3. When you are able to run the specified distance at the correct intensity, you should increase the number of jogging days from 3 to 5. This contributes to a gradual increase in your level of cardiovascular endurance and may help you establish a regular habit of jogging. Continue for several weeks until you feel comfortable running this distance at this speed or until your heart rate drops below your target zone. Because of the anticipated decrease in your heart rate as your heart becomes more efficient, you should get into the habit of checking your heart rate periodically.

Step 4. Keeping the number of workouts between 3 and 5 per week, gradually increase your running distance until you accumulate approximately 15 miles each week. Remember, however, that the number of miles you accumulate is not as important as maintaining the correct intensity of exercise. You will experience little improvement if your level of intensity does not allow your heart rate to remain in the target zone.

SWIMMING

Swimming is one of the best aerobic exercises for the development of cardiovascular endurance. Following are several advantages it has over other activities:

- More musculature is involved in swimming than in jogging, and movement of the arms in each of the strokes occurs through a full range of motion. It should therefore contribute to the development of flexibility in addition to cardiovascular endurance.
- When swimming, people can achieve a complete workout with the body in a non-weight-bearing position. This means that less stress is placed on the joints, and fewer muscular problems result. Those who are unable to participate in other activities because of structural problems with the joints can usually participate in a swimming program.

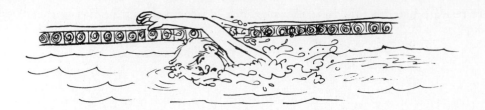

The same principles that apply to jogging apply to swimming. Success depends on your ability to adjust the intensity of your workout so that you maintain your heart rate in the target zone for 20 to 30 minutes of continuous activity. Intensity of the work can be adjusted by the speed at which you swim or by the stroke used. Some strokes require much more vigorous activity than others. For example, except for competitive swimming, the crawl stroke almost always results in a higher heart rate than the breaststroke does. It is important to know the intensity of strokes so that you can alternate a less vigorous stroke with a more vigorous one, which will enable you to swim continuously for 20 to 30 minutes. Few people can begin a program by swimming the crawl stroke continuously for 20 to 30 minutes.

Of course, swimming involves more skill than most other activities, and it is often difficult to find an uncrowded pool where you can swim continuously without interference. It is interesting to note that most individuals who can swim the crawl stroke continuously for 30 minutes or more had to develop their skill and endurance gradually; most started by swimming one lap at a time. Unless you are an experienced swimmer, start your program by swimming one or two laps using the crawl stroke at a comfortable pace. Stop and take your heart rate to determine if the intensity is correct.

You have several options to initially achieve a continuous workout:

- After each lap or laps, get out of the pool and walk vigorously on the deck to the other end of the pool.
- Walk in the pool back to the opposite end (when it is not too deep to walk the entire distance).
- Use a less vigorous stroke, such as the sidestroke, breaststroke, or elementary backstroke, to return to the other end.

Gradually, you will increase the time spent swimming continuously using the crawl stroke. Make sure from time to time, though, that your heart rate remains in the target zone. Eventually, you will be able to swim continuously for 20 to 30 minutes and will have an excellent aerobic program.

CROSS-COUNTRY SKIING

Many experts claim that cross-country skiing is the best aerobic activity. Certainly it is *one* of the best for the development of cardiovascular endurance. As in swimming, the upper body is used extensively, and it is true that the highest maximal oxygen consumption figures for both men and women have been obtained from cross-country skiers. Many people who jog or run in the summer often turn to cross-country skiing for their aerobic workout in the winter. The same basic guidelines presented for walking and jogging can be used to develop a cross-country skiing program.

Cross-country skiing is one of the few sports in which the skill level of the participant is not an important consideration. Fig. 3-7 shows that heart rate responses for those classified as skilled and beginners are similar. Each group of participants was able to keep the heart rate in the desired target zone regardless of skill.

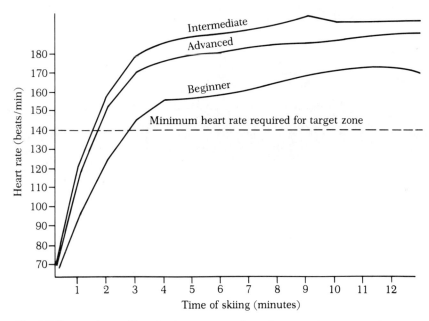

Fig. 3-7 Comparison of heart rate responses for college-aged cross-country skiers according to skill level. Note that even for those classified as beginners, the activity was sufficient to elevate the heart rate above the level necessary to reach the target zone.

BICYCLING

Bicycle riding is an excellent aerobic activity preferred by many over jogging and running. It certainly can be used for the development of cardiovascular fitness. Equipment is important. A good, lightweight 10-speed bicycle is best. It is important that the height of the seat is adjusted correctly. If the seat is at the correct height, there will be a slight bend at the knee when the pedal is in the down position.

Intensity of the task depends on a number of factors. Probably the two most important ones are pedaling speed and gear ratio. All aerobic activities should be rhythmic, and bicycling is no exception. A steady rhythm should be maintained throughout with a constant rate of pedaling from 70 to 90 revolutions per minute. The highest gear ratio at which you can maintain this rate of pedaling should be selected. Of course, you should constantly check your heart rate to make sure it is maintained within the target zone. It has been estimated that to receive the same benefits as from jogging, you must cover about three to five times the distance. However, the distance covered and the speed vary with each person and are influenced by factors such as fitness level, age, and skill.

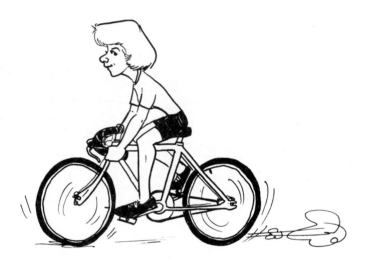

The 4-month beginning program described in Table 3-1 is designed for those with little or no experience. Those who have been involved in other aerobic programs and who find this program too easy should start with the program recommended for the second or third month.

TABLE 3-1 Training program for beginning bicycle riders

Month	Weekday		Weekend day	
	Miles	Exercise days	Miles	Exercise days
1	4-5	3	5-10	1
2	5-7	3	10-20	1
3	8-10	3	20-30	1
4	10-12	3	40-50	1

TABLE 3-2 Objectives for 10, 15, and 20 miles for designated age-groups

Age range	Time goal for 10 miles (min)	Time goal for 15 miles (min)	Time goal for 20 miles (min)
20-30	36	55	75
31-40	40	60	84
41-50	44	65	93
51-60	48	70	102

Most people who exercise regularly are interested in setting objectives and measuring progress. Both have been stressed in planning a good program. Realistic goals for different age-groups are presented in Table 3-2.

These figures are different time goals to be achieved for distances of 10, 15, and 20 miles, either while you are participating in the program or after you have completed the recommended training program. To measure your progress, you might include a 10-, 15-, or 20-mile time trial once or twice each month. As your fitness level improves, you should see a decrease in the time it will take you to cover the designated distance.

Stationary bicycle riding

To some people stationary bicycle riding seems to be the most boring form of exercise. It does, however, have advantages. You can work out in a comfortable environment; it is possible to read, watch television, or listen to a stereo while exercising; and you do not have to worry about traffic or hazards in the road while exercising. It is a safe and convenient way to get a good aerobic workout.

Many of the electronic bikes that are available have features to increase motivation. Several of these automatically adjust the intensity so that you appear to be riding up and down hills. Others present a digital display of your heart rate and caloric expenditure throughout the task. There are even bikes that have a color television and also those that allow you to race against one or more competitors while providing a graphic feedback of the race (Fig. 3–8 on p. 88).

The secret to improving your aerobic fitness level while using a stationary bicycle is the same as for other forms of aerobic training. You must exercise at the right intensity. Intensity is determined by increasing the resistance or pedaling at a faster speed. If you use the correct resistance, one added advantage of stationary cycling is that you will increase the strength and tone of the muscles in your legs. With at least two types of stationary bikes it is also possible to exercise the arms at the same time (Fig. 3–9 on p. 88).

AEROBICS TO MUSIC—AEROBIC DANCE

Exercises or dance routines performed to music have become popular. Such programs are often called "aerobic dance" or simply "aerobics" and are an excellent means of developing your aerobic fitness level. It is estimated that over 23 million Americans participate in aerobic dance.

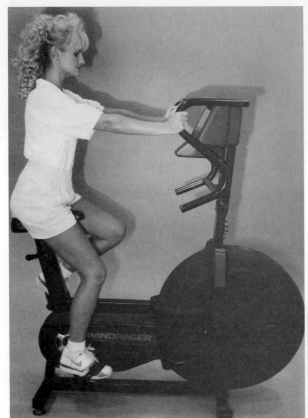

Fig. 3-8 A stationary bicycle that allows you to "race" against one or more competitors.

Fig. 3-9 A stationary bicycle designed so that you can use your upper body while pedaling.

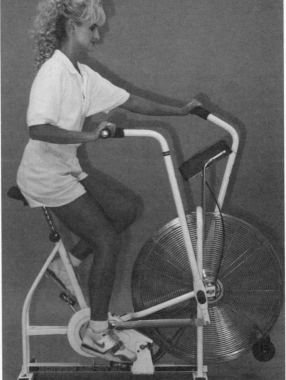

There has been recent concern over the number of injuries associated with high-impact aerobics.[33] Research reports show a 10% to 55% injury rate among participants, depending on how injury is defined. Common types of injuries include shin splints, stress fractures, and tendinitis. It would appear that the number of injuries is dependent on the type of footwear used and the surface involved. It is also evident that many of the injuries are caused by overuse—exercising too frequently.

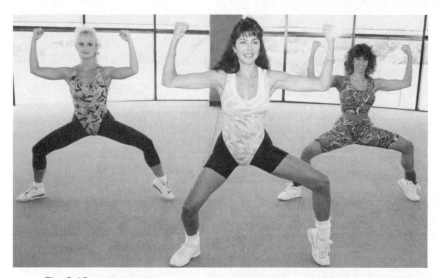

Fig. 3-10 **Aerobics to music is a very popular form of aerobic exercise.**

Because of concern relating to injuries, low-impact aerobics has emerged as an alternative.[17] With low-impact aerobics at least one foot must remain in contact with the floor at all times, and the stress placed on the feet, legs, and knees is reduced significantly. To compensate for this, the large upper body movements are accentuated, and the intensity level of the exercise can still remain high enough to produce aerobic benefits. Research has shown that the low-impact classes can be as much fun and demanding as the high-impact classes (Fig. 3–10).

JUMPING ROPE

Jumping rope is a popular exercise that can effectively develop aerobic fitness. The skill level of the participant and the type of jumping motion obviously affect the intensity of the exercise.

REBOUND RUNNING

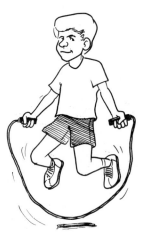

Rebound running (using a mini trampoline) is an exercise used by many individuals to develop aerobic capacity. Although conflicting results exist, it would appear that if the exercise is performed at the rate of 120 to 140 steps per minute, with an accentuated knee lift, this exercise can be used for the development of aerobic fitness. Accen-

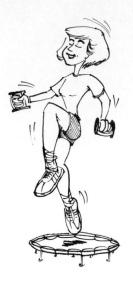

tuated arm movement with hand-held weights may be necessary for those who have a high level of aerobic fitness if they are to achieve the desired heart rate.

STATIONARY ROWING

Stationary rowing is at least as good a form of aerobic exercise as stationary bicycling. It is possibly better because it uses more musculature. The many benefits associated with stationary bicycle riding also apply to stationary rowing. It is easy to maintain your heart rate within your target zone while using such a machine. If it is not high enough, you simply row at a faster pace or increase the resistance. However, additional stress is placed on the lower back, and those with back problems should be cautious when performing this activity.

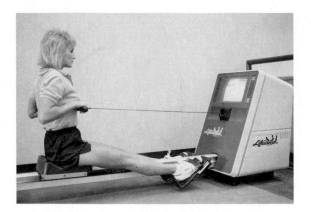

STAIR CLIMBING

At most exercise facilities across the country, stair climbers are fast becoming one of the most popular exercise machines. Since 1980 over 480,000 stair-stepping machines have been sold. The earliest models of stair-climbing machines, which were introduced in the early 1980s, featured stairs that continually rotated, similar to a treadmill. Newer models soon evolved that were pedal-powered, where your feet stay in contact with the pedals, and you step up and down, keeping up with the pedals; your body weight acts as a resistance to the stepping motion (Fig. 3-11).

These machines are often referred to as *steppers*. The height of each step can be "set" in many of these machines so that you step a set distance each time. This will usually range from 2 to 20 inches. In other machines *you* can vary the height that you step. In most cases the faster you step, the shorter the range of motion.

Many people prefer stair steppers to treadmills. One advantage of the stair stepper is that individuals with a limited range of motion can take shorter steps to reduce stress on their joints. There is less stress on the lower legs because your feet stay in contact with the pedals. One study comparing treadmill running with stair stepping showed that the injury rate was much lower when the stair stepping machines were used and that both these machines were equally effective in the development of aerobic fitness.

As with many of the stationary bicycles, computerized screens provide information to the user relating to calories burned, flights of stairs completed, and distance accumulated.

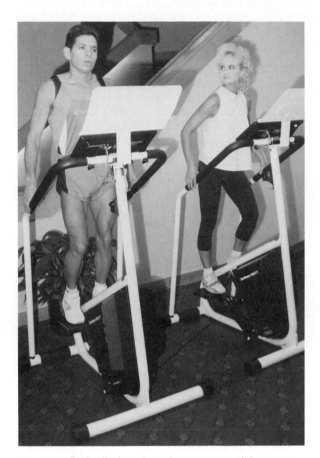

Fig. 3-11 Stair climbers have become one of the most popular exercise machines at health clubs and exercise facilities.

BENCH AEROBICS

A new trend in aerobic exercise is bench aerobics. It has been referred to as "the poor man's stair climber." This is a low-impact, high-intensity workout where participants step up to and down from a bench ranging in height from 4 to 12 inches. They use a variety of step combinations "set" to music[20] (Fig. 3-12 on p. 92). The following guidelines may be beneficial in helping you get started[11]:

- Start out with a bench that is from 4 to 6 inches high.

- Unlike walking or jogging, step up with a flat foot, making sure that you place your entire foot on the bench.
- Do not land on the ball of your foot or bounce. Bouncing will cause you to remain on the ball of your foot.
- When you step down, step directly down and not back too far. Stepping too far back places extra stress on the lower back and on the back of the legs.
- Modify the intensity by varying the step height, increasing the range of motion at the joints, or by varying the footwork to maintain your heart rate in the desired target zone.

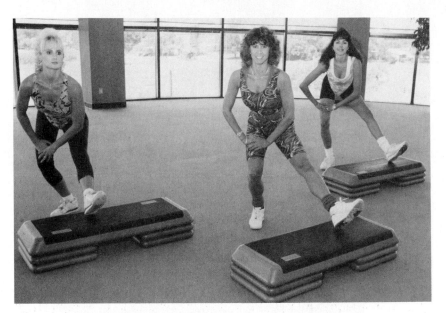

Fig. 3-12 Bench aerobics is a new form of aerobic exercise.

RACQUET SPORTS

Racquet sports, such as tennis, squash, and racquetball, have become popular in the United States, with an estimated 30 million or more participants. As mentioned previously, these activities are not as continuous as most of the other aerobic activities, and the question is whether they can be played at a high enough intensity to qualify as an aerobic activity.

It is easier to develop your skill level with racquetball and squash than it is with tennis, and these are certainly more continuous activities than tennis. Much higher heart rates have been obtained for racquetball and squash than for tennis.

Skill level is important in determining the strenuousness of such activities. Your skill level and that of your opponent are important. A study involving 24 college students enrolled in a beginning racquetball class showed that for most, the activity was strenuous enough to raise and maintain the heart rate to the target zone.[7] Singles matches rather than doubles are recommended for the racquet sports as an aerobic activity. If possible, try to compete with someone of about the same skill level or slightly better.

COMPARISON OF AEROBIC ACTIVITIES

The summary in Table 3-3 compares the advantages and disadvantages of certain aerobic activities and may be helpful to you in determining which activities are best for you.[16]

AEROBIC EXERCISE PROGRAMS

Several different aerobic exercise programs have been developed and can be used for the development of cardiovascular endurance.

Aerobics program

An aerobics program was developed by Dr. Kenneth H. Cooper after 4 years of research on more than 15,000 United States Air Force personnel.[5] The program uses common activities, such as walking, running, tennis, and golf. What is different about this program is the point system developed as a result of the research. This system allows an individual to categorize activities according to energy expenditure. One can determine which activities are best and how long he or she must participate to attain beneficial results. This program appears to be designed specifically for development of the cardiovascular system.

Procedures for initiating the aerobics program. The following list enumerates the procedures to use to receive maximum benefit from this program:

1. You must know exactly how long you need to participate in an activity to gain a particular number of points. This is determined by consulting the charts presented by Cooper.
2. You should earn 30 points per week by selecting the work level from any of the activities. If you have an initially low level of physical fitness, start by earning only 10 or 15 points per week and increase the work load gradually until you can safely earn 30 or more points each week.
3. A minimum of three or four workouts per week is necessary. Earning all 30 points in one exercise session is not acceptable.
4. Keep an accurate record of points earned each day.
5. Make a periodic evaluation of your progress. Performing the 12-minute run test periodically allows you to measure your progress. This test, of course, can be used to earn points for any day you choose to use it.

Typical point values for activities. Cooper's findings show that the most beneficial activities for the development of aerobic fitness are running, swimming, cycling, stationary running, handball, and basketball. The amount or rate of work that would need to be performed for several of these activities to achieve certain points is presented in Table 3-4.

Cooper's findings also indicate that activities such as weight lifting, calisthenics, and isometrics did not contribute to the development of cardiovascular endurance, whereas sports such as golf, tennis, and volleyball produced only minimal contributions. Point values assigned to performance in several of these activities are presented in Table 3-5.

The exercise logging program, which is part of the computer software package available with this book, can be used to quantify the amount of exercise. It calculates the aerobic points for 15 commonly-used aerobic activities and will provide a daily, weekly, monthly, or yearly summary.

TABLE 3-3 Comparison of aerobic activities

Activity	Advantages	Disadvantages	Comments
Walking	• This is a good aerobic activity for people of all ages. • You can walk almost anywhere. • No expensive equipment is needed. • This is a low-impact activity resulting in very few injuries.	• This activity may not be intense enough for those who have a high aerobic fitness level. • Walking in some neighborhoods may not be safe.	• Those who walk tend to exercise more frequently than those who use some other form of aerobic exercise.
Jogging	• This is a slow form of running that can be done at a comfortable pace. • No exercise facility or expensive equipment is needed.	• This is a high-impact activity. • This is not a good activity for those who are extremely overweight or obese. • Not everyone has the fitness level required to jog continuously.	• Many of the injuries associated with running are caused by exercising too frequently.
Swimming	• This is a good non-weight-bearing aerobic activity that is not stressful to the joints. • It involves both the upper and lower body. • It can contribute to an increase in flexibility in the arms and shoulders.	• A high skill level is required. • It is often difficult to find a pool that is not crowded where you can swim laps without interference.	• This is an excellent activity that you can often use when recovering from certain injuries to the lower leg or the knee.
Aerobic dance	• Lively music can make this fun to participate in. • It can be either high impact or low impact. • Group activity increases motivation. • A knowledgeable instructor is available to help you.	• There is a high rate of injuries associated with high-impact aerobics. • A certain level of coordination is necessary.	• Many participants do not realize just how high the level of intensity is with aerobics to music because they are having so much fun.

Activity	Advantages	Disadvantages
Cross-country skiing	• It is one of the most strenuous aerobic activities. • It involves upper and lower body. • It is a very relaxing activity for those who have a high level of stress. • Regardless of your skill level, you get a good aerobic workout.	• A high level of skill is required. • You can only participate at certain times of the year and in certain parts of the country. • Equipment is needed.
Stair stepping	• It is a high-intensity aerobic activity. • There is a lower rate of injuries than there is with jogging. • You can read or watch television while you work out. • Stair-stepping machines are one of the most popular pieces of aerobic equipment in health clubs and fitness facilities, and they are also available for home use.	• Some people become bored easily with the repetitive motion. • It may not be a suitable activity for those with knee problems.
Bicycling	• It is a good nonimpact aerobic activity. • Computerized stationary cycles provide added motivation. • You can read or watch television while using a stationary cycle. • Stationary cycling is a safe convenient way to get a good aerobic workout.	• Outdoor bicycling in a busy neighborhood may be dangerous. • It requires finding a comfortable seat.
Racquetball/ Squash	• Although these activities are noncontinuous, for most individuals, they are strenuous enough to get a good aerobic workout. • These are a good way to relieve stress and tension, particularly for a very competitive individual. • Racquetball is probably the easiest of all the racquet sports to learn to play.	• You need to find an opponent of comparable skill level. • You need an adequate level of skill.

TABLE 3-4 **Point values for selected activities in the aerobics program**

Running (time in minutes for 1 mile)	Running (time in minutes for 2 miles)	Handball or basketball* (time in minutes)	Swimming (time in minutes for 400 yards)	Cycling (time in minutes for 3 miles)	Points
More than 20	—	Less than 8	—	18 or longer	0
$14^1/_2$-20	40 or longer	8	$13^1/_2$ or longer	12-17	1
12-$14^1/_2$	29-40	15	10-$13^1/_2$	—	2
10-12	—	20	7-9	9-11	3
8-10	24-28	28	—	—	4
$6^1/_2$-8	—	35	Less than 7	Less than 9	5
Less than $6^1/_2$	20-24	40	—	—	6

*The times for handball or basketball are for continuous activity and do not include breaks; it must also be full court basketball.

TABLE 3-5 **Point values for additional exercises in the aerobics program**

Activity	Amount of activity	Points
Golf (no motorized carts)	18 holes	3
Hockey*	20 minutes	3
Rope skipping (continuous)	5 minutes	1.5
Skating*	15 minutes	1
Skiing*	30 minutes	3
Tennis	1 set	1.5
Volleyball*	15 minutes	1
Wrestling*	5 minutes	2

*Only the time that is spent actually participating is to be counted.

CIRCUIT TRAINING

Circuit training is a form of general fitness training designed to appeal to participants while increasing their level of fitness. The term **circuit** refers to a given number of exercises arranged and numbered consecutively in a given area. Each numbered exercise in the circuit is a *station*. The type of circuit that is set up depends on the time, space, facilities available, and objectives of the program. The stations are usually located at about equal distances from each other and are designated by signs on the walls or bleachers that might surround it. These signs state the sequence of activities and the prescribed number of repetitions at each station.

Objectives

In circuit training you progress at your own rate from one station to the next, performing a prescribed amount of work at each, until the entire circuit has been completed. Usually, the single circuit is repeated several times, and the time for the total performance is recorded. Proceed from station to station without resting as you attempt to reduce the time taken for a given number of laps around the circuit. You can progress by decreasing the time required to complete a given number of laps of the circuit, by increasing the number of repetitions performed at each station, or a combination of both.

Advantages

The major advantage of circuit training over many other exercise programs is that circuit training stresses continuous activity. It has been shown that continuous activity is a prerequisite for developing the cardiovascular system. Unfortunately, many exercise programs stress only muscular endurance and flexibility and place little emphasis on developing cardiovascular endurance.

Following is a list of advantages of circuit training:

- Each participant is able to start the program at an easy pace and experience success early.
- Circuit training can be organized to involve a large number of participants in a relatively confined area.
- Added motivation is provided by seeing progress from day to day.
- Progression is ensured if the participant exercises regularly.
- The exercise is continuous; thus stress is placed on the cardiovascular system.
- Circuit training provides individualized self-competition. Each participant is competing only against himself or herself and works at his or her own rate.

Organization

Circuit training may be organized in a variety of ways. An example of the organization of a circuit consisting of 10 stations designed to develop each of the components of physical fitness is presented. This circuit is for both men and women. A list of the activities and repetitions required for each are presented in Table 3-6. The specific activities are described later in this chapter.

Four progression levels have been established, although more may be added if needed. Your initial starting level can be determined by your performance on the 12-minute run test. Table 3-7 presents the criteria you can use to determine your

TABLE 3-6 Circuit training activities

Activity	Level I	Level II	Level III	Level IV
Lateral jump	25	30	35	50
Hip raiser	10	12	16	25
Bent-leg curl-ups	10	15	20	30
Rope jump	40	50	60	80
Lateral leg raise	8	10	20	30
Burpee	8	10	20	30
V-sits	10	14	18	24
Push-ups	8	12	20	26
Bench jump	10	16	20	26
Sprinter	20	30	40	50

TABLE 3-7 Criteria for determination of the initial starting level for circuit training

Classification for 12-minute run test	Distance covered (miles)		Initial circuit level
	Men	Women	
Very poor or poor	Less than 1.60	Less than 1.26	Level I
Average	1.60-1.77	1.26-1.43	Level II
Good	1.78-1.94	1.44-1.60	Level III
Excellent	More than 1.95	More than 1.61	Level IV

starting level. If you have not taken this test, starting at the lowest level and progressing from there is probably best.

Description of activities in the circuit*

Lateral jump. Jump laterally across any line on the floor as fast as possible, keeping both feet together and parallel to the line. This activity develops muscular endurance of the legs as well as overall cardiovascular endurance.

Hip raiser. Assume the start position as shown in Fig. 3-13. The hips are elevated as high as possible and then lowered as low as possible without the buttocks touching the floor. This exercise will develop the muscular endurance of certain hip and thigh muscles and the abdominal muscles. It can be a good exercise to correct drooping shoulders.

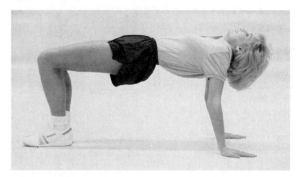

Fig. 3-13 Start position for the hip raiser exercise.

Bent-leg curl-ups. Bent-leg curl-ups strengthen the abdominal muscles and increase their endurance. Lie down with your feet flat on the floor about shoulder width apart. Your knees should be flexed at a right angle. Your arms are folded across your chest with your chin held as close to your chest as possible. Curl up until your elbows touch the upper part of your thighs and then return until your lower back is in contact with the floor.

---

*Several of these exercises are adapted from or are similar to those suggested by Robert Sorani in his book *Circuit Training*.[29]

Rope jump. The rope jump is designed for development of cardiovascular endurance. A regular jump rope is used and you must propel it in a counterclockwise direction so that it passes under your feet and over your head. Each time the rope passes under the feet is one repetition.

Lateral leg raise. Assume a position on the floor lying on either side with legs and lower arm completely extended, using the other arm to maintain your balance (see Fig. 5-18). The upper leg is raised as high as possible, kept straight, and is then returned slowly to the start position. This is one repetition. This exercise is designed to develop the muscles responsible for abduction of the leg. If the circuit is completed more than one time, the sides should be reversed so that the leg that is raised is changed each time around the circuit.

Burpee. The burpee is also called the squat-thrust or the agility four-count exercise. Start in a standing position with the legs straight. Assume the squat position, extend the legs backward so that you are in the push-up position, then reverse this procedure back to the squat position and finally back to the upright position. This completes one repetition. Because this exercise involves many large muscle groups, it contributes to overall muscular endurance.

V-sits. Lie on the floor on your back with your arms fully extended behind your head. Then curl your head toward the chest as your arms and legs are raised simultaneously. A V-position is then attained (Fig. 3-14). Reverse these procedures until the starting position is reached. This exercise is good for development of the abdominal muscles, particularly if the V-position is maintained for a few seconds each time.

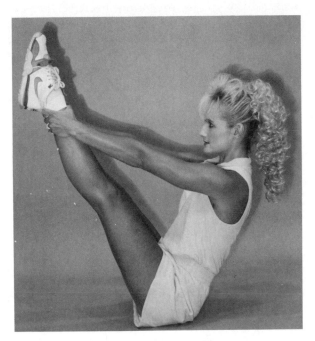

Fig. 3-14 **The V-sit position.**

Push-ups. Men should perform the regular push-up, starting from the front-leaning rest position with the head, back, hips, and legs in a straight alignment. The body is slowly lowered so that the chest lightly touches the floor. The body should remain straight throughout this exercise. The arms are then extended as the body is raised to the starting position. This exercise will develop muscular endurance and strength of the extensors of the forearm. Women should perform the modified push-up (Fig. 3-15).

A 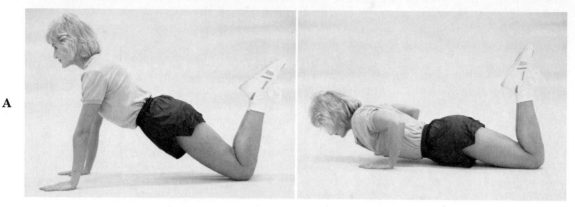 **B**

Fig. 3-15 Start (**A**) and finish (**B**) positions for the modified push-up.

Bench step. For the bench step, face a bench about 12 to 16 inches high. The lowest row of bleachers is usually satisfactory for this exercise. Step up to and down from the bench. This completes one repetition. This exercise is designed to develop cardiovascular endurance and strength and endurance of the leg extensors.

Sprinter. Assume a position similar to a sprinter's starting position, with the weight on the hands and feet with one leg extended straight back and the other flexed with the knee pulled under the chest (Fig. 3-16). The position of the feet is then reversed and reversed again as you return to the starting position. This completes one

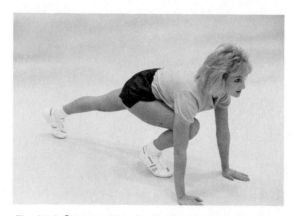

Fig. 3-16 Start position for the sprinter exercise.

repetition. This exercise contributes to the development of strength and endurance of the shoulder and arm extensors and leg flexors and extensors.

Instructions for running a circuit

The following should be used as guidelines for beginning the circuit:

- Practice each exercise before starting the circuit.
- Fifteen minutes will be allowed for men and 18 minutes for women to complete two laps of the circuit.
- If two laps around the circuit are completed before the allocated time has elapsed, the remainder of the time can be spent jogging in place.
- If you complete the two laps of the circuit within the time limit, the next time you attempt the circuit you should move up to the next level.
- If you fail to complete the two laps of the circuit in the prescribed time and are not working at the first level, you should move back one level.
- To measure progress each day, you should record the time taken to complete two laps of the circuit.

An alternative procedure for the organization of circuit training is to allow a specific time (usually 45 seconds or 1 minute) for each exercise. You perform as many repetitions as possible at each station. This is an effective way to show improvement.

CIRCUIT WEIGHT TRAINING

Development of strength and muscular endurance may be combined with development of cardiovascular endurance by using circuit training and weight training. Carefully selected weight training exercises can be used in a predetermined sequence to provide a total workout for each major muscle group.

The following suggestions may be beneficial:

- Exercises should be arranged so that you alternate between upper and lower body.
- Perform 12 to 15 repetitions at each station, working at 40% to 60% of maximal capacity.
- Each set of repetitions should be continuous and not take more than 30 seconds.
- Fifteen to thirty seconds are allowed between each exercise, during which time you should move to the next station and select the resistance.
- The objective is to work continuously for 30 minutes and to complete as many circuits as possible during this time.

THE SUPER CIRCUIT

The super circuit was developed to concentrate even more on the development of cardiovascular endurance while developing strength and muscular endurance. In the super circuit the 15- to 30-second rest period is replaced by a 30-second aerobic activity. Aerobic activities that might be used for each 30-second exercise are running, using an indoor jogger or stationary bicycle, jumping rope, or running in place. All other procedures as outlined previously for circuit weight training can be applied.

Results from a recent research study show dramatic changes after participation in circuit weight training and in the super circuit program.[13] The study involved 36 women and 41 men randomly assigned to one of the following three groups:

- Circuit weight training group

TABLE 3-8 Percentage of improvement in designated variables as a result of circuit weight training and super circuit training

Variable	Super circuit group		Circuit weight training group		Control group (*men and women*)
	Men	Women	Men	Women	
Aerobic endurance	+12.0	+17.0	+12.0	+13.0	No change
Body fat	−17.1	−10.9	−13.3	−10.4	No change
Leg strength	+21.0	+26.0	+15.5	+17.7	No change
Bench press	+21.0	+21.0	+14.0	+20.0	No change

- Super circuit group
- Control group

The two exercise groups did assigned activities for 30 minutes a day, 3 days a week, for 12 weeks. A summary of the improvements that occurred in each group for both men and women is presented in Table 3-8. The results indicate that when weight training exercises are organized into a continuous program with no rest between exercises, significant improvements will occur in cardiovascular endurance, strength, and body composition. These results compare favorably with those of other aerobic programs.

SUMMARY

The following summary will help you to identify some of the important concepts covered in this chapter:

- Your overall objectives for your aerobic exercise program will determine how much exercise you really need.
- Most of the good aerobic activities are continuous and involve large muscle groups.
- Brisk walking can be an ideal aerobic activity for most adults.
- Jogging and running are two of the most popular forms of aerobic exercise for those who are less than 30 years of age.
- Swimming and cycling are excellent nonimpact aerobic activities.
- Low-impact aerobics can be as demanding as high-impact aerobics and is preferred by many because of the lower injury rate associated with it.
- Stair stepping has emerged as one of the most popular and effective forms of aerobic exercise.
- Despite the fact that racquetball and squash are not continuous activities, in most cases they are strenuous enough to raise and maintain the heart rate in the target zone.
- Continuous weight training, such as in circuit training, can be an excellent form of aerobic exercise.

KEY TERMS

aerobic dance   A series of exercises or dance routines performed to music. Also referred to as *aerobics to music* or simply *aerobics*.

bench aerobics   A sequence of exercises performed to music where participants step up to and down from a bench, using a variety of step combinations.

circuit   A given number of exercises arranged and numbered consecutively.

circuit training   A series of exercises arranged in a specific sequence so that participants can complete a predetermined number of repetitions as quickly as possible at each exercise "station."

circuit weight training   A combination of circuit training and weight training to develop an aerobic fitness routine.

cool down   A process whereby you gradually slow down following a workout or exercise session rather than stopping abruptly. Walking until your heart rate returns to near your resting value is an example of a cool-down activity.

intensity of exercise   The stress placed on the body by the activity. With aerobic activities, it can be adequately determined by the heart rate response to the work involved.

jogging   A slow form of running.

rebound running   Stepping or bouncing on a mini trampoline.

shin splints   A "catch-all" term that refers to a painful condition that occurs on the anterior portion of the lower leg. This condition often results from exercise performed on hard surfaces.

warm-up   The initial phase of the workout where you exercise at a low level of intensity. You increase your body temperature and the temperature of the muscles involved in the exercise in preparation for a more strenuous level of activity.

REFERENCES

1. Allen TE et al: Metabolic and cardiorespiratory responses of young women to skipping and jogging, *The Physician and Sportsmedicine* 15(5):109-113, 1987.

2. Angsten P: Low impact comes of age, *American Fitness*, pp 44-46, 1987.

3. Buyze MT et al: Comparative training responses to rope skipping and jogging, *The Physician and Sportsmedicine* 14(11):65-69, 1986.

4. Colfer GR, Chevrette JM: *Running for fun and fitness*, ed 2, Dubuque, Ia, 1980, Kendall/Hunt.

5. Cooper KH: *The aerobics program for total well-being*, New York, 1982, M Evans & Co.

6. De Benedette V: Stair machines: the truth about this fitness fad, *The Physician and Sportsmedicine* 18(6):131-134, 1990.

7. Duroe M: *Cardiovascular aspects of racquetball relative to skill level*, master's thesis, Marquette, 1979, Northern Michigan University.

8. Finkelstein A: It's easy to get fit, *Parents*, pp 170-175, July 1989.

9. Francis F: Injury prevention: physics of foot impact, *Consultant*, pp 107-126, March 1980.

10. Gibson SB et al: Writing the exercise prescription: an individualized approach, *The Physician and Sportsmedicine* 11(7):87-110, 1983.

11. Harste A: Bench aerobics: a step in the right direction?, *The Physician and Sportsmedicine* 18(7):25-26, 1990.

12. Henderson J: Jog, run, race, *Runners World*, 1983.

13. Hempel LS, Wells CL: Cardiorespiratory cost of the Nautilus express circuit, *The Physician and Sportsmedicine* 13(4):82-97, 1985.

14. Howell ML, Morford WR: Circuit training for a college fitness program, *Journal of Health, Physical Education, and Recreation* 35:30, 1964.

15. Katch VL, Villanucci JF: Energy cost of rebound running, *Research Quarterly for Exercise and Sport* 52(2):269,1981.

16. Klug GA, Letternick J: *Exercise and physical fitness*, Guilford, Conn, 1992, Dushkin Publishing Co.

17. Koszuta LE: Low-impact aerobics: better than traditional aerobic dance?, *The Physician and Sportsmedicine* 14(7):156-161, 1986.

18. Koszuta LE: Can fitness be found at the top of the stairs? *The Physician and Sportsmedicine* 15(2):165-169, 1987.

19. Kravitz L, Deivert R: The safe way to step, *Idea Today*, p 59, March 1992.

20. LaForge R: Step exercise, *Idea Today*, p 32, September 1991.

21. Loy SF, Holland GJ: Stair climbing as a training modality, *Wellness Newsletter* 3:1, 1991, Randall Sports Medical Products.

22. Morgan RE, Adamson GT: Circuit training, London, 1957, G Bell & Son.

23. Morgan LF et al: Heart rate responses during singles and doubles tennis competition, *The Physician and Sportsmedicine* 15(7):67-74, 1987.

24. Porcari J et al: Is fast walking an adequate aerobic training stimulus for 30- to 69-year-old men and women? *The Physician and Sportsmedicine* 15(2):119-129, 1987.

25. *Prevention Index '91:* Emmaus, Penn, 1992, Rodale Press.

26. *Prevention Index '86:* Emmaus, Penn, 1987, Rodale Press.

27. *Aerobic Fitness Program Starter,* Chicago, 1988, Schwinn Air Dyne.

28. Solis K et al: Aerobic requirements for the heart rate responses to variations in rope jumping techniques, *The Physician and Sportsmedicine* 16(3):121-128, 1988.

29. Sorani R: Circuit training, Dubuque, Ia, 1966, Wm C Brown Co.

30. Stamford BS: Can you get fit playing racquet sports, *The Physician and Sportsmedicine* 14(1):206, 1986.

31. Stuller J: Considering the stationary cycle, *The Physician and Sportsmedicine* 13(10):161-165, 1985.

32. Stuller J: Terrestrial rowing, *The Physician and Sportsmedicine* 14(3):272-275, 1986.

33. Weaver S: The ABC's of training for touring, *Bicycling,* p 35, April 1983.

34. Wolf MD: Avoiding aerobic injuries, *Athletic Business,* pp 10-14, March 1985.

Determining Your Correct Pace for Walking or Jogging

Purpose

To determine the pace at which you should be walking or jogging to maintain your heart rate in your target zone.

Procedures

You need to first calculate your target-zone heart rate according to the procedures outlined in Chapter 2.

$$\text{Maximum heart rate} = 220 - \text{Age}$$

$$= 220 - \underline{\hspace{1cm}}$$

$$= \underline{\hspace{1cm}} \text{ beats/min}$$

Target-zone heart rate:
$$\text{Upper limit} = \text{Maximum heart rate} \times 0.85$$

$$= \underline{\hspace{1cm}} \times 0.85$$

$$= \underline{\hspace{1cm}} \text{ beats/min}$$

$$\text{Lower limit} = \text{Maximum heart rate} \times 0.7$$

$$= \underline{\hspace{1cm}} \times 0.7$$

$$= \underline{\hspace{1cm}} \text{ beats/min}$$

$$\text{Target-zone heart rate} \underline{\hspace{1cm}} \text{ to } \underline{\hspace{1cm}} \text{ beats/min}$$

You will need to measure a 1-mile course or use a measured track so that you know exactly what constitutes 1 mile. Start by walking as fast as you can and try to cover the mile without stopping. Record the time it takes, and determine your heart rate immediately after completing the walk.

Results

Record your results in the spaces provided below:

Time to walk 1 mile _____ minutes
Heart rate at completion of walk _____ beats/min

Compare your heart rate at the end of the walk to your target-zone heart rate, which you calculated and recorded above and check the correct response below:
My heart rate at the end of the mile walk was:

_____ Below my target zone
_____ Within my target zone
_____ Above my target zone

If your heart rate at the end of the walk was within your target zone, you know that the pace you were walking is the correct pace for you and that if you decide to include walking in your exercise program, this is the speed at which you need to walk.

If your heart rate was above your target zone at the end of the 1-mile walk, you need to walk the same distance again at a slower pace and repeat the above procedures until you find the correct pace to walk at so that your heart rate remains at the desired level.

At the end of the 1-mile walk, if your heart rate was below your target zone and you have no medical problems, you need to repeat the above procedures, jogging slowly rather than walking. By trial and error and making adjustments each time it should not take you long to determine the speed at which you need to jog in order to achieve and maintain your desired heart rate.

Strength and Muscular Endurance

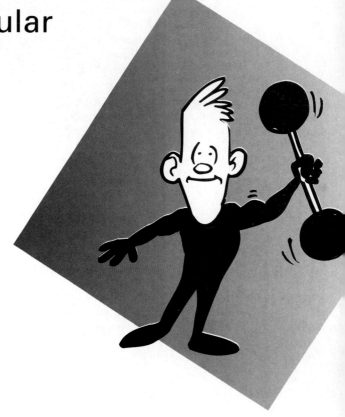

CHAPTER OBJECTIVES

When you understand the material in this chapter, you will be able to:

- Differentiate clearly between strength and muscular endurance and understand their importance
- Identify and define the three types of muscle contraction
- Evaluate the different procedures for development of strength and muscular endurance
- Identify the major muscles and muscle groups in the body and know which exercises can be used to develop each of these

- Design and implement a strength/muscular endurance program based on your specific needs
- Explain why "overload" is important in the development of strength and muscular endurance
- Discuss muscle soreness and know what steps you can take to avoid it
- Evaluate your level of strength and muscular endurance for specific muscle groups

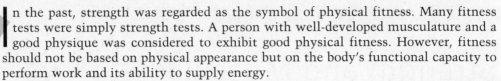

In the past, strength was regarded as the symbol of physical fitness. Many fitness tests were simply strength tests. A person with well-developed musculature and a good physique was considered to exhibit good physical fitness. However, fitness should not be based on physical appearance but on the body's functional capacity to perform work and its ability to supply energy.

Today many people believe that strength and muscular endurance are important only for athletes and for those doing heavy physical work. Certainly these people require a high level of strength and muscular endurance if they are to perform efficiently. However, these physical fitness components are also important to the average person.

Increasing strength and muscular endurance should make it easier to perform everyday tasks. Carrying a suitcase, moving furniture, pushing a stalled vehicle, or mowing the lawn will become easier if you develop the strength and endurance of the muscles involved in each task.

In addition, increased strength and muscular endurance should contribute to the following:
- Maintenance of correct posture
- Improved personal appearance
- Decreased risk of muscle injuries
- Prevention and alleviation of low back pain
- Increased joint flexibility

DEFINITION OF TERMS

Strength and muscular endurance are important health-related physical fitness components that are often confused. It is important to clearly differentiate between them.

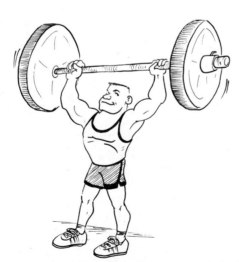

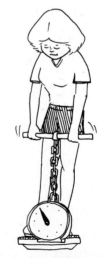

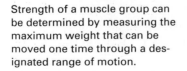

Strength of a muscle group can be determined by measuring the maximum weight that can be moved one time through a designated range of motion.

Strength can also be measured by applying a maximum force against a resistance. With this procedure, little or no movement takes place because the magnitude of the force is usually measured by using a dynamometer.

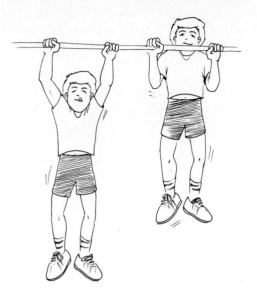

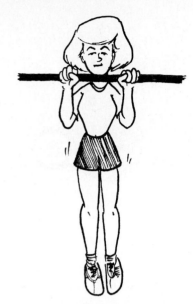

Muscular endurance of a muscle group can be determined by the number of repetitions performed by that muscle group.

Muscular endurance can also be determined by measuring the time a contraction can be sustained. Body weight and gravity often act as the resistance.

Strength is the amount of force a muscle or muscle group can exert against a resistance in one maximum contraction.

Muscular endurance is the ability of a muscle or muscle group to apply force repeatedly or to sustain a contraction for a period of time.

TYPES OF MUSCLE CONTRACTION

All body movements depend on the contraction of muscles. Your neurological system acts as a communication network between the muscular and skeletal systems. Messages are sent from the central nervous system to the muscles telling them to contract and how strongly they should contract to perform specific movements.

Skeletal muscles possess four unique properties:
- Excitability—the ability to receive and respond to stimulation from the nervous system
- Contractibility—the ability to develop internal force or tension
- Extensibility—the muscle's ability to stretch past its normal resting length
- Elasticity—the muscle's ability to return to its normal resting length

The force generated by a muscle or muscle group will depend on your sex and body weight and the number of active fibers recruited by the nervous system to perform a task.

When a muscle contracts, tension is created within the muscle and it may shorten, lengthen, or remain the same. There are two types of muscle contractions—isometric and isotonic.

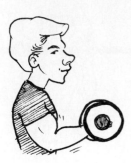 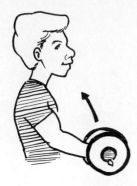

With this isometric contraction the force generated by the muscle is equal to the resistance. Since no movement occurs, the force necessary to sustain the resistance will depend on the angle at the joint.

If sufficient force is generated by the biceps muscle as it contracts, the muscle will shorten and the forearm will move up as the weight is lifted. This then becomes an isotonic contraction.

Isometric contraction

Isometric contractions occur when the force exerted by the muscle as it contracts is equal to or less than the resistance. Tension develops in the muscles as an isometric contraction occurs. The muscles involved do not noticeably shorten or lengthen, and little or no movement takes place at the joint. This is often called a static contraction.

Isotonic contraction

Isotonic contractions are often called dynamic contractions and occur when the force generated by the muscle as it contracts is greater than the resistance. Movement occurs at the joint, and the muscles involved shorten and lengthen (Fig. 4-1).

Each isotonic contraction consists of two phases:

- Concentric phase (positive work)—the muscle shortens and works against gravity.
- Eccentric phase (negative work)—the muscle lengthens as it returns to its original position.

Force applied to the weight varies at different points throughout the range of motion. This happens because of gravity's effect against the rotary movement of the segment and because of the system of levers that exist in the body. For example, consider the two-arm curl. Once you have overcome the initial resistance, lifting the weight may be easy or difficult depending on the position of the weight in relation to your body (Fig. 4-2).

Fig. 4-1 Position of the biceps muscle in relation to the elbow joint.

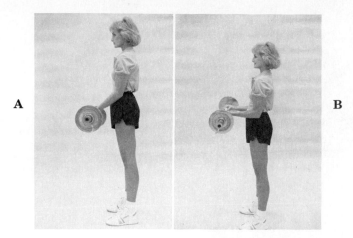

Fig. 4-2 Relationship between joint angle and difficulty of a task. **A,** At an angle of about 120 degrees, the force that can be generated by this muscle group is greatest and the task will appear to be easy. **B,** At an angle of 90 degrees, muscles involved in this movement are at a disadvantage and the task may appear to be difficult.

The point at which force applied to the weight is weakest is often called the ***sticking point***. The force necessary to move the weight is often insufficient at this point, and the task cannot be completed. If the weight can be moved past this point, the task gets easier again. It can then usually be completed, because less force is needed for the remainder of the task.

During an isotonic task the muscles are not working at or near their capacity except at one point in the range of motion. For this reason, several companies have produced isotonic machines that vary the resistance throughout the range of motion to match the functional strength of the muscles. These are called variable resistance isotonic machines. These machines change the resistance by using a leverage system, so that at the point where the muscle is weakest, the load is the lightest and where the muscle is strongest, the load is the heaviest. Muscles therefore have to exert maximum effort throughout the range of motion if the correct resistance is used.

The most common equipment using this technique is the Nautilus brand (Fig. 4-3 on p. 112). It is a system of chains and variable-shaped cams that provide a balanced resistance over a full range of movement.

With isotonic equipment, momentum can also influence the task's difficulty. It is important to perform isotonic contractions slowly to minimize the contribution that movement makes to task performance.

Isokinetic contraction

As noted in the previous section, in an isotonic contraction the muscle's functional strength varies at different angles, and speed of movement can influence the task's difficulty. In an isokinetic contraction, speed of motion is controlled so that resistance is varied to match the force applied by the muscles. The most popular machines using this technique are the Cybex and Orthotron machines. You

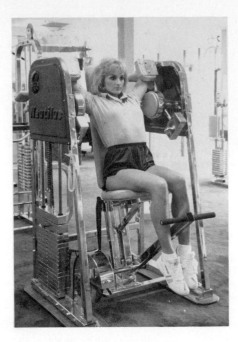

Fig. 4-3 Use of the Nautilus Super Pullover machine for development of the upper body.

Fig. 4-4 An Orthotron machine, which controls the speed of motion.

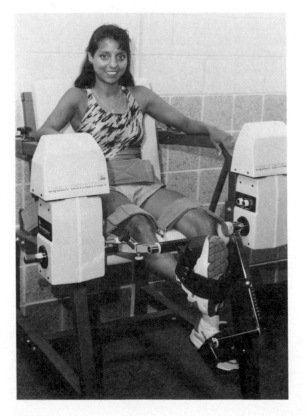

apply a maximum effort, and the isokinetic device automatically controls the speed at which you can move through the full range of motion. At the points at which muscular force and mechanical advantage are greatest, the resistance will also be greatest, resulting in a constant speed. This provides maximum resistance throughout the range of motion (Fig. 4-4).

WEIGHT-TRAINING GUIDELINES AND SAFETY

These guidelines should be followed when you participate in weight training:

Warm-up: Each training session should be preceded by a 5- to 10-minute warm-up. The warm-up should include stretching exercises for each muscle group involved.

Breathing: While executing each exercise, make sure that you breathe correctly. You should breathe out while performing the lift and breathe in while returning to the starting position.

Range of motion: Make sure that each exercise is performed correctly through the full range of motion. Exercises performed incorrectly or with too much resistance are likely to reduce flexibility and could cause muscle injury.

Spotting: When using free weights it is important to work out with a partner who can be a spotter when you are performing exercises. This is particularly important when working with heavy weights in such exercises as the bench press.

Weights and collars: When using free weights, make sure that the collars are tight and fastened securely so that weights do not fall off.

Speed: Each exercise should be performed slowly with a steady application of force. This is important with the lowering phase (negative work). It is recommended that the lowering phase take about twice as long (4 seconds) as the lifting phase (2 seconds).

Sequence: The order in which major muscle groups should be exercised is important. The largest muscle groups should be exercised first, and the same muscle groups should not be exercised successively.

Symmetry: As mentioned previously, muscles are usually grouped in sets that oppose one another. In many cases, because of what we do, the body favors specific muscle groups, and quite frequently, one muscle group will be naturally strong while the opposing group will be much weaker. For example, because we constantly lift and carry various items, the biceps muscle in the front of the arm will usually be well developed. However, because we seldom do much to develop the muscles at the back of the arm, the triceps will usually be much weaker.

To maintain balance and symmetry, when muscles on one side of a joint are exercised, then the opposing muscle group should also be exercised. When an imbalance occurs between muscle groups, it can negatively affect your posture, reduce the flexibility of the joint, and possibly increase the risk of injury.

A good example of increased risk of injury relates to shin splints, which are often caused by muscle imbalance. The large muscle in the back of the leg—the gastrocnemius—is usually well developed, whereas the muscle in the front of the lower leg—the tibialis anterior—is usually not well developed and in most cases needs to be strengthened.

The major muscle groups in the body are identified in Figs. 4-5 and 4-6 on p. 114.

Opposing muscles or muscle groups that often create problems are listed below[15]:

Quadriceps (front of thigh)	Hamstrings (back of thigh)
Adductors (inner thigh)	Abductors (outer thigh)

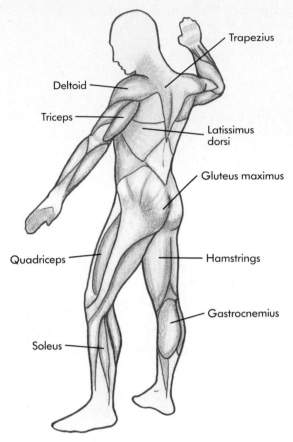

Fig. 4-5 Major muscles of the body—a posterior view.

Fig. 4-6 Major muscles of the body—an anterior view.

Pectorals (chest)	Rhomboids (upper back)
Abdominals (stomach)	Erector spinae (lower back)
Gastrocnemius (back of lower leg)	Tibialis anterior (front of lower leg)
Biceps (front of upper arm)	Triceps (back of upper arm)

If a particular muscle or muscle group is stronger than what it should be, it often needs to be stretched. If it is weaker than its opposing muscle or muscle group, it needs to be strengthened. Exercises for the development of the major muscle groups in the body are included later in this chapter. Stretching exercises for each of the major muscle groups in the body are included in Chapter 5.

BASIC TERMINOLOGY

To understand the following procedures, three terms need to be defined:

Repetition: A repetition is the completion of a designated movement through a full range of motion.

Set: A set is a designated number of repetitions attempted without a rest.

Resistance: Resistance is the workload you are attempting to move.

PRINCIPLES FOR WEIGHT TRAINING USING NAUTILUS EQUIPMENT

These guidelines are recommended when using Nautilus equipment:

- Select a resistance for each exercise that allows performance of between 8 and 12 repetitions.
- Perform only one set for each exercise during each exercise session.
- Use this equipment no more than three times each week.
- Continue each exercise until no more repetitions can be performed, up to a maximum of 12. When this number can be performed, add one additional weight.
- For maximum results the position of the body in relation to the machine is important. For all single-joint rotary machines the axis of the cam must line up with the joint that is being exercised (Fig. 4-7).
- The first two or three repetitions of each exercise should be performed at a slightly slower pace than the rest as you concentrate on moving through the entire range of motion.
- The lowering portion of each exercise should be accentuated. It should take about 2 seconds to lift the weight and about 4 seconds to lower it.
- On machines that have two-part exercises, it is important to move quickly from the first to the second task.

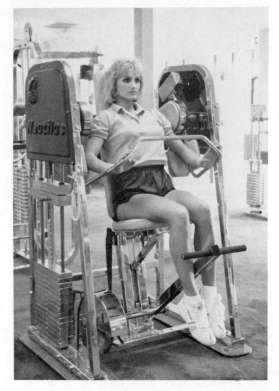

Fig. 4-7 **Use of the Nautilus Super Pullover machine. Note how the axis of the cams lines up with the shoulder joint.**

BASIC PRINCIPLES OF WEIGHT-TRAINING PROGRAMS

When you participate regularly in a good weight-training program, you will increase the strength and endurance of muscles involved. There may also be a corresponding increase in muscle size. This is called muscle hypertrophy and results from an increase in size of the cross-sectional area of fibers that make up the muscle.

A basic principle involved in weight-training programs is the **overload principle**. This states that muscular strength, endurance, and size will increase only if muscles are systematically subjected to workloads greater than those to which they are accustomed. As your muscle group becomes stronger, your body will adapt to the increased resistance. If further improvement is to occur, the workload must be progressively increased. For each exercise, each muscle must perform at or near its strength and endurance capacity if maximum gains are to occur.

Overload may be achieved by any combination of the following:

- Increasing the amount of weight lifted
- Increasing the repetitions in a set
- Increasing the number of sets
- Increasing the speed with which repetitions are performed
- Decreasing the time for rest between sets (if more than one set is attempted)

Note that if the speed of movement is increased, you must perform the exercise correctly and move through the full range of motion.

Many resistance training programs are available. They manipulate the training variables to maximize strength, endurance, or size. The best procedures have not been clearly established. For this reason, only general guidelines are presented.

DEVELOPMENT OF STRENGTH AND MUSCULAR ENDURANCE

The same criteria that apply to development of cardiovascular endurance also apply to the development of strength and muscular endurance. These relate to intensity, duration, and frequency.

Intensity

In weight training, intensity of the workout relates to the extent muscles are overloaded. Programs can be specifically designed for the development of either strength or muscular endurance. Differences between these programs relate to the number of repetitions and the amount of resistance. As a general rule, a strength program will involve a low number of repetitions (usually 8 or less) with a heavy resistance. For those wishing to develop muscular endurance, a greater number of repetitions must be performed (usually 12 to 20) with less resistance.

Most people involved in a weight-training program are interested in both strength and endurance. Performing between 8 and 12 repetitions is probably ideal for this. These concepts are summarized in Fig. 4-8. The amount of weight that will create an adequate resistance for each of these programs will vary among people and programs. The suggested percentages in Fig. 4-8 can be used as a starting point to determine what might be best for you. Additional procedures for planning such a program are presented in a later section in this chapter.

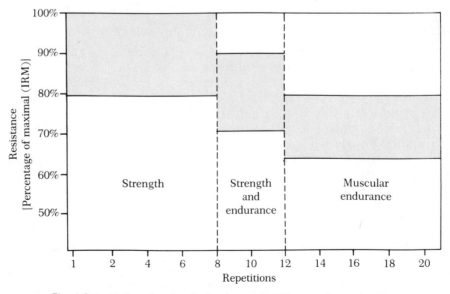

Fig. 4-8 Guidelines for developing strength and muscular endurance.

Duration

The duration of each training session will vary, depending on the person's level of strength and muscular endurance and his or her objectives. Several weight-training programs are available using different procedures and pieces of equipment. Your program will depend on the equipment available and how much time you have. If the weight-training program is to supplement an aerobic program, the exercises may need to be selected so that they can be completed in 15 to 20 minutes. Procedures for circuit weight training and the super circuit have been set up so that each of these programs can be completed in about 30 minutes (see Chapter 3). Research indicates that each of these programs can be used to combine your weight training and aerobic workout.

Frequency

When the muscular system has been stressed, it must be allowed to rest. It needs time for recovery and to adapt to a higher physiological level. It is not wise to perform exercises for the same muscle groups on successive days. A good weight-training program should be performed 3 or 4 days per week on every other day.

GUIDELINES FOR DEVELOPMENT OF STRENGTH AND MUSCULAR ENDURANCE

The following procedures can be followed for setting up a basic weight-training program.

- Select the muscle groups you wish to develop. There are several major muscle groups that you may want to include in a training program. These include the following:

  The anterior muscles in the upper legs
  The muscles in the chest and upper arms
  The posterior muscles in the upper legs
  The muscles in the shoulders and upper back
  The posterior muscles in the lower legs
  The abdominal muscles

- Select exercises for each of the muscle groups you wish to develop. Exercises for development of each of these muscle groups are described in a later section in this chapter.

- Determine the maximum weight you can lift one time for each of these exercises. It is necessary to determine your absolute strength for each of these exercises. This is called *1 RM (repetition maximum)*. This allows you to measure your progress. It is also used to determine the initial resistance for each exercise.

- Start with a resistance equal to 70% of your maximum strength for each of the exercises selected, and determine how many repetitions you can perform using this weight. If you cannot perform 8 repetitions continuously, the weight is too heavy and should be reduced.

- The objective of the program is to increase your strength to where you can perform three sets of 12 repetitions with a short period of rest between each set. When you can do this, you need to increase the resistance.

- If you want a program directed more toward either strength or muscular endurance, adjust the number of repetitions and the resistance to incorporate the information previously presented.

TABLE 4-1 Sample weekly recording sheet for individualized weight-training program

NAME _____
WEEK NUMBER ___1___

BODY WEIGHT
DAY 1 _____ lb
DAY 2 _____ lb
DAY 3 _____ lb

Exercise	1 Rm	Day 1			Day 2			Day 3		
		Date _____			Date _____			Date _____		
		Resistance	Reps/sets		Resistance	Reps/sets		Resistance	Reps/sets	
Two-arm curl	____	____	____ / ____		____	____ / ____		____	____ / ____	
Bench press	____	____	____ / ____		____	____ / ____		____	____ / ____	
Quadriceps lift	____	____	____ / ____		____	____ / ____		____	____ / ____	
Leg curl	____	____	____ / ____		____	____ / ____		____	____ / ____	
Lateral pull-down	____	____	____ / ____		____	____ / ____		____	____ / ____	
Upright rowing	____	____	____ / ____		____	____ / ____		____	____ / ____	

- Perform each exercise three times per week. Make sure that you alternate exercise and rest days.
- Retest every 2 to 4 weeks to measure your progress.

A sample weekly recording sheet that can be used for weight training is included in Table 4-1.

ISOTONIC EXERCISES FOR DEVELOPMENT OF STRENGTH AND MUSCULAR ENDURANCE

The following procedures may be helpful in organizing and implementing an isotonic exercise program without the use of weights.

- Select the exercises you wish to incorporate in your program. Some test items included in this chapter are excellent exercises that can be included. Other good exercises are described in the section on circuit training in Chapter 3, or you may include exercises of your own.
- Determine the maximum number of repetitions you can perform in 1 minute for each exercise. This is important so that you can measure improvement.
- For the first week, use half of the maximum number of repetitions for each exercise and perform two sets on each of 3 nonconsecutive days. Make sure that you complete the first set for all the exercises before starting the second set.
- For the second and third weeks, use half the maximum number of repetitions for each exercise and perform three sets on each of 3 nonconsecutive days.
- For the fourth week, do one set using the maximum number of repetitions on each exercise day.
- Starting the fifth week, add 1 to 3 repetitions per week to each exercise.
- Retest every 4 to 8 weeks and determine the maximum number of repetitions that you can perform for each exercise. By doing this, you will be able to measure improvement.

A sample recording sheet that you can use is included in Table 4-2.

TABLE 4-2 **Sample weekly recording sheet for isotonic exercise program without the use of weights**

NAME _____

WEEK NUMBER _____

BODY WEIGHT
DAY 1 _____ lb
DAY 2 _____ lb
DAY 3 _____ lb

Exercise	Max number of repetitions/ minute	DAY 1 Date_____ Reps/sets	DAY 2 Date_____ Reps/sets	DAY 3 Date_____ Reps/sets
_____	_____	___ / ___	___ / ___	___ / ___
_____	_____	___ / ___	___ / ___	___ / ___
_____	_____	___ / ___	___ / ___	___ / ___
_____	_____	___ / ___	___ / ___	___ / ___
_____	_____	___ / ___	___ / ___	___ / ___
_____	_____	___ / ___	___ / ___	___ / ___
_____	_____	___ / ___	___ / ___	___ / ___
_____	_____	___ / ___	___ / ___	___ / ___
_____	_____	___ / ___	___ / ___	___ / ___
_____	_____	___ / ___	___ / ___	___ / ___

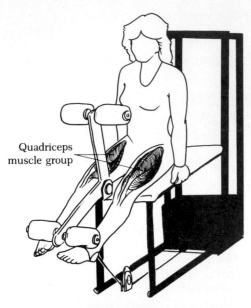

Fig. 4-9 Location of the quadriceps muscle group.

Quadriceps muscle group

WEIGHT-TRAINING EXERCISES FOR THE DEVELOPMENT OF STRENGTH AND MUSCULAR ENDURANCE

Six major muscle groups have previously been listed. In this section the major muscles in each of these groups will be identified and exercises that you can use for their development will be explained. Most exercises use free weights or equipment such as the Universal or Nautilus, which are available at many institutions and health clubs. The equipment you have available may not be quite the same, and you may need to adapt the procedures slightly for the exercises described.

Anterior muscles in the upper legs

The four main muscles located in front of the upper legs are collectively called the quadriceps group (Fig. 4-9). The muscles that make up this group are the rectus femoris, vastus intermedius, vastus lateralis, and vastus medialis. Weight-training exercises for their development include the quadriceps lift and leg press.

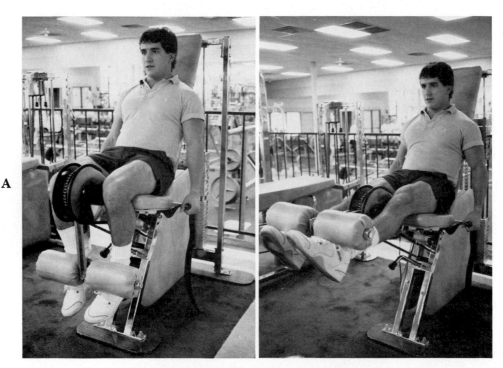

Fig. 4-10 Start **(A)** and finish **(B)** positions for quadriceps lift exercise.

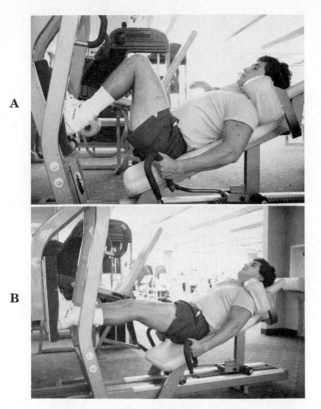

Fig. 4-11 Start **(A)** and finish **(B)** positions for the leg press exercise.

Quadriceps lift. Sit with your lower leg at right angles to your thighs and the front of your ankles against the bar (Fig. 4-10). Extend your legs until they are parallel with the floor, and then return to the starting position. The upper body must remain in an upright position, and the back of the knees should remain in contact with the end of the bench.

Leg press. Sit at the leg press machine with legs bent at 90 degrees or less at the knee joint. Place both feet firmly on the pedals, and grasp the handles on the seat. Press the feet forward until the legs are straight, and then bend them slowly to return to the starting position (Fig. 4-11).

Muscles in chest and upper arms

The main muscles located in front of the chest and the upper arms are the pectoralis major and minor, the anterior deltoid, and the biceps and triceps (Fig. 4-12). Exercises for their development include the bench-

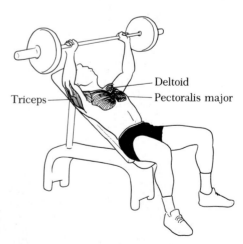

Fig. 4-12 Location of muscles in the chest and upper arms.

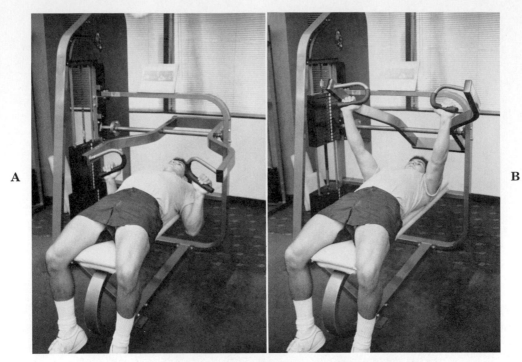

Fig. 4-13 Start **(A)** and finish **(B)** positions for the bench press.

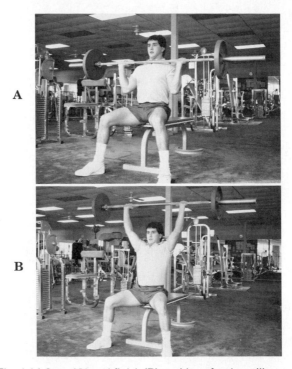

Fig. 4-14 Start **(A)** and finish **(B)** positions for the military press.

press, standing press, parallel dips, biceps curl, shoulder flexion, and shoulder adduction.

Bench press. Lie flat on a bench with your knees bent and your feet flat on the floor (Fig. 4-13). The handles are held with the palms-forward grip at about the width of your shoulders. The weights are then pressed directly upward until your arms are fully extended and then returned to the starting position to complete one repetition. Your back should remain straight throughout.

Military press. This exercise may be performed while sitting or standing upright. The palms-forward grip should be used with the hands slightly more than shoulder-width apart. Push the bar overhead until the arms are fully extended, and then lower it slowly until it touches the chest (Fig. 4-14).

Parallel dips. Support your body in an upright position with your arms straight and with your feet off the floor. Bend your arms and lower your body until there is a right angle or less at the elbow joint. Push up with your upper arms until you return to the start position (Fig. 4-15).

Two-arm curl. Stand with your feet shoulder-width apart in an upright position. A barbell is held with the palms-forward grip and your arms extended. With elbows close to your body, the bar is curled to the shoulder/neck area and then returned to the starting position. This constitutes one repetition (Fig. 4-16 on p. 124). This exercise may also be performed using a machine (Fig. 4-17 on p. 124).

Shoulder flexion. Stand with your feet together and legs straight. Hold a hand weight with the right hand with the overhand grip in front of the thigh. Keeping the arm straight, lift the arm up until it is shoulder height. Hold this position momentarily, and return to the starting position. Repeat this exercise using the left hand (Fig. 4-18 on p. 125).

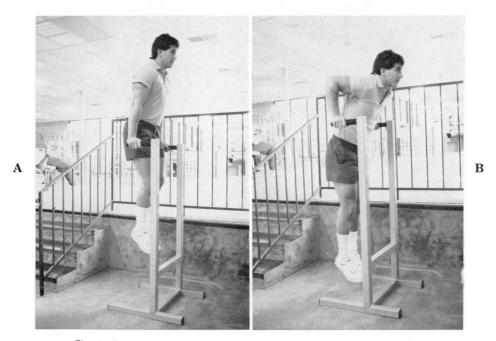

Fig. 4-15 Start **(A)** and finish **(B)** positions for the parallel dip exercise.

A 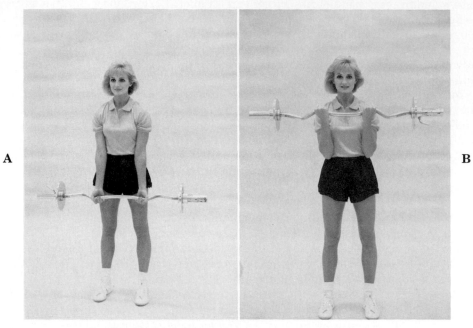 B

Fig. 4-16 Start **(A)** and finish **(B)** positions for two-arm curl exercise.

A 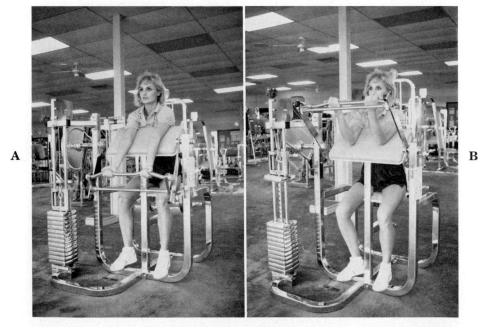 B

Fig. 4-17 Start **(A)** and finish **(B)** positions for the two-arm curl using a biceps machine.

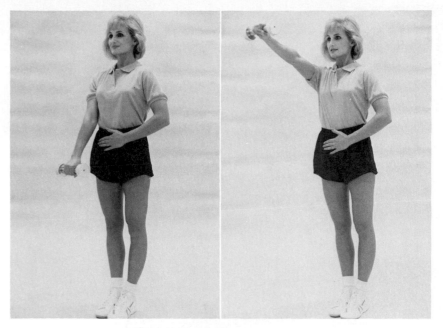

Fig. 4-18 Shoulder flexion exercise using hand weights.

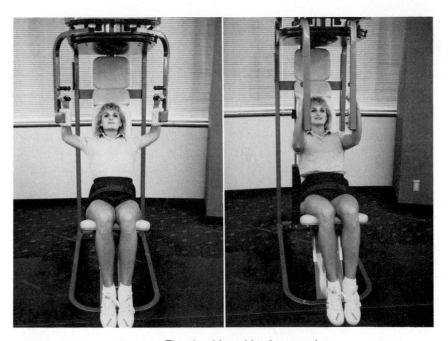

Fig. 4-19 The shoulder adduction exercise.

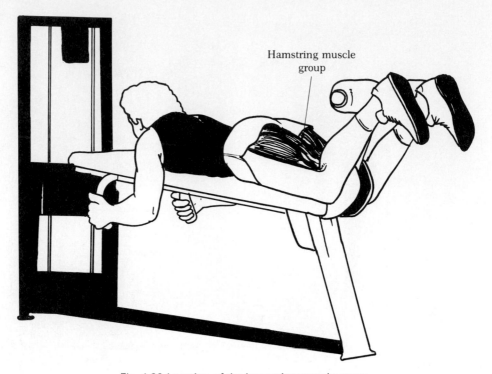

Hamstring muscle
group

Fig. 4-20 Location of the hamstring muscle group.

Shoulder adduction. This is often called horizontal adduction. Sit with your forearms and palms against the pads in the machine. Your elbows should be at about shoulder height. Slowly push the pads together until they meet, and then return to the start position (Fig. 4-19).

Posterior muscles in upper legs

The large muscle group at the back of the legs that crosses both the hip and knee joints is the hamstring muscle group. It consists of three muscles—the semimembranosis, semitendinosus, and the biceps femoris (Fig. 4-20). Exercises for development of the hamstring muscles are leg curls and hip extension.

Leg curls. Lie face down with legs extended and the back of your heels against the bar. Your feet are then lifted upward until they touch your buttocks. They are then returned to the starting position (Fig. 4-21).

Hip extension. Stand sideways to the machine, placing the roller behind the bent knee and holding the bar for support. Press the roller back until both knees are together, making sure that you do not lean forward or arch your back. Return to the start position (Fig. 4-22).

Muscles in the shoulders and upper back

The major muscles associated with the shoulders and the posterior aspect of the upper arms are the rhomboids, triceps, trapezius, latissimus dorsi, and deltoid (posterior head) (Fig. 4-23 on p. 128). Exercises for development of these muscles are the lateral pull-down, bent-over rowing, triceps curl, seated rowing, shoulder elevation, and shoulder abduction.

Lateral pull-down. Kneel and grasp the bar with the palms-forward grip or sit on a bench as shown in Fig. 4-24. The bar is pulled down until it touches the base of your neck and then returned to the starting position to complete one repetition. Your body must be kept straight throughout. If the weight lifts you off the floor, the effectiveness of this exercise is reduced. If this happens, you must be held down by another person.

Bent-over rowing. Stand in the bent-over position with your back straight and slightly above parallel to the floor. Your feet should be shoulder-width apart, with your knees comfortably bent. The bar should be grasped with the overhand grip, with the hands slightly wider apart than the shoulders. Pull the bar up slowly until it touches the chest, and lower it to the start position with the arms completely extended (Fig. 4-25, p. 129).

Triceps curl. Grip the bar with the overhand grip. Keeping your upper arms and elbows motionless and close to your sides, push the bar down in front of your thighs until your arms are straight. Return to the start position (Fig. 4-26, p. 129). This exercise can also be performed using free weights (Fig. 4-27, p. 130).

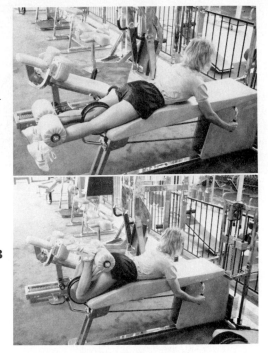

Fig. 4-21 Start **(A)** and finish **(B)** positions for the leg curl exercise.

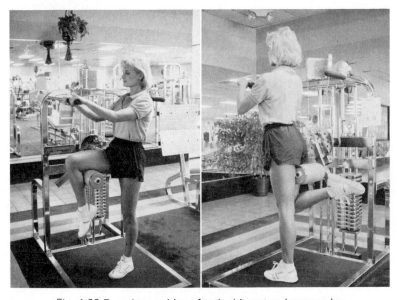

Fig. 4-22 Exercise positions for the hip extension exercise.

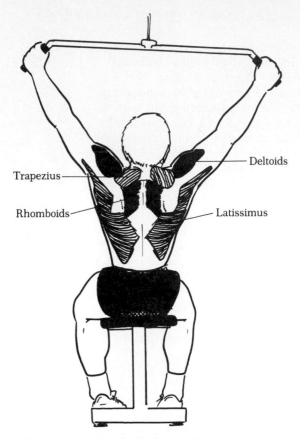

Trapezius

Deltoids

Rhomboids

Latissimus

Fig. 4-23 Muscles associated with the shoulders and the upper back.

A 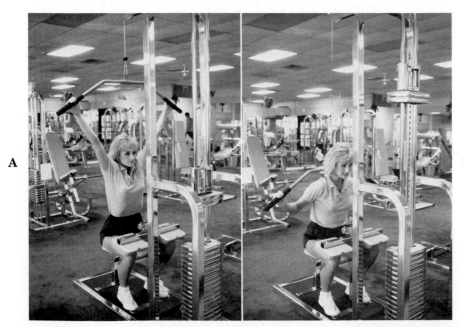 B

Fig. 4-24 Start **(A)** and finish **(B)** positions for the lateral machine pull-down exercise.

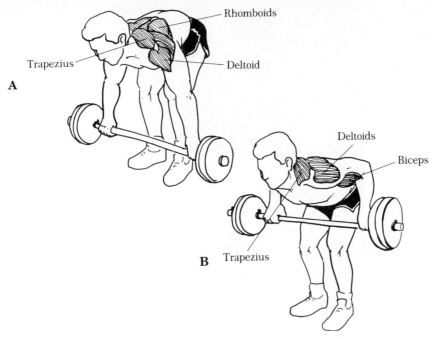

Fig. 4-25 Start **(A)** and finish **(B)** positions for bent-over rowing.

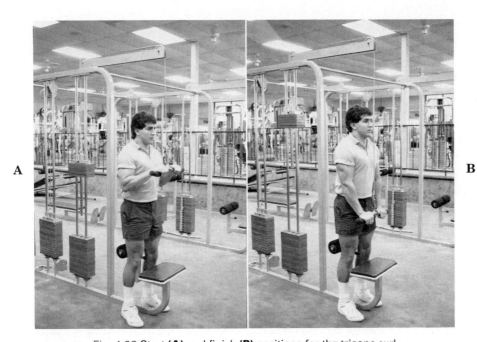

Fig. 4-26 Start **(A)** and finish **(B)** positions for the triceps curl.

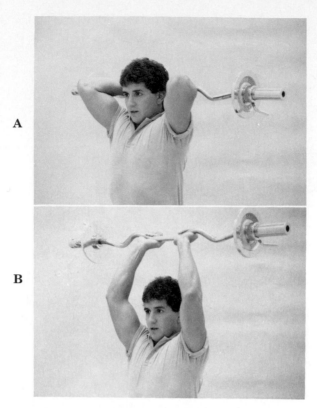

Fig. 4-27 Start **(A)** and finish **(B)** position s for the triceps curl using free weights.

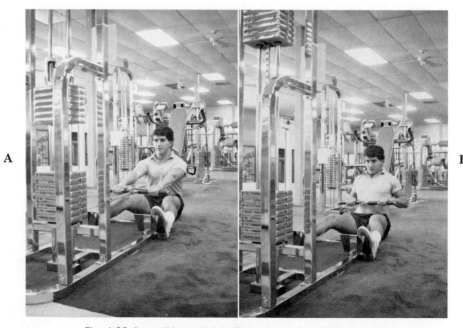

Fig. 4-28 Start **(A)** and finish **(B)** positions for seated rowing.

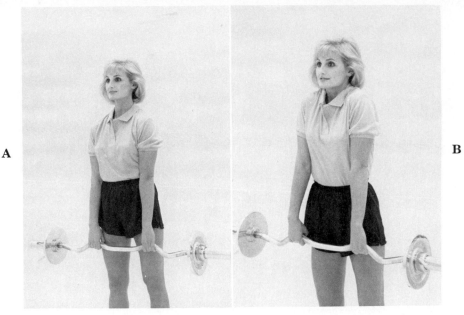

Fig. 4-29 Start **(A)** and finish **(B)** positions for shoulder elevation exercise.

Seated rowing. Use the overhand grip with the hands about shoulder-width apart. Pull the bar to the chest, extend the arms, and lower the weight (Fig. 4-28).

Shoulder elevation. This is commonly called the shoulder shrug. Start with the bar at the rest position in front of the thigh. Use the overhand grip, and keeping the arms straight, elevate the bar by contracting the trapezius and then lower the bar to the rest position (Fig. 4-29).

Shoulder abduction. Sit in the machine with your elbows by your sides and with your forearms resting against the arm pads. Press up against the pads until they are at shoulder height and then slowly lower them to the start position (Fig. 4-30 on p. 132).

Posterior muscles in lower legs

The two major muscles in back of the lower legs are the gastrocnemius and the soleus, which is beneath the gastrocnemius (Fig. 4-31 on p. 132). The calf raise exercise develops these muscles.

Calf raise. Stand on your toes on a 2-inch × 4-inch board with the bar on your shoulders behind your neck. Raise to full extension, lifting your heels as high as possible while keeping your toes in contact with the board, and then lower your heels so that they are as close as possible to the ground (Fig. 4-32 on p. 133).

Abdominal muscles

There are three major muscles in the abdominal muscle group. These are the rectus abdominis, and the internal and external oblique muscles (Fig. 4-33 on p. 133). Two exercises are given for their development.

Curl-ups with weights. The arms are folded across the abdominal area, and a weight is held there. Use a sit-up bench set at about 40 degrees. The feet are tucked

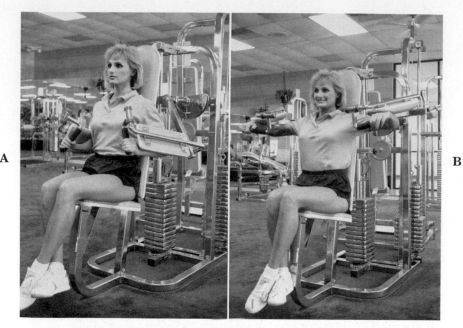

A   B

Fig. 4-30 Start **(A)** and finish **(B)** positions for the shoulder abduction exercise.

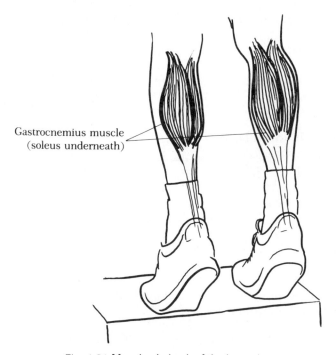

Gastrocnemius muscle
(soleus underneath)

Fig. 4-31 Muscles in back of the lower leg.

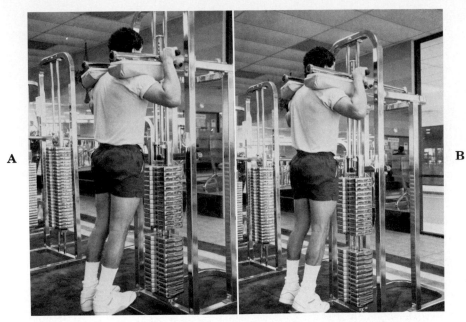

Fig. 4-32 Start **(A)** and finish **(B)** positions for the calf raise exercise.

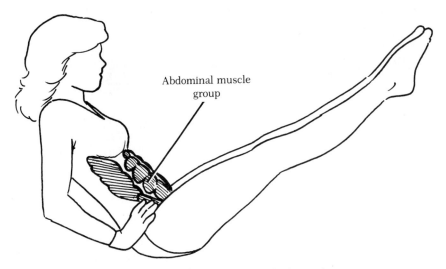

Fig. 4-33 Position of the abdominal muscles.

under the support, and the head is tilted forward with the chin close to the chest. Curl up slowly, touching the elbows to the upper leg, and return to the start position (Fig. 4-34 on p. 134). This exercise can be made more difficult by moving the weight farther away from the abdominal area toward the head or by increasing the amount of weight.

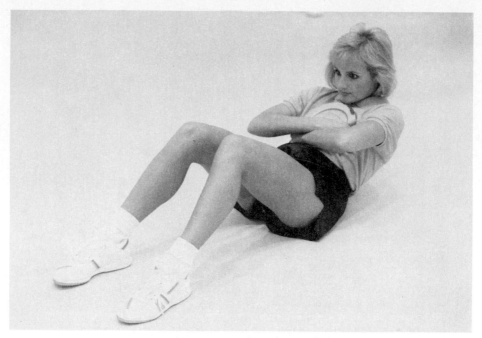

Fig. 4-34 The curl-up exercise using additional weight.

A

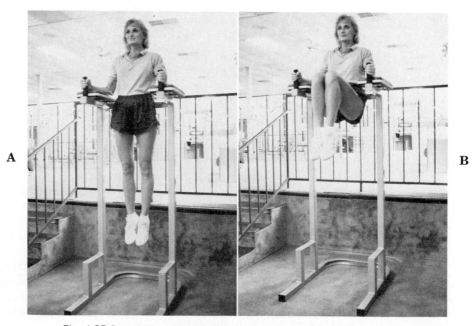

B

Fig. 4-35 Start **(A)** and finish **(B)** positions for the hip flexion exercise.

Hip flexion. For this exercise, support yourself on your forearms so that you hang vertically, making sure that you keep your shoulders parallel to the floor. With your legs held together, bend your knees and raise them until they are perpendicular to the waist. Hold this position for 2 seconds, and then lower them slowly back to the start position (Fig. 4-35).

MUSCLE SORENESS

Muscle soreness often occurs as a result of participation in an exercise program. It may occur during, immediately after, or 24 to 48 hours after the exercise session. The cause of this pain is not fully understood. However, it is believed that the acute pain that occurs during exercise is caused by accumulation of metabolic by-products created by insufficient blood flow. This type of pain usually disappears soon after exercise stops.

Delayed muscle soreness is usually the result of repetitive strenuous muscle contractions, such as in isotonic programs involving weight training or calisthenics. The cause is unknown, although it is believed that microscopic tears may occur where muscles attach to bones.[3] Delayed muscle soreness is usually felt at the start of an exercise program or during an exercise program when you increase the intensity of the workload. It is suggested that it can be avoided by the following:

- Warming up properly
- Starting an exercise program at a low level of intensity
- Increasing the workload gradually throughout the program
- Cooling down correctly after each exercise session

If delayed muscle soreness does occur, static stretching combined with the use of heat may help alleviate the pain.

USE OF ANABOLIC STEROIDS

An anabolic steroid is a synthetic drug that functions similar to the male hormone testosterone. It was developed for use by physicians in the treatment of disorders in which protein synthesis was important.[22] Unfortunately, in recent years considerable interest has arisen among athletes concerning its use for increasing their athletic performance and also among high-school students who may use it to enhance physical appearance.[7]

Anabolic steroids are taken most frequently in conjunction with a high-intensity strength/weight-training program. Evidence suggests that this combination can result in rapid gains in muscle size and strength. However, it would appear that such a practice is potentially dangerous and can create a health hazard.

The American College of Sports Medicine has conducted a comprehensive survey of the literature and carefully evaluated the claims made for and against the use of anabolic steroids for improving human physical performance.[2] Following is a summary of some of their conclusions:

- Anabolic steroids in the presence of an adequate diet can contribute to an increase in body weight.
- An increase in muscle strength achieved through high-intensity exercise and proper diet can be enhanced by the use of anabolic steroids in some individuals.
- The use of anabolic steroids does not increase aerobic power or capacity.
- The use of anabolic steroids has been associated with adverse effects on the liver, cardiovascular system, reproductive system, and psychological status in limited research with athletes.

- The use of anabolic steroids is contrary to the rules and ethical procedures of athletic competition as set forth by most sports-governing bodies. The American College of Sports Medicine supports these ethical procedures and deplores the use of anabolic steroids by athletes.

It should be noted that anabolic steroids are not used just by athletes. A recent study estimated that approximately 1 in 15 high-school students have used steroids, and athough the most common reason given for their use was improved athletic performance, there were 25% who used steroids simply for "enhanced appearance."[7]

Of particular concern is recent evidence that shows that the use of steroids[8,14]:

- Significantly lowers high-density lipoprotein (HDL) levels
- Elevates low-density lipoprotein (LDL) levels
- Increases total cholesterol levels

These three changes are associated with an increased risk of coronary artery disease and are explained in detail in Chapter 10.

> It would appear that the use of anabolic steroids is unethical, unhealthy, and—in most cases—illegal. The possibility of developing severe and harmful side effects would appear to far outweigh any potential gains in athletic performance.

MEASUREMENT OF STRENGTH AND MUSCULAR ENDURANCE

Principle of specificity

Cardiovascular endurance is a general component and can be measured by one test. However, this is not the case with either strength or muscular endurance. Each of these is likely to vary considerably for each of the muscle groups. Because one muscle group has a high degree of strength and muscular endurance does not necessarily mean that other groups will be similarly developed. This is the principle of specificity. A good example is a gymnast who works on the parallel bars. If he or she is to be successful, a high degree of strength and muscular endurance in the upper body must be developed. Because the legs are used much less, strength and muscular endurance in the lower body will be considerably less than in the arms and shoulders.

Because of the principle of specificity, it is necessary to administer many different strength and muscular endurance tests so that different muscle groups can be evaluated.

Strength tests

Strength is measured by determining the maximum force that a muscle or muscle group can exert once and only once. This is referred to as 1 RM (repetition maximum). Strength may be measured by either the isometric or isotonic method. Regardless of which is used, some equipment is necessary.

To measure strength isometrically, a dynamometer or tensiometer is used. A muscle or muscle group contracts, and this force is transmitted by springs or cables to the face of the instrument. The score can be read there. Little or no movement takes place with isometric tests. It is therefore important to standardize the angle for each test, so that consistent results are obtained.

Strength may also be determined isotonically by determining the maximum amount of weight that can be moved once and only once through the designated range of motion. For example, if a person can perform one two-arm curl using 100 lb but cannot move 110 lb through the full range of motion, then the strength of the muscle group being tested (the flexors of the forearm) is approximately 100 lb. A trial and error system must be used with this method, and weights must be added or subtracted with adequate rest between trials in an attempt to determine the maximum weight that can be moved once. It should be emphasized that performing a number of repetitions with the same weight or sustaining a contraction over time measures muscular endurance rather than strength. Procedures for four strength tests are presented in Laboratory Experience 4-1 at the end of this chapter. However, the isotonic method just described can be used with any weight-training exercises to determine the strength of the muscle group involved. You may want to use the specific weight-training equipment that you have available to determine your strength for each muscle group that you exercise. In this way, you will be able to measure your progress.

Muscular endurance tests

For each group of muscles, muscular endurance can be measured by how many repetitions are performed continuously or in a designated period of time (isotonic), or by how long a contraction can be sustained (isometric). Procedures for the muscular endurance tests for men and women are included in Laboratory Experience 4-2 at the end of this chapter.

An alternate procedure for measuring muscular endurance is included in Laboratory Experience 4-3. The results from seven tests are combined to give you an "overall" measurement of muscular endurance.

SUMMARY

The following summary will help you to identify some of the important concepts covered in this chapter.
- The level of strength and muscular endurance that you have will determine the efficiency with which you perform everyday tasks.
- All movements that occur in the body depend on the contraction of muscles.
- Because strength and muscular endurance are specific to each muscle group, you need to include specific exercises for each of the muscle groups that you wish to develop.
- The intensity of a weight-training workout relates to the extent that muscles are overloaded.
- To avoid muscle soreness, you need to warm up, start out at a low level of activity, and gradually increase the amount of work that you do.
- To measure strength, you determine the maximum force that you can exert one time, whereas to measure muscular endurance, you determine how many repetitions you can perform or how long you can sustain a specific contraction.

KEY TERMS

concentric contraction An isotonic contraction where the muscle shortens and works against gravity.

eccentric contraction An isotonic contraction in which the muscle lengthens while it performs work as it returns to its original position.

isokinetic contraction   An isotonic contraction where the speed of motion is controlled, so that a maximum force is applied by the muscle through a full range of motion.

isometric contraction   A contraction where the force exerted by the muscle is equal to or less than the resistance. No movement takes place at the joint, and there is no change in the length of the muscles. Also called static contraction.

isotonic contraction   A contraction where movement occurs at the joint, and there is a shortening and lengthening of muscles involved. Also called dynamic contraction.

muscular endurance   The ability of a muscle or muscle group to apply force repeatedly or to sustain a contraction for a period of time.

one-repetition maximum (1 RM)   The maximum force that can be exerted only once by a muscle or muscle group.

overload   Subjecting a muscle to a workload greater than that to which it is accustomed.

repetition   Completion of a designated movement through a full range of motion.

resistance   The workload you are attempting to move.

set   A specified number of repetitions attempted consecutively.

sticking point   The point in the range of motion in an isotonic contraction where force applied by a muscle is weakest.

strength   The amount of force a muscle or muscle group can exert against a resistance in one maximum contraction.

REFERENCES

1. Allsen PE, Harrison JM, and Vance B: *Fitness for life: an individualized approach*, ed 4, Dubuque, Ia, 1989, Wm C Brown.
2. American College of Sports Medicine: The use of anabolic-androgenic steroids in sports, *Sports Medicine Bulletin* 19:13, 1984.
3. Armstrong RB: Mechanisms of exercise-induced delayed onset muscle soreness: a brief review, *Medicine and Science in Sports and Exercise* 16:6-36, 1984.
4. Berger RA: *Introduction to weight training*, Englewood Cliffs, NJ, 1984, Prentice Hall.
5. Bowers RW, Fox E: *Sports physiology*, ed 3, Dubuque, Ia, 1992, Wm C Brown.
6. Brooks GA, Fahey TD: *Fundamentals of human performance*, New York, 1987, Macmillan.
7. Buckley W et al: Estimated prevalence of anabolic steroid use among male high school seniors, *Journal of American Medical Association* 260:3441, 1988.
8. Costill D et al: Anabolic steroid use among athletes: changes in HDL-C levels, *The Physician and Sportsmedicine* 12:112, 1984.
9. DiGennario J: *The new physical fitness: exercise for everybody*, Englewood, Colo, 1984, Morton.
10. Fox E, Bowers R, and Foss M: *The physiological basis of physical education and athletics*, ed 4, Philadelphia, WB Saunders.
11. Golding LA, Myers CR, and Sinning WE: *The Y's way to physical fitness*, ed 2, Rosemont, Ill, 1982, YMCA.
12. Fleck SJ, Kraemer WJ: *Designing resistance training programs*, Champaign, Ill, 1987, Human Kinetics Publishers.
13. Fleck SJ, Kraemer WJ: Systems of resistance training, *Fitness Management* 4(2):23-25, 1988.
14. Hurley BF et al: HDL cholesterol in body builders vs. power lifters. Negative effects of androgen use, *Journal of American Medical Association* 252:4, 1984.
15. Institute for Aerobic Research: *Common muscle imbalances*, Dallas, Tx, 1988.
16. Kerlan R, MacKenzie RB: Sports medicine: forget old fashioned sit-ups, *Shape* 5:44, 1986.
17. Manz RL: *The hydrafitness manual for omnikinetic training*, Belton, Tex, 1983, Hydra-Fitness Industries.
18. MacArdle WD, Katch FI, and Katch VL: *Exercise physiology, energy, nutrition and human performance*, ed 3, Philadelphia, 1991, Lea & Febiger.
19. McGlynn G: *Dynamics of fitness*, ed 2, Dubuque, Ia, 1990, Wm C Brown.
20. O'Shea JP: *Scientific principles and methods of strength fitness*, ed 2, Reading, Mass, 1976, Addison-Wesley.

21. *Physical fitness training,* Department of the Army, Ft Monroe, Va, 1985, US Government Printing Office.

22. Prentice W: *Fitness for college and life,* ed 3, St Louis, 1991, Mosby–Year Book.

23. Reid JG, Thomson JM: *Exercise prescription for fitness,* Englewood Cliffs, NJ, 1985, Prentice Hall.

24. Stone WJ, Kroll WA: *Sports conditioning and weight training. Programs for athletic competitors,* Newton, Me, 1986, Allyn & Bacon.

25. Shields CL et al: Comparison of leg strength training equipment, *The Physician and Sportsmedicine* 13(2):49-56, 1985.

26. Stamford B: Building bigger muscles, *Physician Sports Medicine* 15(6):266, 1987.

27. *Strength training,* Dallas, Tex, Aerobics Center (printed material).

28. Westcott WL: *Strength fitness: physiological principles and training techniques,* ed 2, Boston, 1987, Allyn & Bacon.

29. Williams MH: *Lifetime physical fitness,* Dubuque, Ia, 1985, Wm C Brown.

30. Yesis M: Body in motion, *Shape* 4:37-49, 1985.

Measurement of Strength

The following tests can be used to measure strength:

- Grip strength
- Back strength
- Bench press
- Leg strength

Grip strength

Grip strength is probably the most common measurement, possibly because the hand dynamometer is available at many universities, health clubs, and schools. Squeeze the dynamometer as tightly as possible, using the musculature of the hand. No part of your upper or lower arm or your hand may push against any object or against any other part of your body. The force exerted may be read from the dial of the dynamometer and should be recorded to the nearest pound (Fig. 4-36).

Results

Record results in the space provided.

Grip strength _____ lb

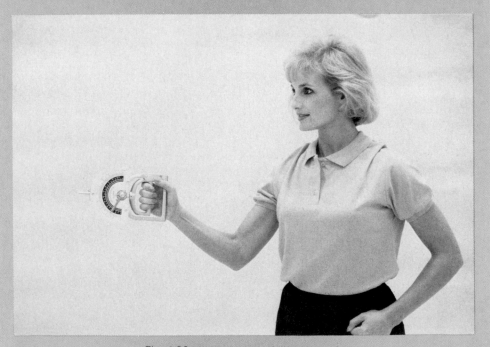

Fig. 4-36 Measurement of grip strength.

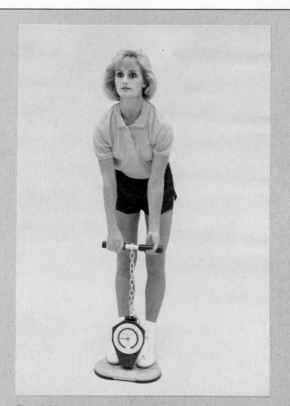

Fig. 4-37 Measurement of back strength: an example of an isometric contraction.

Back strength

For testing back strength (Fig. 4-37), use a back dynamometer. Stand upright on the base of the dynamometer with your feet shoulder-width apart, your arms straight, and your fingers extended downward as far as possible on the fronts of your thighs. The bar is then attached to the chain so that it is 1 to 2 inches below your fingertips. Then, bend forward slightly and grasp the bar. The correct position to lift is with your back bent forward slightly at the hips and your legs straight. Your head should be held upright, and you should look straight ahead. Lift steadily, keeping legs straight and feet flat on the base of the dynamometer. At the completion of the test, your back should be almost straight. If it is perfectly straight, the test should be repeated with the bar slightly lower.

Results

Record results in the space provided.

Back strength _____ lb

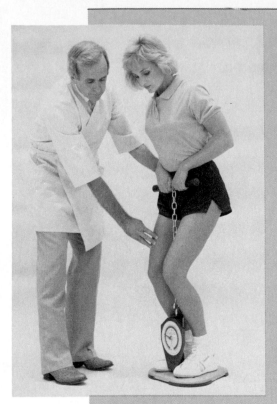

Fig. 4-38 Position for the leg strength test.

Bench press

Either free weights or a bench press machine may be used for this test (Fig. 4-13). Lie flat on the bench with your knees bent and feet flat on the floor. Determine by trial and error the maximum weight that can be lifted once. When lifting the weight, hold the barbell with the palms-forward grip at about the width of the shoulders. Press the bar directly upward until your arms are fully extended. Your back must not be arched during this test; it must remain in contact with the bench. If the bench is wide enough, it will be beneficial to bend your legs so that you have about a 90-degree angle at the knee joint and place your feet flat on the bench rather than on the floor.

Results

Record results in the space provided.

Bench press _____ lb

Leg strength

The bar should be held in the center, with both hands together and with the palms facing toward the body. It should be at a level where the thighs and trunk meet (Fig. 4-38). Your back must be kept straight as you pull as hard as possible on the chain and try to straighten your legs. Maximum performance will result when your legs are almost straight at the end of the lift. This will usually occur if the bar is attached to the dynamometer when the knees are bent at about 120 degrees.

Results

Record results in the space provided.

Leg strength _____ lb

Classification of strength scores

To evaluate the scores for each of the strength tests refer to Table 4-3 (men) or Table 4-4 (women).

TABLE 4-3 **Strength profile chart** *(men)*

Percentile rank	Grip strength (lb)			Back strength (lb)			Bench press (lb)			Leg strength (lb)			Fitness category
	Age (years)			**Age (years)**			**Age (years)**			**Age (years)**			
	<30	30-50	>50	<30	30-50	>50	<30	30-50	>50	<30	30-50	>50	
95	150	135	118	451	406	358	203	183	161	504	454	400	Excellent
90	144	129	114	422	380	335	191	172	151	474	426	326	
80	136	123	108	387	348	307	175	158	139	436	393	346	Good
70	131	118	104	362	325	286	164	148	130	409	369	325	
60	126	114	100	340	306	269	155	139	122	386	348	307	Average
50	122	110	97	320	288	253	146	131	115	365	329	290	
40	118	106	94	300	270	237	137	123	108	344	310	273	
30	113	102	90	278	251	220	128	114	100	321	289	255	Fair
20	108	97	86	253	228	199	117	104	91	294	265	234	
10	100	91	80	218	196	171	101	90	79	256	232	204	Poor
5	94	85	76	189	170	148	89	79	69	226	204	180	
Mean	122	110	97	320	288	253	146	131	115	365	329	290	
Standard deviation	17	15	13	80	72	64	35	32	28	85	76	67	

TABLE 4-4 Strength profile chart (women)

Percentile rank	Grip strength (lb)			Back strength (lb)			Bench press (lb)			Leg strength (lb)			Fitness category
	<30	30-50	>50	<30	30-50	>50	<30	30-50	>50	<30	30-50	>50	
95	84	76	67	266	239	210	105	95	84	301	271	238	Excellent
90	81	73	64	251	226	199	100	91	81	285	257	226	
80	76	69	61	234	210	185	95	86	76	266	240	211	Good
70	73	66	58	221	199	175	91	83	73	252	227	200	
60	71	63	56	210	189	166	88	80	71	241	217	191	Average
50	68	61	54	200	180	158	85	77	68	230	207	182	
40	66	59	52	190	171	150	82	74	66	219	197	174	
30	63	56	50	179	161	141	79	71	63	208	187	164	Fair
20	60	53	47	166	150	131	75	68	60	194	174	153	
10	55	46	44	149	134	117	70	63	55	175	157	138	Poor
5	52	46	41	134	121	106	65	59	52	159	143	126	
Mean	68	61	54	200	180	158	85	77	68	230	207	182	
Standard deviation	10	9	8	40	36	32	12	11	10	43	39	34	

Measurement of Muscular Endurance

Tests recommended for the measurement of muscular endurance for men and women are given in Table 4-5. Note that for women it is necessary to modify the push-up and pull-up tests. The reason for this is the difference in upper body strength between males and females. Many college-aged females lack the strength to do one regular pull-up and/or are unable to perform one regular push-up. The static push-up is offered as an alternate for the push-up or modified push-up, because of the ease of administering the test.

TABLE 4-5 Muscular endurance tests

Test	Suggested for men	Suggested for women
Bent-leg curl-up	Yes	Yes
Push-up	Yes	No
Modified push-up	No	Yes
Static push-up	Yes	Yes
Pull-up	Yes	No
Flexed arm hang	No	Yes
Modified pull-up	No	Yes
Bench jump	Yes	Yes

Bent-leg curl-up

The bent-leg curl-up measures muscular endurance of the abdominal muscles. These muscles are important in maintaining good posture. Poorly developed abdominal muscles also contribute to low back pain. To begin this test, lie on your back on the floor with your feet flat on the floor about shoulder-width apart and held by a partner. Knees should be flexed, forming about a right angle (Fig. 4-39 on p. 146). Fold your arms across your chest, and move the top of your head as far forward as possible while pressing your chin against your chest. This is the start position for this test. Curl up until your elbows touch the upper part of your thighs, and then return until your lower back is in contact with the floor. Perform as many curl-ups as possible in 1 minute.

Results

Record results in the space provided.
Number of curl-ups in 1 minute _____

Push-up (men only)

The push-up measures endurance of the muscle group responsible for extension of the forearm. The largest muscle of this group is the triceps. Assume a prone position on the floor with hands directly under your shoulder joints, legs straight and together, and toes tucked under in contact with the floor. Then push with your arms until they are fully extended. The body is then lowered until your chin or chest touches the floor. At this point there should be a straight line from

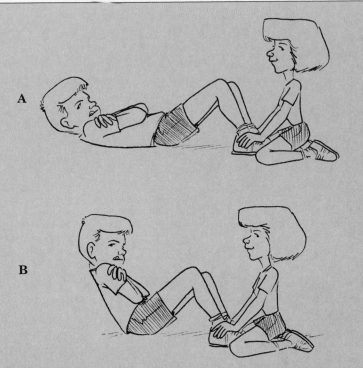

Fig. 4-39 Start (**A**) and finish (**B**) positions for the bent-leg curl-up test.

your head to your toes. All of this movement must be performed by the arms and shoulders, and not by any other part of the body. Perform as many push-ups as possible in 1 minute. You may rest in the up position if desired.

Results

Record results in the space provided.
Number of push-ups _____

Modified push-up (women only)

To start this exercise, assume the push-up position (as for men) but support your weight on your knees and not on your feet. Your legs should be bent upward at the knees (Fig. 4-40). Keeping your body in a straight line from the top of your head to your knees, lower your upper body until your chest just touches the floor and then push back up to the fully extended position. Perform as many repetitions as possible in 1 minute.

Results

Record results in the space provided.
Number of modified push-ups _____

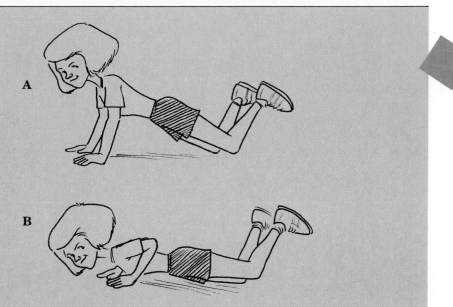

Fig. 4-40 Start **(A)** and finish **(B)** positions for the modified push-up.

Static push-up

The static push-up (Fig. 4-41) is an alternate test for the push-up or modified push-up test. It may be preferred because it is easier to administer and much easier to standardize the procedures. From a straight-arm front-leaning position with your hands directly under your shoulders, lower your body until your elbows are at 90 degrees. Hold this position for as long as possible. The test is terminated when any part of your body other than your hands or toes touches the floor or when you can no longer maintain your body in a straight line parallel to the floor.

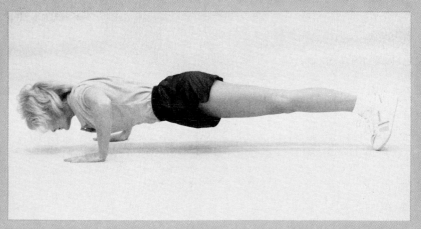

Fig. 4-41 The position to be maintained in the static push-up. Note that the back must be straight, and the elbow joint must be at an angle of 90 degrees or less.

Results

Record results in the space provided.
Time for static push-up _____ seconds

Bench jump

The bench jump determines muscular endurance of the lower extremity. A 16-inch bench is used, and you jump up to the bench as many times as possible in 1 minute. If you are unable to jump, you may step up; however, this takes more time. Your arms may swing freely, but you are not permitted to push down on your thighs with your hands. One repetition is counted each time both feet are planted on the bench and then returned to the floor.

Results

Record results in the space provided.
Number of bench jumps in 1 minute _____

Pull-up (men only)

The pull-up primarily measures endurance of the muscle group responsible for flexion of the forearm. The major muscle of this group is the biceps brachii or, as it is commonly called, the biceps. Grasp the horizontal bar with both hands, palms forward. The "dead hang" position is assumed, with arms fully extended and feet off the ground. Raise your body until your chin is above the top of the bar, and then lower yourself until your arms are fully extended. The pull-up is repeated until you can no longer raise your chin above the bar. The knees may not be raised nor is kicking permitted to perform more pull-ups.

Results

Record results in the space provided.
Number of pull-ups _____

Flexed-arm hang (women only)

The flexed-arm hang measures endurance of the flexors of the forearm. You must use the overhand grip with palms facing forward. Then raise your body off the floor until the chin is level with the bar. This position is maintained for as long as possible. Time is stopped when the chin cannot be maintained level with the bar.

Results

Record results in the space provided.
Time for flexed-arm hang
_____ minutes _____ seconds

Modified pull-up (women only)

For the modified pull-up, the chinning bar is adjusted to the height of the sternum and the feet remain in contact with the floor throughout. Grip the bar with palms forward, and slide your feet under the bar until your arms form a right angle with your body. Your weight must rest on your heels as you attempt to pull up, so that your chin or forehead touches the bar with the body held straight. This is repeated as many times as possible (Fig. 4-42).

Results

Record results in the space provided.

Number of modified pull-ups _____

Evaluation of muscular endurance test scores

To evaluate your score for each of the muscular endurance tests, refer to Table 4-6 (men) or Table 4-7 (women) (pp. 150–151).

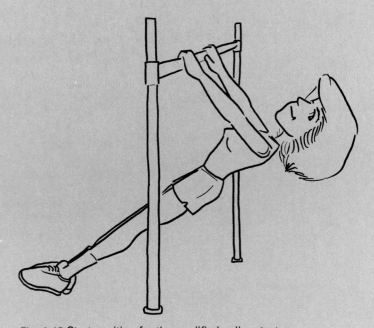

Fig. 4-42 Start position for the modified pull-up test.

TABLE 4-6 Muscular endurance profile chart (men)

Percentile rank	Bent-leg curl-ups (1 minute) Age (years)			Static push-up (Time—seconds) Age (years)			Push-ups (Repetitions) Age (years)			Pull-ups (Repetitions) Age (years)			Bench jump (Repetitions) Age (years)			Fitness category
	<30	30-50	>50	<30	30-50	>50	<30	30-50	>50	<30	30-50	>50	<30	30-50	>50	
95	62	57	49	77	69	60	53	47	41	14	13	11	38	35	31	Excellent
90	59	54	46	72	65	57	50	44	39	12	11	10	36	33	29	
80	54	50	43	67	60	53	46	41	36	10	9	9	34	31	27	Good
70	51	47	40	63	57	50	43	38	34	9	8	8	33	30	26	
60	49	44	38	60	54	47	40	36	32	8	7	7	31	28	25	Average
50	46	42	36	57	51	45	38	34	30	7	6	6	30	27	24	
40	44	40	34	54	48	43	36	32	28	6	5	5	29	26	23	
30	41	37	32	51	45	40	33	30	26	5	4	4	27	24	22	Fair
20	38	34	29	47	42	37	30	27	24	4	3	3	26	23	21	
10	33	30	26	42	37	33	26	24	21	2	1	1	24	21	19	Poor
5	30	27	23	37	33	30	23	21	19	0	0	0	22	19	17	
Mean	46	42	36	57	51	45	38	34	30	7	6	6	30	27	24	
Standard deviation	10	9	8	12	11	9	9	8	7	4	4	3	5	5	4	

TABLE 4-7 Muscular endurance profile *(women)*

Percentile rank	Bent-leg curl-ups (1 minute) Age (years)			Modified push-ups (Repetitions) Age (years)			Static push-ups (Time—seconds) Age (years)			Flexed-arm hang (Time—seconds) Age (years)			Modified pull-ups (Repetitions) Age (years)			Bench jump (1-minute) Age (years)			Fitness category
	<30	30-50	>50	<30	30-50	>50	<30	30-50	>50	<30	30-50	>50	<30	30-50	>50	<30	30-50	>50	
95	50	45	39	45	41	35	39	34	31	19	18	14	41	36	32	28	26	23	Excellent
90	47	42	37	40	37	32	36	32	29	17	16	13	38	33	30	26	24	21	
80	43	39	34	35	32	28	33	29	26	15	14	12	34	30	27	24	22	19	Good
70	40	36	32	31	29	25	30	27	24	14	13	11	31	27	25	23	21	18	
60	37	34	30	28	26	22	28	25	23	13	12	10	28	25	23	21	19	17	Average
50	35	32	28	25	23	20	26	23	21	12	11	9	26	23	21	20	18	16	
40	33	30	26	22	20	18	24	21	20	11	10	8	24	21	19	19	17	15	
30	30	28	24	19	17	15	22	19	18	10	9	7	21	19	17	17	15	14	Fair
20	27	25	22	15	14	12	19	17	16	9	8	6	18	16	15	16	14	13	
10	23	22	19	10	9	8	16	14	13	7	6	5	14	13	12	14	12	11	Poor
5	20	19	17	5	5	5	13	12	11	5	4	4	11	10	10	12	10	9	
Mean	35	32	28	25	23	20	26	23	21	12	11	9	26	23	21	20	18	16	
Standard deviation	9	8	7	12	11	9	8	7	6	4	4	3	9	8	7	5	5	4	

Evaluating Muscular Endurance Using Weights or Weight Machine

An alternate method of evaluating muscular endurance is adapted from Allsen, Harrison, and Vance[1] and is based on the earlier work of DiGennario.[9] Seven exercises are done to evaluate muscular endurance. These are identified in Table 4-8 and are described in detail previously in this chapter.

The resistance to be used in each exercise is a percentage of your body weight. These percentages are identified in Table 4-8. The resistance should be calculated by multiplying this percentage by your body weight and recorded in Table 4-8.

For each exercise, try to perform the maximum number of repetitions possible, consecutively, using the designated resistance. A maximum of 17 repetitions is allowed for men and 15 for women. Points are earned for each exercise based on the number of repetitions completed. These points may be determined by consulting Table 4-9. Points for each exercise should be recorded in Table 4-8, and the total number of points for all seven exercises is then determined. This is your overall score for muscular endurance. This score may be interpreted by consulting Table 4-10.

TABLE 4-8 **Muscular endurance tests using weights**

Exercise	Body weight	Percentage of body weight	Resistance to be used	Repetitions completed	Points earned
Two-arm curl	_____	× 0.33 =	_____	_____	_____
Bench press	_____	× 0.67 =	_____	_____	_____
Lateral machine pull-down	_____	× 0.67 =	_____	_____	_____
Upright rowing	_____	× 0.33 =	_____	_____	_____
Quadriceps lift	_____	× 0.67 =	_____	_____	_____
Leg curl	_____	× 0.33 =	_____	_____	_____
Curl-up	_____	× 0.14 =	_____	_____	_____

TOTAL POINTS EARNED: _____

TABLE 4-9 **Evaluation of muscular endurance tests**

Repetitions			
Men	Women	Points	Muscular endurance category
0-3	0.2	5	Very poor
4	3	7	Poor
5-8	4-7	9	Fair
9-11	8-10	11	Good
12-16	11-14	13	Very good
17	15	15	Excellent

TABLE 4-10 **Overall muscular endurance classification (total points for all seven tests)**

Points	Category
35-48	Very poor
49-62	Poor
63-76	Fair
77-90	Good
91-104	Very good
105	Excellent

Results

Record results in the space provided.

Total points earned: _____
Muscular endurance category: _____

Flexibility

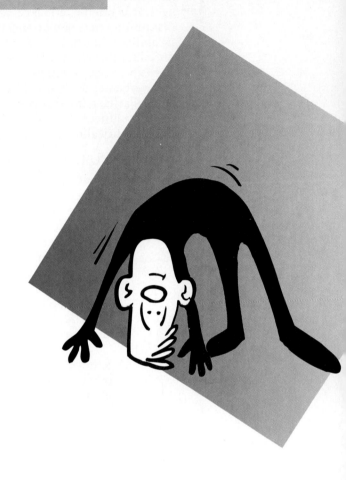

CHAPTER OBJECTIVES

When you understand the material in this chapter, you will be able to:

- Define flexibility, and explain why it is important
- Identify and discuss the factors that limit flexibility
- Evaluate the different procedures used for the development of flexibility
- Develop a flexibility program designed to meet your individual needs
- Discuss the causes of low back pain, and know how to avoid and/or alleviate this problem
- Measure your level of flexibility, and know how to interpret the results
- Define each of the important terms

155

Flexibility is one of the most important health-related components of physical fitness. It is often overlooked and misunderstood. It can be defined simply as the maximum range of motion possible at a joint.

The ability to move each joint through a full range of motion without undue strain is essential for the efficient execution of many everyday tasks. With limited flexibility you may experience "tightness" or "stiffness" at joints and have difficulty performing some movements. Such simple tasks as pulling a shirt or blouse over your head, putting on slacks, tying shoelaces, or getting into or out of the back seat of a two-door car are often difficult for those with a limited range of motion at certain joints. Increased flexibility allows freer and more efficient movement with less resistance.

JOINT STRUCTURE AS IT RELATES TO MOVEMENT

Minimal information about joint structure and the role of muscles is necessary for a basic understanding of flexibility.

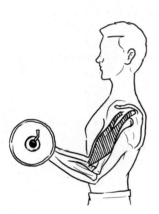

Fig. 5-1 Contraction of the biceps brachii, resulting in flexion at the elbow joint.

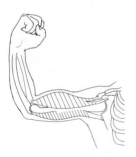

Fig. 5-2 Contraction of the biceps muscle to cause flexion at the elbow joint will result in maximum range of motion only if the triceps muscle relaxes.

A joint is simply a junction of two or more bones where movement takes place. The joint's structure is important, because it will determine what movements can take place at the joint and in some cases will limit the range of motion. For example, the elbow and knee joints are hinge joints that allow movement in only one direction. The only movements possible are flexion and extension. When the forearm and lower leg are fully extended, the bones "lock" into position and the structure of these joints permits no further movement in that direction.

In contrast, joints such as the shoulder and hip are ball-and-socket joints. The rounded head of one bone fits into a hollow cavity of another. This allows movement in many directions and will usually allow a greater range of motion than does a hinge joint.

Flexibility, however, is not limited just by the structure of joints. If it were, we could not improve flexibility because we are unable to change the structure of joints. Soft tissues play an important role and greatly influence the amount of movement possible at a joint. These tissues include muscles, tendons, and ligaments.

Muscles pass across joints and are attached to bones by a tendon. The force exerted by a muscle as it contracts is applied to a bone, and movement will take place at a joint if the force is sufficient to overcome the resistance. In Fig. 5-1 if the force exerted by the biceps brachii is greater than the resistance caused by the weight and the forearm, then movement will take place at the elbow joint.

Muscles are arranged strategically in sets so that when one set contracts and shortens, another set lengthens and must relax. This is demonstrated in Fig. 5-2.

Muscles are protected from overstretching by the stretch reflex. If you try to overstretch a muscle, it will actually contract to prevent this muscle from overstretching.

BASIC FACTS ABOUT FLEXIBILITY

Following are some basic facts concerning flexibility. As you become more knowledgeable about flexibility, you will realize how important it is to maintain an adequate level of flexibility and you will be much more likely to take time to include flexibility exercises in your regular exercise program.

Inactivity contributes to poor flexibility

People who are active tend to be more flexible than those who are not. The reason for this is that flexibility depends on movement. With little or no movement, muscles and other soft tissues tend to become shorter and tighter. They lose elasticity, and flexibility is decreased. This can clearly be seen by observing what happens when, because of an injury, an arm or a leg is placed in a cast. The reason for the cast is to immobilize the limb so that little or no movement takes place. When the cast is removed, the first thing you notice is that the muscles have lost both size and strength and that very little movement is now possible at the joint. Physical therapy is usually prescribed in an attempt to restore normal movement.

When you sit for extended periods, very little movement takes place and muscles can become weaker and joints less flexible. The hamstring muscle group is a good example. This is the large muscle group that crosses both the hip and knee joints at the back of your thighs. When you are sitting for long periods and there is flexion at both of these joints, these muscles are in a shortened position and they become accustomed to that position. The end result is that these muscles become shorter than what they should be, resulting in loss of flexibility at the hip joint, unless time is taken to stretch these muscles.

Decreased flexibility with age is usually caused by physical inactivity

Most people become less flexible as they get older. They have greater difficulty in performing basic skills and also have more aches and pains after physical activity. The reason for this is that most people become less active as they get older. This has some negative implications as far as flexibility is concerned.

The muscles become weaker, they fatigue more easily, and they function less efficiently. In some instances, this results in poor body alignment with a corresponding loss of flexibility. Also, lack of activity can contribute to loss of bone density, which contributes to osteoporosis. As joints become weaker, there is a significant loss of flexibility. A good flexibility program is important to decrease the loss of flexibility that occurs as you get older.

Females are usually more flexible than are males of the same age

During adolescence, when flexibility reaches its highest level, the difference between males and females is most pronounced. Girls have a much greater range of motion than do boys. The norms for college students and adults indicate that women have slightly higher scores than do men. The reason may be that they tend to participate more in activities that promote flexibility, such as dance and gymnastics (Fig. 5-3 on p. 158).

Excessive body fat usually limits flexibility

Obese people usually have difficulty moving efficiently, and their range of motion at certain joints is often restricted. Fat deposits act as a wedge between moving parts of the body, thus restricting movement.

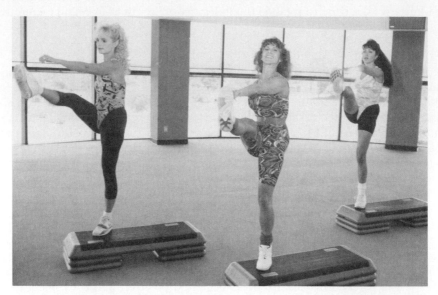

Fig. 5-3 Bench aerobics develops flexibility and is a good form of aerobic exercise.

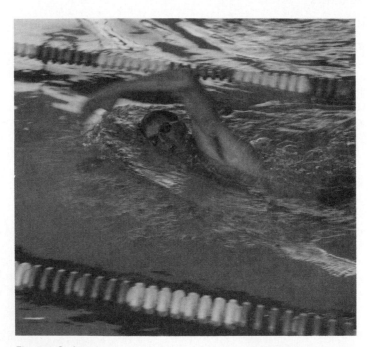

Fig. 5-4 Swimming is another good aerobic exercise that develops flexibility.

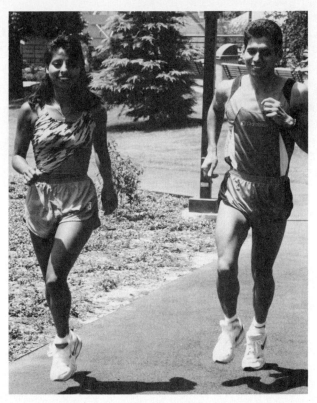

Fig. 5-5 With walking or jogging, there is flexion at both the hip and knee joints. For this reason, it is important to stretch the hamstring muscle group at the end of each exercise session.

Participation in some activities improves flexibility

Regular participation in physical activities that involve a full range of movement at a joint will help prevent loss of movement and increase flexibility. A good example is the crawl stroke in swimming. The elbow joint moves through a full range of motion, and flexibility will be developed (Fig. 5-4).

Some activities use a limited range of motion and will possibly decrease flexibility. For example, with jogging there is slight flexion at the hip and knee joints most of the time. This can result in a shortening of muscles in the back of the leg. Unless they are stretched, particularly after each exercise session, decreased flexibility can occur (Fig. 5-5).

Flexibility is specific to each joint

Flexibility is not a general component of physical fitness. Instead, it is specific to each joint. This means that you may have a good range of motion in some joints and a poor range of motion in others. Flexibility is not a single characteristic, because it is not uniformly present in each joint. Because of this, you must include specific exercises for each movement at each joint for which you want to increase flexibility.

Poor flexibility can contribute to poor posture

Poor flexibility is often caused by muscles that are shorter and tighter than they should be. It may also be a result of an imbalance of development of opposing pairs of muscles. These conditions often contribute to poor posture.

Poor flexibility is often associated with increased tension and pain

It has been known for a long time that stretching is beneficial for alleviation of stress and tension. Those who are under prolonged stress often have pain in the neck, shoulders, and back. One reason is that with constant tension and stress, muscles are tighter than they should be. We have already seen that this can contribute to poor flexibility.

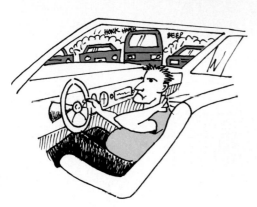

Stress often creates tension in the neck and shoulders.

Too much flexibility may be harmful

It is important to stretch within the normal limits of your body and not exceed this range of motion. When joints are overstretched, ligaments and muscles tend to lose elasticity and may remain lengthened rather than returning to their original size. If this happens, a joint may become less stable and become more prone to injury. This condition often occurs with basketball players who frequently land off balance on the side of their feet after jumping. Ligaments holding the ankle joint in place become stretched and lose their elasticity.

Muscle imbalance may reduce flexibility

We have seen that muscles are arranged in pairs and that as one muscle shortens and contracts, another will lengthen and relax (Fig. 5-2). It is important to maintain a strength and flexibility "balance" between opposing pairs of muscles. For example, if weight training strengthens one group of muscles and neglects the opposing group, a loss of flexibility at that joint will occur.

Skill often depends on a high level of flexibility

Participants in sports recognize the importance of flexibility and are aware that good performance depends on adequate flexibility. A flexible joint increases your ability to reach and stretch during performance and allows you to move more easily and efficiently from one position to another. The importance of this can be seen in such sports as racquetball, tennis, and soccer. In other sports and activities, an extremely high level of flexibility is essential for success. These include dancing, gymnastics, figure skating, diving, sprinting, and cheerleading. Participants in these activities need to work at maximum development of flexibility (Fig. 5-6).

Increased flexibility helps prevent muscle-related injuries

Joints are constantly stressed during activities when muscles contract repeatedly. Injuries often occur when a short, tight muscle contracts vigorously. Increased flexibility can reduce injuries by allowing body parts to move more freely. This is particularly true in activities involving agility and/or speed.

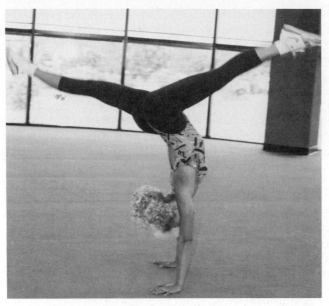

Fig. 5-6 Skill in gymnastics requires a high degree of flexibility.

Increased flexibility helps reduce muscle soreness

A good stretching program, particularly after an exercise session, can reduce the muscle stiffness and soreness that often results from a vigorous workout.

DEVELOPMENT OF FLEXIBILITY

Flexibility may be developed using several techniques. The three most common are the ballistic, static, and contract-relaxation methods.

Ballistic stretching technique

Although the ballistic stretching technique is successful in the development of flexibility, most authorities no longer recommend its use, particularly for those simply interested in the development of an adequate level of flexibility. In addition, it is not recommended for those who are suspect to frequent muscle injuries.

This method uses momentum generated from bouncing and jerking movements to produce the force necessary to stretch muscles. The alternate toe-touch exercise is an example of a ballistic stretching exercise. With this exercise you assume a standing posi-

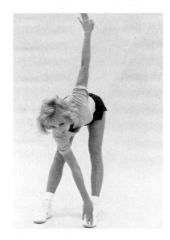

Fig. 5-7 The alternate toe-touch exercise. This is an example of a ballistic stretching exercise.

tion with the legs straight, feet shoulder-width apart, and arms extended above your head. Keeping your legs straight, reach down to touch the left foot with your right hand, then return to the starting position before reaching down again to touch the right foot with your left hand (Fig. 5-7).

The major concern relative to this method of stretching is that the force generated by the body's momentum may overstretch the muscles involved. When this occurs the stretch reflex is activated, whereby a signal is sent to the muscle to contract, preventing it from stretching even further. Tension is therefore created in the muscle, and there is a greater chance that soreness and/or injury will occur.

It should be noted that many movements that occur during several different physical activities are ballistic-type movements. In racquetball and fencing, for example, vigorous movements often create undue tension in muscles. When you participate in these activities, "extra time" should be taken to warm up and stretch before you participate. Because of the nature of activities such as these, there are still some participants who use the ballistic stretching technique.

Static stretching technique

In the static method the stretch position is assumed slowly and gently and then held for a period of time. Care must be taken to move through a full range of motion until tightness is felt in the muscle or muscle group involved. However, the position must not be forced to the extent that it causes pain. Flexibility exercises are designed to relieve pain, not to create it.

Guidelines for performing static stretching exercises

The following guidelines are suggested for the development of flexibility using static stretching exercises:

- Movement should occur slowly through the full range of motion until tightness is felt. The position should then be held for 10 to 30 seconds.
- Care must be taken not to force joints beyond their normal range of motion.
- As you hold the position, you should be able to feel the muscles involved relax. As the muscles relax the position should become easier to hold. If this does not occur it may be an indication that you are forcing your joint to move too far. Reduce the stretch and find a more comfortable position.
- Relaxation must be part of a good stretching program. The more relaxed a muscle is, the less likely it is to be injured during the stretch. To help you relax, breathe slowly and deeply while holding the stretch. As you exhale, try to reach just a little farther and sustain the contraction.
- Exercises that are performed using only one side of the body must be repeated with the other side of the body.
- A minimum of five repetitions should be performed for each exercise.
- Because flexibility is specific to the various joints, exercises must be included for each movement at each joint for which flexibility is to be developed or maintained.
- Exercises need to be alternated in the routine to stretch different muscle groups.
- Correct execution of each exercise is important. Unless movement occurs through the full range of motion, the exercise will be ineffective.
- Flexibility exercises should be included at the beginning and the end of each exercise session.

The contract-relaxation method for development of flexibility

The secret of a good stretching program is to ensure that the muscles involved are completely relaxed. A procedure to increase the ability of muscles to relax is the contract-relaxation method. It is based on the fact that muscles are arranged in pairs and that when one set contracts and shortens, the opposing set lengthens and relaxes.

Guidelines for using the contract-relaxation technique

These guidelines are suggested for development of flexibility using the contract-relaxation method:

- You must first contract the opposite muscle group to the one you are trying to stretch. As this occurs a signal to relax is sent from the central nervous system to the muscle group that you eventually wish to stretch. This contraction should be sustained for at least 5 seconds.
- You then perform a static stretch, with movement occurring slowly through a full range of motion following the same procedures as the static stretch technique. You should find that the muscles involved are more relaxed and that you can move through a greater range of motion.

EXAMPLE OF CONTRACT-RELAXATION TECHNIQUE FOR DEVELOPMENT OF TRUNK FLEXION

For trunk flexion, performance will depend on your ability to stretch hamstring and lower back muscles. Maximum performance will result only if you are able to relax these muscles. To achieve this, you must first contract the opposing muscles—the abdominal and quadriceps muscles. This can probably best be achieved by performing a sit-down exercise against resistance.

Step 1

Contraction of the abdominal and quadriceps muscles using a sit-down exercise against resistance.

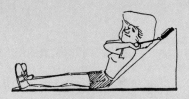 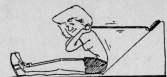

The second step involves performance of the trunk flexion exercise as you try to relax the lower back and hamstring muscles.

Step 2

Performance of trunk flexion with relaxation of lower back and hamstring muscles.

By following these procedures, you should be able to increase your score significantly on the trunk flexion test.

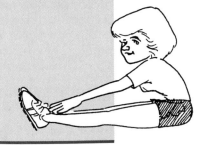

FLEXIBILITY PROGRAM

Regardless of which technique is used for the development of flexibility, it must be recognized that it is a gradual process and, to be successful, exercises must be performed regularly—preferably every day and certainly not less than 3 days per week.

As progress occurs, and if time permits, it may be advantageous to increase the number of repetitions from 5 to 10 and to increase the time that each contraction is held. There is evidence to suggest that maximum development will occur when each contraction is held for 30 seconds. Remember that as you sustain a contraction, it should become easier if you relax the muscles involved.

Flexibility and warm-up

Flexibility and warm-up exercises are not the same and should not be confused. If flexibility exercises are performed before you participate in an exercise program, they should be preceded by warm-up activities. A warm-up is any activity that increases the circulation of the blood and increases the total body temperature, as well as the temperature of the muscles involved in movements to follow.

Activities that are continuous and rhythmic in nature and that involve large muscle groups are ideal for warm-up activities. Care must be taken to perform them by starting at a slow gentle pace and gradually increasing the intensity until your target-zone heart rate is approached. Many activities meet these criteria and can be used. Jogging in place, riding a stationary bicycle, or jumping rope are examples of activities that can be performed slowly and continuously and that involve sufficient musculature to increase your heart rate and muscle temperature.

Stretching exercises are important but should not substitute for the warm-up. The reason is that each stretching exercise is designed to increase the range of motion at a specific joint. They do little to increase the circulation of the blood or to raise the body temperature or temperature of muscles.

Warming up first before performing flexibility exercises will result in the following:
- A greater range of motion at the joint
- Reduced likelihood of injury and soreness
- Maximum increase in the elasticity of the muscle

Flexibility and weight training

It is a common misconception that weight training reduces flexibility and will contribute to a decrease in the range of motion possible at joints. This will not occur in a weight-training program where each exercise is performed correctly through a full range of motion and where exercises for opposing muscle groups are included. A good weight-training program should supplement a good flexibility program. Not only will it increase flexibility, but it will also strengthen the muscles that cause movement at each of the joints. This additional strength should assist in avoiding injury during any activity, but particularly in those such as football, soccer, basketball, and racquetball, which involve contact or sudden vigorous bursts of movement.

EXERCISES FOR DEVELOPMENT OF FLEXIBILITY

The following exercises can be used to develop the range of motion at specific joints.

Sitting hamstring stretch

Start this exercise by sitting on the floor with one leg extended and the sole of the other foot against the thigh of the extended leg (Fig. 5-8). Bend slowly from the waist making sure that you keep your lower back straight, and slide both your hands slowly

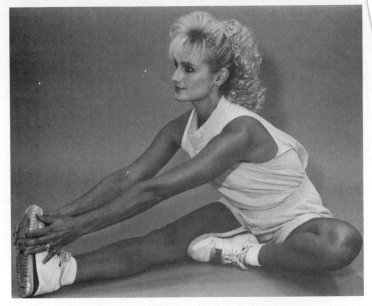

Fig. 5-8 Sitting hamstring stretch.

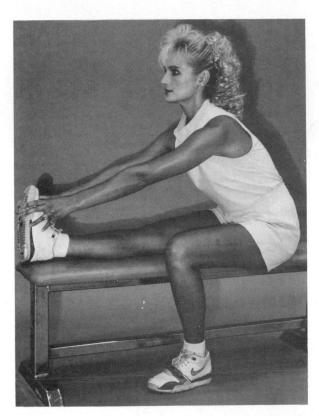

Fig. 5-9 Sitting hamstring stretch performed while sitting on a bench. Care should be taken to make sure your back remains straight.

down the extended leg until you feel tightness in the back of your leg. If you can reach your toes, grasp them and pull them toward you to exert a stretch in the calf and the hamstring muscles. Hold this position. Repeat the movement with the opposite leg. This exercise can also be performed while sitting on a bench (Fig. 5-9 on p. 165).

Lying hamstring stretch

Start this exercise by lying on your back with your left leg bent at the knee and your left foot flat on the floor. Grasp behind the right thigh, and pull your right knee to your chest. Straighten your right leg until you feel tension in the hamstrings. Hold this position (Fig. 5-10).

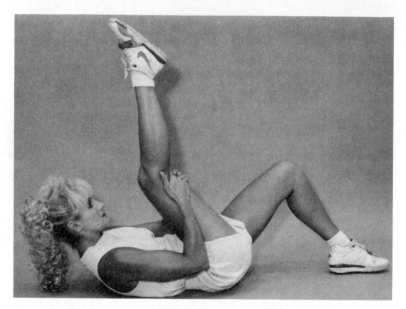

Fig. 5-10 Lying hamstring stretch.

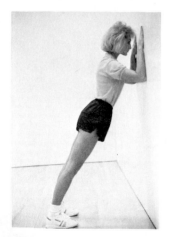

Fig. 5-11 Achilles tendon and calf stretcher.

Achilles tendon and calf stretcher

Stand facing the wall with your feet about 12 inches apart, 2 to 3 feet from the wall (Fig. 5-11). Lean forward and place the palms of your hands flat against the wall. Slowly bend forward, bringing the elbows closer to the wall, making sure that your body and legs remain straight and your heels remain in contact with the floor. Bend forward until you feel tightness in the calf and in the tendons that attach to your heel. Hold this position.

This exercise may also be performed by stretching one leg at a time. If this is preferred, place one foot in front of the other foot, with the front foot approximately 9 inches from the wall, and follow the same procedures as outlined previously. If this stretch is to be effective, the heel of the back foot must remain in contact with the floor (Fig. 5-12).

Low back stretcher

Start the low back stretcher (Fig. 5-13) by lying on your back with your left leg bent at the knee and your left foot flat on the floor. Your right leg should be straight, and your arms should be by your sides. Slowly flex your right leg and, grasping it just below the knee, pull your knee toward your chest. At the same time, tuck your chin in and bring your forehead as close to your knee as possible. Hold this position. This stretch should be felt in the lower back. Care must be taken to keep the flat of your back in contact with the floor at all times. This exercise may also be performed by pulling both knees toward your chest at the same time (Fig. 5-14).

Lateral bend

The lateral bend (Fig. 5-15 on p. 168) is designed to stretch the lateral muscles of the trunk and upper body. Start in the front standing position, with the feet shoulder-width apart and the left arm extended upward and the right arm down with the palm touching the outer right thigh. Bend your trunk to the right by sliding the right hand down the side of the right thigh as far as possible. At the same time, lift the left side of your body toward the ceiling so that the stretch is felt in the left side above your waist. Hold this position.

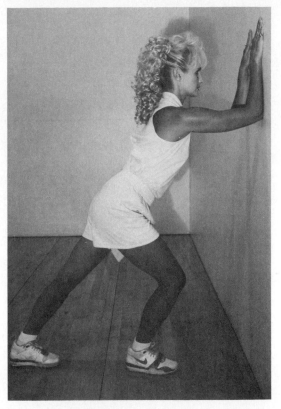

Fig. 5-12 Achilles tendon and calf stretcher. Stretch one leg at a time.

Quadriceps stretch

The quadriceps stretch (Fig. 5-16 on p. 168) is designed to stretch the quadriceps muscle group—the large set of muscles located in the front of the thigh. Start by standing 2 to 3 feet away from a wall, and support yourself by placing your left hand

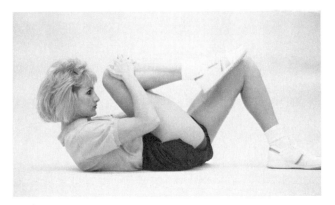

Fig. 5-13 Low back stretcher.

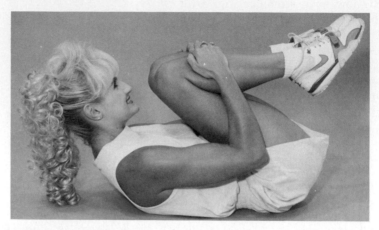

Fig. 5-14 Low back stretcher, pulling both knees toward your chest.

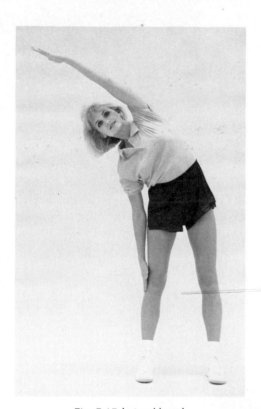

Fig. 5-15 Lateral bend.

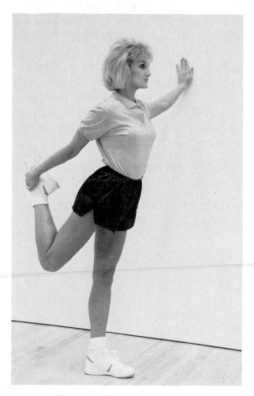

Fig. 5-16 Quadriceps stretch.

against the wall. Supporting your weight on your left foot, flex your right knee, lift it up in front of you, and grasp the front of your right ankle with your right hand. Slowly move your bent right knee downward and backward, and at the same time push your right foot slowly away from your buttocks while resisting this movement with your hand. You should feel tension in your right front thigh. Hold this position.

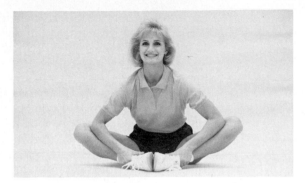

Fig. 5-17 Groin stretch.

Groin stretch

The groin stretch (Fig. 5-17) is designed to stretch the muscles in the inner thighs. Start by sitting on the floor with the knees flexed, with the bottoms of your feet touching each other, and attempt to reach a position in which your heels are no more than 9 inches from your buttocks. Grasp your ankles with both hands, and pull your head and chest forward and downward as you push your knees toward the floor, until the stretch is felt in the upper thigh area. Make sure that you keep your back straight at all times. Hold this position. The elbows may be used to press on the inside of the thighs to add to the stretch.

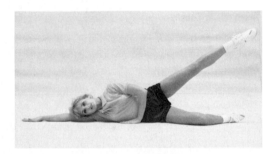

Fig. 5-18 Lateral leg raise.

Lateral leg raises

Lateral leg raises (Fig. 5-18) are designed to contract the lateral hip muscles and stretch the adductor muscles on the medial side of the leg. Start by lying on your right side with your right leg bent slightly at the knee and in contact with the floor. Your left leg should remain straight. Your right arm should be extended above your head and in contact with the floor, and your head should rest comfortably on your right arm. Your left arm should be positioned so that your left hand rests on the floor in front of your chest to maintain balance. Move your left leg upward slowly as far as possible with the leg straight and the knee facing frontward. Your foot should be extended with your toes as far away from the ankle as possible. Hold this position.

Arm circles

Arm circles (Fig. 5-19) increase the flexibility of the shoulder joint. Start this exercise by standing with your feet shoulder-width apart. Let your arm describe a circle from front to back, initiating the movement at the shoulder joint and making sure it moves through a full range of motion. This exercise may be performed with one arm at a time or with both arms at the same time and may be done by moving the arm(s) front to back or back to front. If it is performed with

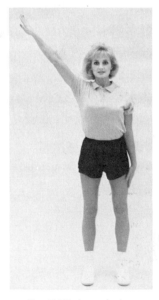

Fig. 5-19 Arm circles.

one arm, the body should give slightly with it; there will be a slight body rotation. If it is performed with both arms together, the circles will come closer to the front of your body, and there will be no body rotation.

Hip circles

Hip circles (Fig. 5-20) develop flexibility of the hip joint. Start this exercise by standing 2 to 3 feet away from a wall, and place your right hand against the wall to maintain balance. Support your weight on the right leg. Bend the left knee comfortably and describe a circle, starting with the thigh in front of the body and moving it through the full range of motion to where it is level with or even slightly behind the hips. This movement may also be performed in the opposite direction.

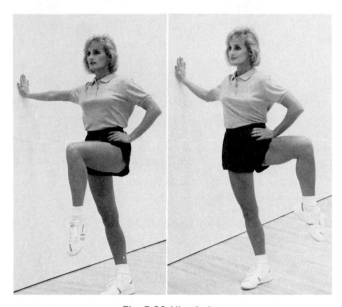

Fig. 5-20 Hip circles.

LOW BACK PAIN

Low back pain is one of the most common complaints among adults in the United States. If you have difficulty in straightening up after sitting all morning, if you feel pain in your back when you bend over to pick something up, or if you have difficulty bending to tie your shoelaces, there is a strong possibility that you are one of the 85 million Americans who suffer from low back pain each year. It is estimated that 80% of us will experience low back pain sometime during our lives.

Low back pain is a hypokinetic disease—one that is caused by lack of activity—and it appears that more than 80% of the low back pain problems are caused by inadequate muscular development. Low back pain occurs most often between the ages of 25 and 50, a time when many people become less active as they spend more time on family and occupational activities.

Causes of low back pain

As previously stated, the major cause of low back pain is inadequate muscular development. Development and maintenance of muscle function depend on its use. The strength of a muscle is directly related to the amount of work it does. As a muscle works against a resistance, the strength of that muscle will increase. If the muscle does not perform work, a loss of strength will result. In an inactive person, many of the large muscle groups are not used often enough. They therefore lack enough strength to maintain correct body alignment, which is one of their specific tasks.

Poor abdominal development is one of the most common causes of low back pain. The pelvis should be tipped up in the front, but if the abdominal muscles are weak, they are unable to exert enough pressure to keep the pelvis in place, and it drops down in the front, causing a forward pelvis tilt. This in turn causes the vertebrae in the low back region to be slightly displaced, and their articular processes press against one another, causing the ache in the lower area of the back.

Another group of muscles associated with low back pain is commonly referred to as the hamstring muscle group. This group consists of three large muscles that are located at the back of the thigh, and all are associated with movement at both the hip and the knee joints.

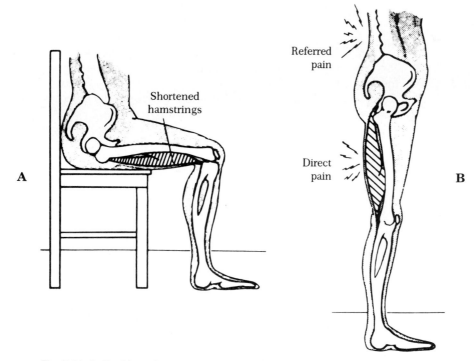

Fig. 5-21 **A,** Position of the hamstring muscle group in relation to the bone structure when sitting. If much of the time is spent sitting, this muscle group may become much shorter than it should be. **B,** Effect that a shortening of the hamstring muscles has on the pelvis when you assume an upright standing position.

The difficulty experienced by most persons in touching their toes with the fingertips without bending the knees is caused by the fact that the hamstring muscles often are not long enough to permit such extreme stretching. This shortening of the hamstring muscle group often occurs in those who spend a lot of time sitting (Fig. 5-21, *A*). If these muscles are not given stretching exercises, and if they are constantly held in positions that tend to shorten them, they become adjusted to this position. When a person stands, both the knee and hip joints are fully extended (Fig. 5-21, *B*). If the hamstring muscles are shorter than they should be, this will cause both direct pain in the immediate area of the muscles and referred pain in the low back region.

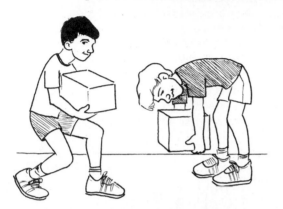

The correct and incorrect way to lift objects.

LOW BACK PAIN AND PERFORMANCE OF EVERYDAY TASKS

If you have already experienced low back pain or if you want to reduce your chances of suffering from it in the future, it may be necessary to change the way you perform everyday activities. How you sit, stand, rest, or sleep can be extremely important. The following suggestions may help:

- When sitting, if possible, have your knees slightly higher than your hips and sit upright rather than with your shoulders forward.
- When sitting at a desk, move the chair in as close as possible so that you are more upright rather than bent over your work.
- When standing, try to keep your knees slightly bent and one foot slightly in front of the other.
- When lifting objects, bend at the knees and hips and make sure the object is as close to your body as possible when both lifting and carrying it.
- At least once a day try to lie flat on the floor or other flat surface with your knees bent at right angles and legs resting on the top of a chair or coffee table.

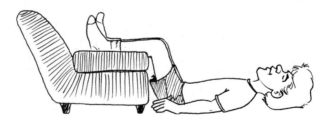

- When sleeping on your back, place a pillow under your knees so that they are raised slightly.

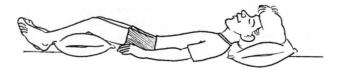

EXERCISES FOR ALLEVIATING LOW BACK PAIN

Most of those who suffer from low back pain can relieve the problem if they perform a few simple exercises each day. These can also be done for prevention of low back pain.

Exercises need to be selected that will place a minimal amount of stress on the lower back and that will strengthen the abdominal muscles and stretch the hamstring muscles. The following six exercises can be used for these purposes. It is suggested that two sets of each be performed each day, starting with 5 repetitions per set and gradually increasing to 10.

Pelvic tilt

Lie on your back on the floor with your knees bent, your feet on the floor, and your arms resting comfortably by your sides (Fig. 5-22). Tighten your stomach muscles, and consciously tilt your pelvis so that your lower back is flat against the floor. Hold this position for a minimum of 10 seconds, then relax.

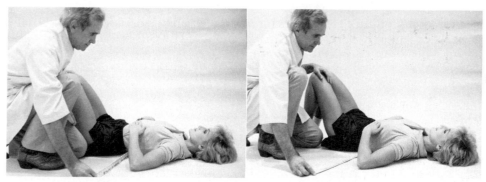

Fig. 5-22 **Pelvic tilt.**

Partial curl-up

Lie on your back with your knees bent at about 90 degrees, with your feet flat on the floor and your arms crossed comfortably across your chest (Fig. 5-23). Slowly curl your head, shoulders, and trunk toward your knees without jerking, until you can feel the contraction of your abdominal muscles. Your lower back should remain in contact with the floor. Hold for a minimum of 10 seconds, and return to the floor.

Partial wall slide

Stand with your back toward a wall and your feet shoulder-width apart, about 3 to 6 inches from the wall (Fig. 5-24 on p. 174). Lean against the wall, and slide your buttocks down slowly until you can feel your lower back flat against it. Hold this position for 10 seconds. (NOTE: For those wishing to develop the quadriceps at the same time, the buttocks should be moved farther down until the thighs are parallel to the floor, and this position should be held.)

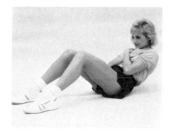

Fig. 5-23 **Partial curl-up.**

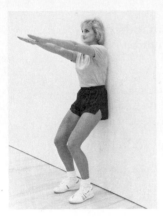

Fig. 5-24 Partial wall slide.

The following three additional exercises can be used for relief or prevention of low back pain:

- Lying hamstring stretch (Fig. 5-10)
- Low back stretcher (Fig. 5-13)
- Sitting hamstring stretch (Fig. 5-9)

MEASUREMENT OF FLEXIBILITY

Because flexibility is specific to each joint, it is not possible to measure it with one test. Each movement possible at a joint must be measured if all aspects of flexibility are to be evaluated (Fig. 5-25).

A number of indirect tests requiring little or no equipment have been developed for classroom use that measure movement at certain joints. The three most common tests are the following:

- Trunk flexion—sit and reach
- Trunk extension
- Shoulder lift

The procedures for these tests are included in Laboratory Experiences 2-1 to 2-3 at the end of this chapter. Norms are also included so that you can evaluate your results.

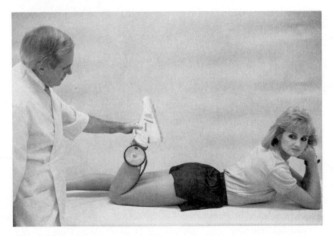

Fig. 5-25 An instrument such as a flexometer can measure joint flexibility.

SUMMARY

The following summary will help you to identify some of the important concepts covered in this chapter.

- Your level of flexibility will be reflected by the range of movement that is possible at each of the joints.
- If you do not exercise and/or you sit for long periods, your flexibility at certain joints is likely to be less than adequate.
- Poor flexibility is often associated with poor posture, muscle soreness, and increased incidence of muscle-related injuries, tension, and pain.

- The two best methods for the development of flexibility appear to be static stretching and the contract-relaxation method. The ballistic method is not recommended.
- Flexibility exercises need to be included in each exercise session, in addition to warm-up activities and your aerobic workout.
- Possibly 80% of the lower back pain problems are directly related to improper muscular development.
- Flexibility exercises are designed to reduce pain and muscle soreness, not to create them.

KEY TERMS

ball-and-socket joint A joint where the rounded head of one bone fits into the hollow cavity of another.

ballistic stretching A series of bouncing and jerking movements, where force generated by the moving segment provides the force necessary to stretch the muscle.

contract-relaxation stretching technique A stretching technique to increase the ability of muscles to relax.

elasticity (muscle) The ability of a muscle to regain its original shape after being stretched.

flexibility The maximum range of motion possible at a joint or joints.

hamstring The large muscle group located at the back of the thigh that crosses both the hip and knee joints.

hinge joint A joint that allows movement to take place in one direction and where the only movements possible are flexion and extension.

joint A junction of two or more bones.

ligament A tough band of tissue that holds bones together.

quadriceps The large muscle group at the front of the thigh responsible for extension at the knee joint.

static stretching Movement of a joint that occurs slowly and gradually through the maximum range of motion.

stretch reflex A mechanism that prevents overstretching of a muscle by forcing the muscle to contract.

tendon Fibrous tissue that connects muscle to bone.

REFERENCES

1. Alter J: *Stretch and strengthen*, Boston, 1986, Houghton Mifflin.
2. Alter J: *Surviving exercise*, Boston, 1983, Houghton Mifflin.
3. Anderson B: *Stretching for everyday fitness*, Bolinas, Calif, 1980, Shelter Publications.
4. Beaulieu JE: Developing a stretching program, *The Physician and Sportsmedicine* 9:59, 1981.
5. Boyer Company: *Care for your back*, 1983, New York, Boyer.
6. Brehm BA: Flexibility: the importance of mind and muscle, *Fitness Management*, p. 16-18, Sept/Oct 1987.
7. Brehm BA: How to warm up and why, *Fitness Management*, p. 18, Nov/Dec 1987.
8. Brehm BA: Stretching, *Fitness Management*, p. 15, Sept/Oct 1987.
9. Brehm BA: The warm-up: its physiological contribution to safe and effective exercise, *Fitness Management*, p. 19-20, Nov/Dec 1987.
11. Corbin CB: *Concepts of physical fitness*, ed 7, Dubuque, Ia, 1991, Wm C Brown.
12. Fox EL, Kirby TE, and Fox AR: *Bases of fitness*, New York, 1987, MacMillan.
13. Greenberg JE, Pargman D: *Physical fitness: a wellness approach*, Englewood Cliffs, NJ, 1987, Prentice Hall.
14. Heywood VH: *Designs for fitness*, Minneapolis, 1984, Burgess.
15. Jampal H: Get flexible, *Shape*, p. 32, May 1983.

16. Johnson PE et al: *Physical education: a problem solving approach to health and fitness,* New York, 1966, Holt, Rinehart & Winston.

17. Kahnert JH: *Excellence in physical fitness,* ed 2, Dubuque, Ia, 1981, Kendall Hunt.

18. Kusinitz I, Fine M: *Your guide to getting fit,* Palo Alto, Calif, 1987, Mayfield.

19. Leighton JR: Instrument and technic for measurement of range of joint motion, *Archives of Physical Medicine and Rehabilitation* 36:571, 1955.

20. Miller DK, Allen TE: *Fitness: a lifetime commitment,* ed 3, Edina, Minn, 1986, Burgess.

21. Nieman DC: *Fitness and sports medicine: an introduction,* Palo Alto, Calif, 1990, Bull.

22. Prentice WE: *Fitness for college and life,* ed 3, St Louis, 1991, Mosby–Year Book.

23. Rosato FD: *Fitness and wellness,* St Paul, 1987, West.

24. Rushing S: *Exercises for people who hate to exercise: exercises for flexibility, muscle tone and relaxation,* San Antonio, Tex, 1982, Rushing Productions.

25. Shellock FG: Physiological benefits of warm-up, *Physician and Sports Medicine* 11(10):134, 1983.

26. Stamford B: Flexibility and stretching, *Physician and Sports Medicine* 12(25):171, 1984.

27. Stamford B: How do muscles work? *The Physician and Sportsmedicine* 14:10, 1986.

28. The First Aider: Stretching to win: basic facts to share with your athletes, Cramer Products, Inc. 57(3):1, Nov/Dec 1987.

29. White AH, Kunse P: Oh my aching back, *Nation's Business,* p. 78, Oct 1983.

Measurement of Flexibility: Trunk Flexion—Sit and Reach Test

Purpose

The purpose of this test is to measure trunk flexion. This will be determined by your ability to stretch the lower back and hamstring muscles.

Equipment

Equipment needed is a flex box with a measuring scale marked in inches or centimeters. (NOTE: A yardstick taped to either the lowest row of bleachers or to a bench turned on its side can be used.)

Procedure

1. Remove your shoes and sit with your knees fully extended and the bottom of your feet flat against the surface of the flex box.
2. Your arms are extended forward, with one hand placed on the top of the other.
3. With the instructor or partner holding your knees straight, steadily reach as far forward as possible and maintain this position for 3 seconds. (NOTE: No bouncing or jerking movements are allowed, and it is important that the knees remain absolutely straight. Slight flexion at the knee joint will greatly influence the results.)

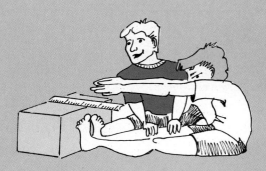

Sit and reach flexibility test.

Scoring

The distance in front of or beyond the edge of the board that can be sustained is measured and recorded. Measurements in front of the board are negative, whereas those beyond are positive. Record your score in the space provided below.
Trunk flexion—sit and reach
_____ inches
(Be sure to indicate + or −.)

Classification of scores

To evaluate your score, refer to Table 5-1.

TABLE 5-1 **Trunk flexion: sit and reach test**

Classification	Percentile rank	Men	Women
Excellent	95	9.5	10.5
	90	8.0	9.0
Good	80	6.5	7.5
	70	5.0	6.0
Average	60	4.0	5.0
	50	3.0	4.0
	40	2.0	3.0
Fair	30	1.0	2.0
	20	−0.5	0.5
Poor	10	−2.0	0.0
	5	−3.5	−2.5

LABORATORY EXPERIENCE 5–2

Measurement of Flexibility: Trunk Extension

Purpose
The purpose of this test is to determine the range of motion when the back is arched from the prone position.

Procedures
1. Lie face down on the floor, with a partner applying pressure on the back of the thighs.

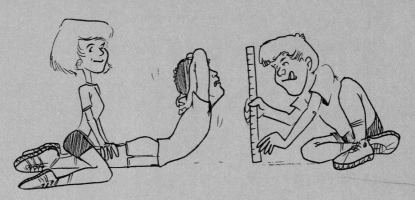

Fig. 5-26 Trunk extension test of flexibility.

2. With fingers interlocked behind your neck, gently raise your head and shoulders as far as possible from the floor.
3. This position must be held for 3 seconds (Fig. 5–26).

Scoring

The distance from the floor to the chin is measured to the nearest $1/2$ inch. Record your score in the space provided below.
Trunk extension _____ inches

Classification of scores

To evaluate your score, refer to Table 5-2.

TABLE 5-2 **Trunk extension flexibility test**

Classification	Percentile rank	Men	Women
Excellent	95	23.5	26.0
	90	22.0	24.0
Good	80	20.0	22.0
	70	19.0	20.5
Average	60	18.0	19.0
	50	17.0	18.0
	40	16.0	17.0
Fair	30	15.0	15.5
	20	14.0	14.0
Poor	10	12.0	12.0
	5	10.5	10.0

LABORATORY EXPERIENCE 5–3 _____

Measurement of Flexibility: Shoulder Lift Test

Purpose

The purpose of this test is to measure flexion at the shoulder joint.

Procedure

1. Lie face down with your chin on the floor and your arms fully extended and parallel.
2. Hold a stick or ruler horizontally with both hands. Keep elbows and wrists straight.
3. Raise your arms upward as far as possible, with your chin remaining in contact with the floor. (NOTE: Make sure your chin remains in contact with the floor and that you do not extend the wrists to increase your score.) (Fig. 5-27 on p. 180.)

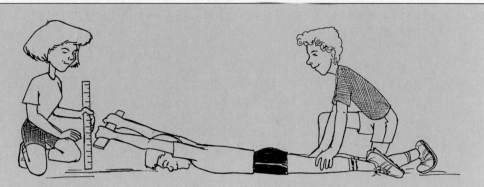

Fig. 5-27 Shoulder life test of flexibility.

Scoring

The distance is measured from the bottom of the stick or ruler to the floor. Record your score in the space provided below.

Shoulder lift _____ inches

Classification of scores

To evaluate your score, refer to Table 5-3.

TABLE 5-3 Shoulder flexion test

Classification	Percentile rank	Men	Women
Excellent	95	28.0	29.0
	90	26.0	27.0
Good	80	24.0	25.0
	70	22.0	23.0
Average	60	21.0	21.5
	50	19.0	20.0
	40	17.0	18.5
Fair	30	16.0	17.0
	20	14.0	15.0
Poor	10	12.0	10.0
	5	10.0	11.0

Nutrition and Fitness

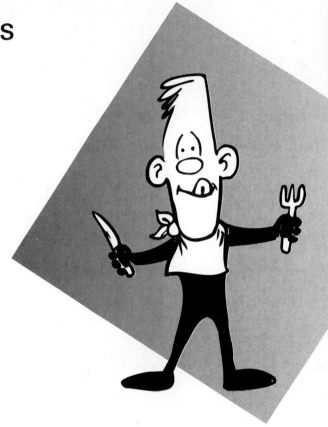

CHAPTER OBJECTIVES

When you understand the material in this chapter, you will be able to:

- Describe what it means to "eat well" and be able to analyze and evaluate your eating habits
- Identify the six major categories of nutrients that you need to be healthy, and know how to plan a nutritionally balanced diet to include appropriate amounts of each of them
- Differentiate between simple and complex carbohydrates, and know how to increase your intake of complex carbohydrates without getting an excessive amount of fat
- Differentiate between complete and incomplete protein, and know how to select foods to ensure an adequate protein intake
- Explain why an excessive amount of fat is more fattening than is the same amount of protein and carbohydrates, and be able to identify foods low in fat
- Analyze your food intake using the exchange lists or other appropriate technique, evaluate your obtained scores, and know how to incorporate necessary changes

"I would like to exercise regularly and eat better, but I just can't get myself to do it." This is a statement that I hear just about every day from students who are usually fighting to control their weight and/or body fat, who seldom find time to exercise, and who have constantly been on one diet or another. Most of these students recognize the importance of regular exercise and good nutrition, but they either do not know what to do or else they lack the motivation to do it.

The average person in today's world is confused and does not really know what constitutes a healthful diet and has a hard time establishing a consistent healthful eating pattern. There are several reasons for this:

In America our nutritional habits have changed during recent years.
- The average American adult eats almost half of his or her meals away from home.
- Only 39% of adults eat the traditional three meals each day.
- Less than 50% of the entire population eat breakfast each day.
- Over 40% of the people who eat out eat at fast-food restaurants.

Skipping meals and eating out make it difficult to be successful at developing good, consistent eating habits.

The large variety of foods now available makes it difficult to make good choices. Although there are many healthful foods available, they are frequently outnumbered by less nutritious foods that are often advertised more frequently and made to look more attractive. Consider the following facts:

On a typical day in the United States:
- The average person will drink more soft drinks than milk. (NOTE: Coca-Cola spends $500,000 per day on advertising.)
- Half of the food consumed each day is processed rather than fresh.
- Almost two thirds of the total calories each day comes from fat and sugar.
- One quarter of the vegetables eaten each day are potatoes, with the majority of these in the form of French fries or potato chips.

Because there are so many different food choices now available, we really do not know which ones are best and we become confused (Fig. 6-1). We often choose foods that are more convenient or those which are advertised most frequently. These are often the foods that are *least* healthful.

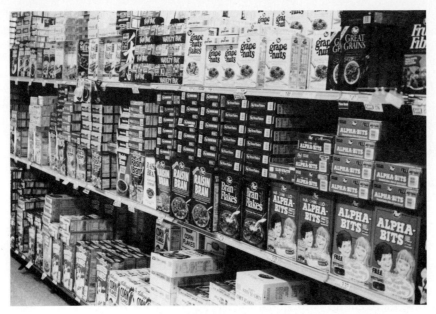

Fig. 6-1 So many breakfast cereals are now available that the average person has a hard time deciding which one is best.

The nutritional information that is available is often confusing and contradictory. Each day we either see on television or we read about different diets, different health foods and supplements, and conflicting research reports. These add to the confusion, and the average person has a hard time knowing what to believe. Even the information on food labels is very confusing. This has forced the Federal Drug Administration to initiate new standards for food labeling. Unfortunately, these will not go into effect until 1993.

Because of the confusion and conflicting information that is available, it is no wonder that in a recent national survey, almost 80% of the American adult population admitted that they need "help" if they are to make a commitment to permanently change their eating habits.

A major problem is that a large percentage of the people fail to realize the importance of everyday decisions that they make. Another problem is that there is so much conflicting information available, most people have a hard time knowing what to believe. By understanding the material in this chapter and the next chapter, you will become more knowledgeable concerning nutrition and exercise and you will understand the role of each of these relative to weight management. In addition to learning what to do, you must be willing to implement changes in your lifestyle. Eleven important guidelines are listed in Chapter 8. These should help you to identify which changes you need to make. A simple self-evaluation is included with these guidelines, so that you can evaluate the consistency of your eating and exercise habits. It will take motivation and dedication if you are to be successful.

EATING WELL

In theory, eating well is not difficult. All you need to do is to eat a sufficient portion of the foods that supply adequate amounts of all the essential nutrients, and learn how you can eat all of these foods without gaining weight or getting fat.

If you eat well, you should not always feel hungry, consistently be lacking in energy, or constantly be craving certain foods. Because no one food contains all the essential nutrients, it is important to eat well-balanced meals consisting of a variety of different foods. You must also learn how to limit the foods that are high in calories and which provide very few of the essential nutrients.

What we eat can significantly affect our health, how we develop and grow, and how efficiently we can perform our everyday tasks. Specifically, by eating well you can:

- Reduce your body weight
- Have less body fat
- Have more energy throughout the day
- Look and feel better
- Lower your cholesterol level
- Reduce your chances of cardiovascular disease, certain types of cancer, and osteoporosis
- Enhance your performance of everyday tasks

NUTRIENTS

A **nutrient** is simply defined as a basic substance that the body uses for a variety of important functions. In more simple terms, it can be defined as anything you eat for which your body has a use. Nutrients are needed by the body for a variety of reasons:

- For normal growth and development of the body
- To supply energy for the performance of everyday tasks
- For resistance to infection and disease
- To regulate the functions of the body's cells

The six major categories of nutrients are as follows:

- Carbohydrates
- Fats
- Proteins
- Vitamins
- Minerals
- Water

Most plants and animals that we use for food, as well as our own bodies, consist primarily of these six nutrients. All nutrients are composed of elements or atoms bonded together by energy. The composition of the six classes of nutrients is shown at the top of p. 185.

Note that all of the nutrients, except minerals, contain hydrogen and oxygen, the elements of which water is made. Four of the nutrients contain carbon and are there-

	Hydrogen	Oxygen	Carbon	Nitrogen
Carbohydrate	X	X	X	
Fat	X	X	X	
Protein	X	X	X	X
Vitamins	X	X	X	
Minerals				X
Water	X	X		

fore classified as **organic.** This means that they can be oxidized, or burned, to produce energy. However, only three of these—carbohydrates, fats, and protein—can be oxidized in the body to yield energy. Vitamins help in the oxidation process, but they do not yield energy for human use.

Unlike minerals, vitamins are organic and can be easily destroyed by heat and light. To maintain the maximum level of vitamins, be careful not to overcook the foods that contain them.

Energy nutrients

The energy derived from foods is measured in kilocalories, or as they are more commonly known, calories. One **calorie** is the amount of heat that is necessary to raise 1 kg of water 1° C. It can be used to express the potential energy of food and the amount of energy used by the body in performing everyday activities.

The energy equivalent of 1 lb of fat is 3500 calories. If a person takes in 3000 calories per day from the food he or she eats and uses only 2500 calories each day, he or she will accumulate 500 excess calories per day. This adds up to 3500 calories per week, which is the equivalent of 1 lb of fat.

Energy can be derived from only three of the nutrients—carbohydrates, fats, and proteins. Vitamins, minerals, and water have no calories. It is also important not to forget one other organic compound—alcohol. Alcohol is not a nutrient because it is not essential to the functioning of the body, but it does contain calories. Alcohol basically contains no nutrients, and the calories obtained from this are often referred to as "empty" calories. Because of this, you must be careful to limit your intake of calories coming from alcohol.

The four sources of calories are compared here. Note that there are approximately 28 g in 1 oz.

Energy equivalents for fats, protein, carbohydrates, and alcohol

Fat	9 calories/g
Protein	4 calories/g
Carbohydrate	4 calories/g
Alcohol	7 calories/g

Practically all foods contain mixtures of fats, proteins, and carbohydrates. If you know how many grams of each is contained in the food you eat, you can determine the numbers of calories.

EXAMPLE:

Following is the nutritional information given by McDonalds Corporation for their McLean Deluxe Hamburger with cheese:

Protein	24 g
Carbohydrates	35 g
Fat	14 g

The energy equivalent is calculated as follows:

Protein	24 g	×	4	=	96 calories
Carbohydrates	35 g	×	4	=	140 calories
Fat	14 g	×	9	=	126 calories
TOTAL CALORIES				=	362 calories

The percentage of calories derived from each of the energy nutrients can now be calculated as follows:

Protein	96/362	=	26%
Carbohydrates	140/362	=	39%
Fat	126/362	=	35%

In any nutritional plan, these percentages are very important. The recommended percentages for each of these nutrients are discussed later in this chapter.

To calculate these percentages for an entire day, you need to record the amounts of each of the foods consumed. The total number of grams for each of these nutrients can then be obtained by consulting a table showing the nutritional content of foods, by getting this information from food labels, or by using the food exchange lists that are explained later in this chapter. The following example should help you to understand how this is done:

EXAMPLE:

Suppose that your caloric consumption for the day was as follows:

Proteins	75 g
Carbohydrates	400 g
Fats	100 g

You must now convert these figures to calories

Proteins	75 g	×	4	=	300 calories
Carbohydrates	400 g	×	4	=	1600 calories
Fats	100 g	×	9	=	900 calories
TOTAL				=	2800 calories

The percentages for each of the nutrients can now be obtained as follows:

Proteins	=	300/2800	= 11%
Carbohydrates	=	1600/2800	= 57%
Fats	=	900/2800	= 32%

Do not forget that if alcohol is consumed, this must be figured into the calculations. Each gram of alcohol contributes 7 calories.

Essential nutrients

Your body is capable of making some of the specific nutrients from others. However, certain nutrients are absolutely indispensable to your body's functioning and cannot be made by your body. These are termed **essential nutrients.** Note that the term "essential" means more than "necessary," because many of the nutrients that the body makes for itself are necessary. For example, cholesterol is necessary for the efficient functioning of the body, but it is not an essential nutrient because sufficient amounts can be manufactured within the body. An essential nutrient is a necessary nutrient that can be obtained only from the food you eat. There are at least 42 nutrients that are considered to be essential. These are as follows:

ESSENTIAL NUTRIENTS _____

Fat—2 essential fatty acids

Linoleic acid
Linolenic acid

Protein—9 essential amino acids

Leucine
Isoleucine
Lysine
Methionine
Phenylalanine
Threonine
Tryptophan
Valine
Histidine

Carbohydrate—2

Glucose
Fiber

Vitamins—13

FAT-SOLUBLE

Vitamin A
Vitamin D
Vitamin E
Vitamin K

WATER-SOLUBLE

Vitamin C (Ascorbic acid)
B Complex
  B1 (Thiamin)
  B2 (Riboflavin)
  Niacin
  B6 (Pyridoxine)
  Pantothenic acid
  Folacin
  B12
  Biotin

Minerals—15

Calcium
Chlorine
Chromium
Cobalt
Copper
Iodide
Iron
Magnesium
Manganese
Phosphorus
Potassium
Sodium
Sulphur
Selenium
Zinc

Water

This might seem like a lot to worry about to ensure that you take in all of these in the appropriate amounts. However, the use of the eating right pyramid and the exchange lists makes it possible to plan a balanced diet from a variety of foods that usually will meet all your nutritional needs.

RECOMMENDED DIETARY ALLOWANCES

If you choose to think in terms of nutrients, it will be necessary to use a standard such as the **Recommended Dietary Allowances** (RDA) to evaluate your nutritional intake. These are determined by a committee funded by the U.S. government. They represent the amounts of essential nutrients that are considered adequate to meet the

TABLE 6-1 Recommended dietary allowances, revised 1989

Category	Age (years) or condition	Weight (kg)	Weight (lb)	Height (cm)	Height (in)	Protein (g)	A (μg RE)*	D (μg)†	E (mg a-TE)‡	K (μg)
							Fat-soluble vitamins			
Males	15-18	66	145	176	69	53	1000	10	10	65
	19-24	72	160	177	70	58	1000	10	10	70
	25-50	79	174	176	70	63	1000	5	10	80
	51 +	77	170	173	68	62	1000	5	10	80
Females	15-18	55	120	163	64	44	800	10	8	55
	19-24	58	128	164	65	46	800	10	8	60
	25-50	63	138	163	64	50	800	5	8	65
	51 +	65	143	160	63	52	800	5	8	65
Pregnant						60	800	10	10	65
Lactating	1st 6 months					65	1300	10	12	65
	2nd 6 months					62	1200	10	11	65

C (mg)	Thiamin (mg)	Riboflavin (mg)	Niacin (mg NE)§	B6 (mg)	Folate (μg)	B12 (μg)	Calcium (mg)	Phosphorus (mg)	Magnesium (mg)	Iron (mg)	Zinc (mg)	Iodine (μg)	Selenium (μg)
	Water-soluble vitamins						**Minerals**						
60	1.5	1.8	20	2.0	200	2.0	1200	1200	400	12	15	150	50
60	1.5	1.7	19	2.0	200	2.0	1200	1200	350	10	15	150	70
60	1.5	1.7	19	2.0	200	2.0	800	800	350	10	15	150	70
60	1.2	1.4	15	2.0	200	2.0	800	800	350	10	15	150	70
60	1.1	1.3	15	1.5	180	2.0	1200	1200	300	15	12	150	50
60	1.1	1.3	15	1.6	180	2.0	1200	1200	280	15	12	150	55
60	1.1	1.3	15	1.6	180	2.0	800	800	280	15	12	150	55
60	1.0	1.2	13	1.6	180	2.0	800	800	280	10	12	150	55
70	1.5	1.6	17	2.2	400	2.2	1200	1200	320	30	15	175	65
95	1.6	1.8	20	2.1	280	2.6	1200	1200	355	15	19	200	75
90	1.6	1.7	20	2.1	260	2.6	1200	1200	340	15	16	200	75

From Recommended Dietary Allowances, 10th Edition, 1989, National Academy of Sciences, Washington, DC, National Academy Press.

The allowances, expressed as average daily intakes over time, are intended to provide for individual variations among most normal persons as they live in the United States under usual environmental stresses. Diets should be based on a variety of common foods to provide other nutrients for which human requirements have been less well defined. Weights and heights of reference adults are actual medians for the U.S. population of the designated age, as reported by NHANES II. The use of these figures does not imply that the height-to-weight ratios are ideal.

*Retinol equivalents 1 retinol equivalent-1 μg ß-carotene.

†As cholecalciferol. 10 μg cholecalciferol 5400 ru of vitamin D.

‡a-Tocopherol equivalents, 1 mg d-a tocopherol = 1 a-TE.

§1 NE (niacin equivalent) is equal to 1 mg of niacin or 60 mg of dietary tryptophan.

known nutritional needs of most healthy persons in the United States. It should be noted that they are recommendations, not requirements and certainly not minimal requirements. They are based on the concept that there is a range within which most healthy persons' intake of nutrients probably should fall. Different people have different requirements, and because of this, these recommended allowances are set at a reasonably high point so that the majority of the population would be covered. It is probably wise to aim at getting 100% or more for each nutrient. The RDAs for each of the essential nutrients are listed in Tables 6-1 to 6-3.

In addition to an RDA for each of the essential nutrients, there is also a recommendation for total caloric intake. In setting this recommendation, the committee took a different approach. In establishing the RDA for the nutrients, it was agreed that it would be sensible to set generous allowances so that a little extra would provide insurance against deficiencies. However, with total caloric intake, extra calories will eventually lead to obesity or overweight. Thus the RDA for caloric intake was set at the mean, not at the upper end of the curve as it was for the individual nutrients. The Recommended Energy Intakes for males and females is presented in Table 6-4.

It should be noted that these are the recommendations for healthy individuals who are trying to *maintain* their body weight. Those trying to lose weight will need to take in considerably fewer calories. Males require more calories than do females

TABLE 6-2 Estimated safe and adequate daily dietary intakes of selected vitamins and minerals for adults*

Vitamins		Trace elements†				
Biotin (µg)	Pantothenic acid (mg)	Copper (mg)	Manganese (mg)	Flouride (mg)	Chromium (mg)	Molybdenum (mg)
30-100	4-7	1.5-3.0	2.0-5.0	1.5-4.0	50-200	75-250

*Because there is less information on which to base allowances, these figures are not given in the main table of RDA and are provided here in the form of ranges of recommended intakes.
†Since the toxic levels for many trace elements may be only several times the usual intakes, the upper levels for the trace elements given in this table should not be habitually exceeded.

TABLE 6-3 Estimated sodium, chloride, and potassium minimum requirements of healthy persons

Age	Weight (kg)*	Sodium (mg)*,†	Chloride (mg)*,†	Potassium (mg)‡
10-18	50	500	750	2000
>18§	70	500	750	2000

*No allowance has been included for large, prolonged losses from the skin through sweat.
†There is no evidence that higher intakes confer any health benefit.
‡Desirable intakes of potassium may considerably exceed these values (~3500 mg for adults).
§No allowance included for growth. Values for those below 18 years assume a growth rate at the 50th percentile reported by the National Center for Health Statistics and averaged for males and females.

TABLE 6-4 **Recommended daily energy intake**

Age (years)	Men Recommendation (calories)	Men Range (calories)	Women Recommendation (calories)	Women Range (calories)
11-14	2700	2000-3700	2200	1500-3000
15-18	2800	3100-3900	2100	1200-3000
19-22	2900	2500-3300	2100	1700-2500
23-50	2700	2300-3100	1800	1400-2200
51-75	2400	2000-2800	1600	1200-2000
>75	2050	1050-2450	1600	1200-2000

each day, simply because the average male weighs more than does the average female. Your body weight significantly affects how many calories you will use each day in performing your everyday tasks (see Chapter 7).

How many calories you *use* each day will obviously determine the number of calories you can consume if you are trying to maintain your body weight. Note that for a 20-year-old male, the recommendation is 2900 calories per day. For a 20-year-old female it is 2100 calories per day.

CARBOHYDRATES

As the name implies, carbohydrates are simply compounds composed of carbon, hydrogen, and oxygen. The most basic form is glucose, which is produced by green leafy plants through a complex process known as photosynthesis. Carbohydrates have traditionally been categorized in two groups—simple and complex. However, this classification is misleading. A further breakdown is presented in Fig. 6-2. Note that the simple carbohydrates are often referred to as "sugars," and the complex carbohydrates are referred to as "starches" and "fiber."

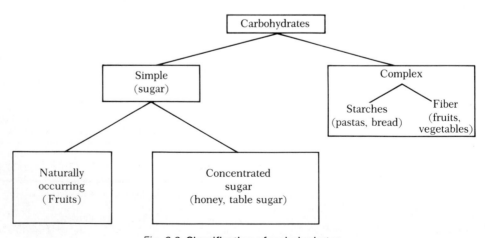

Fig. 6-2 Classification of carbohydrates.

Simple sugars

With the **simple sugars** it is important to distinguish between those that occur naturally in fruits and those which are classified as concentrated sugar. This further classification of the simple sugars is very important. The naturally occurring simple carbohydrates in fruits usually come packaged with vitamins, minerals, and possible fiber. The concentrated sugar that is in cakes and cookies is often referred to as "empty calories" and is of limited nutritional value. It is also important to note that sugar has been added to many other products. Canned fruits and vegetables, soft drinks, and many breakfast cereals contain large amounts of simple sugar. The following comparison of nutritional information for two different breakfast cereals will clearly show this.

TOTAL RAISIN BRAN		NABISCO SHREDDED WHEAT	
Serving Size—1 oz		Serving Size—1 oz	
Calories—86		Calories—90	
Carbohydrates	22 g	Carbohydrates	23 g
Fiber	3 g	Fiber	3 g
Simple sugar	10 g	Simple sugar	0 g
Complex carbohydrates	9 g	Complex carbohydrates	20 g

NOTE: There are 10 g of simple sugar in Total Raisin Bran, whereas Nabisco Shredded Wheat does not contain any. Of the 23 g of carbohydrates in Nabisco Shredded Wheat, 20 come from complex carbohydrates. Clearly from a nutritional standpoint, Nabisco Shredded Wheat is the better choice.

Table 6-5 shows the sugar content of selected foods. The equivalent teaspoon measurement of sugar is given for each of the foods listed. Each teaspoon of sugar is equivalent to 5 g of carbohydrates and is approximately equal to 20 calories.

Despite the widespread use of artificial sweeteners, the consumption of simple refined sugar has continued to rise. In 1992 the average American consumed 148 lb of simple refined sugar as compared with 124 lb in 1975. Simple refined sugars now contribute approximately 19% of the total calories consumed by the average person. Because sugar is of little nutritional value, this means that he or she must rely on 81% of the total calories consumed to provide 100% of the essential nutrients needed each day.

The recommendation is that we get no more than 10% of our calories from simple refined sugar. For a person eating 2000 calories per day this would mean that he or she should get no more than 200 calories from simple refined sugar. This is the equivalent to approximately 10 tsp of sugar per day. The average American presently consumes approximately 36 tsp of sugar per day.

Extra sugar also means that we get extra calories. For example, for a person eating 2000 calories per day with 19% of these calories from simple refined sugar, he or she will be getting 180 extra calories per day from sugar, compared with a person who limits his or her intake of sugar to 10%. If this occurs each day, over a period of 1 year this is the equivalent of approximately 18 lb of fat, which this person is likely to accumulate as a result of this "extra" sugar intake.

TABLE 6-5 Sugar content for selected foods

Food	Portion size	Teaspoons of added sugar
Beverages		
Wine	3.5 oz	3.0
Gatorade	8 oz	3.5
Lemonade (Country Time)	8 oz	6.0
Tonic Water	8 oz	8.4
Sprite	12 oz	9.0
Most other soda	12 oz	8.0
Dairy products		
Ice cream—vanilla	1 cup	6.0
Lowfat yogurt (Dannon)	1 cup	6.0
Sherbet ice cream	1 cup	11.0
Yogurt—fruit flavored	1 cup	8.0
Chocolate milkshake	1 cup	6.0
Hot-fudge sundae	1 dish	16.0
Cakes, pies, desserts, snacks		
Apple pie	1 slice (6 oz)	6.5
Strawberry shortcake	1 serving	12.0
Popsicle	1	4.5
Cupcake (with icing)	1 (2½″ diam.)	3.2
Twinkies	2	9.6
Chocolate cake	1 piece (2.3 oz)	5.3
Cookies and doughnuts		
Doughnut—plain	1 large	3.0
Doughnut—glazed	1 large	6.0
Brownie	1 (2 oz)	4.6
Sugar cookie	1 (2 oz)	6.0
Candy		
M&M Peanuts	14	3.0
Milk chocolate with almonds	1 oz	3.2
Peanut butter cup	1	4.8
Breads/grains		
Hot dog bun	1	3.0
Hamburger bun	1	3.0
Bread—white	1 slice	2.5
Cinnamon bun	1 medium	10.5
Breakfast cereals		
Sugar Frosted Flakes	1 oz	2.8
Fruitful Bran—Kelloggs	1 oz	1.8
Fruit & Fiber—Post	1 oz	1.6
Grape Nuts—Post	1 oz	.6
Raisin Bran—Total	1 oz	2.0
Fruit Loops	1 oz	3.3

Modified from *How Sweet Is It?* Center for Science in Public Interest, Washington, DC, 1985, and *Hidden Sugar In Familiar Foods*, Texas Agricultural Extension Services, College Station, Tex, 1985.

TABLE 6-6 Wendy's baked potato with toppings

Item	Calories	Fat (g)	Percent of calories from fat
Baked potato with sour cream and chives	460	24	47
Baked potato with cheese	590	34	52
Baked potato with chili and cheese	510	20	35
Baked potato with bacon and cheese	570	30	47
Baked potato with broccoli and cheese	500	25	45

Starches

Starches are made of long chains of glucose molecules that are linked together. They are found in the following:

Grain products	Starchy vegetables
Rice	Corn
Pasta	Potatoes
Bread	Peas
Cereals	Beans

Other vegetables and fruits contain lesser amounts of complex carbohydrates.

Many people mistakenly think that carbohydrates are fattening. The reason that they think this is that they frequently combine carbohydrates with large amounts of fat. For example, we often add whole milk to breakfast cereal; add large amounts of butter to foods such as bread, baked potatoes, and corn; and add rich, high-fat sauces or dressings to pasta. When this happens, you frequently finish up getting more calories from the fat than you get from the carbohydrates. For example, a large baked potato usually contains approximately 200 calories, with almost all of these calories coming from carbohydrates. Toppings such as butter, margarine, cheese, and chili can often increase the caloric value to 500 or 600 calories. Table 6-6 contains information pertaining to some of the baked potatoes available at one of the leading fast-food restaurants:

The secret to eating well is to learn how to eat lots of complex carbohydrates without adding large amounts of fat.

Fiber

The term **fiber** is used by most people as if it represented a single entity. Actually there are many compounds, mostly carbohydrates, that make up fiber. Fiber is defined as any part of a food plant that cannot be broken down and digested by the human body. It includes the parts that give the plant shape, structure, and strength. It has been referred to as "roughage" or "bulk." Fiber is contained in vegetables, fruits, legumes, grains, and seeds. There are two different types of fiber—insoluble and soluble.

Insoluble fiber. This type of fiber does not dissolve in water. It is the fiber that gives plants their firm structure. It is found in the cell walls of many grains, vegetables, and fruits. Insoluble fiber helps to prevent constipation, hemorrhoids, and diverticulosis and may also help to prevent certain types of cancer.

Soluble fiber. This is the second type of fiber. It is soluble in water and forms a gel from the water that it absorbs. It is the nonstructural materials in plant cells such as pectins and gums. It is found in oats, barley, kidney beans, and most vegetables. Soluble fiber has been shown to lower cholesterol levels in some people and can be used by diabetics to help stabilize their blood glucose levels. Foods that contain soluble fiber are also more likely to satisfy your appetite. When fiber combines with water it swells and expands, creating a feeling of fullness.

How much fiber should you eat? The average fiber intake in the United States is 15 g per day. This is much less than what you need. Although there is no RDA value for fiber, the American Dietetic Association recommends that we increase our fiber intake to 25 to 35 g per day to ensure the maximum health benefits. Many well-known nutritionists are suggesting that you need 30 to 40 g or more each day.

A listing of the fiber content for selected foods is included in Laboratory Experience 6-1. You can evaluate your fiber intake and determine whether it is adequate.

Getting more fiber in your diet. Following are some suggestions for getting more fiber in your diet:

- Eat more fruits, vegetables, and grain products.
- Increase your consumption slowly—digestive discomfort can be reduced if fiber is added gradually.
- Because of the different types of fiber and their different functions, make sure that you get your fiber from a variety of different sources.
- The peelings of fruits and vegetables are often high in fiber. Try to eat these as often as possible.
- If you increase your fiber intake, be sure to increase your intake of water. Fiber removes water from your body.
- If your fiber intake is consistently low, you may want to include a high-fiber cereal with your breakfast. The following breakfast cereals have 7 or more grams of fiber:

Cereal	Serving size (oz)	Dietary fiber (g)
Kellogg's All Bran with extra fiber	1	14
General Mills Fiber One	1	13
Kellogg's All Bran	1	10
Nabisco 100% Bran with oat bran	1	8
U.S. Mills Uncle Sams	1	7

NOTE: Kellogg's All Bran and Fiber One have the most fiber. If you do not like the taste of these, you may want to try mixing ¼ cup of one of these with 1 cup of your regular cereal. This will still increase your fiber intake considerably.

Foods high in fiber are usually good for those trying to control their weight. They are foods that are typically low in fat; they generally take longer to chew, therefore slowing down your food intake; and they often promote a feeling of fullness.

Functions of carbohydrates

Carbohydrates perform a number of important functions in the body:

- They are the primary source of energy for the body, because they can provide energy more efficiently than do the other energy nutrients.
- Glucose is the simplest form of carbohydrates. The body must maintain a normal level of glucose in the blood, because the brain and central nervous system constantly require glucose.
- An adequate intake of carbohydrates is necessary for the complete metabolism of fat.
- Carbohydrates are stored in the body in the muscles and the liver in the form of glycogen. An adequate intake of carbohydrates is necessary if these stores are to be replenished. The more glycogen you have stored, the more you will have available as fuel for the body. This is particularly important for those who participate regularly in endurance-type activities such as jogging, running, cycling, and swimming.

Carbohydrate intake: How much do you need?

It is apparent that Americans need to change their eating habits in relation to their carbohydrate intake. A comparison of the current habits and the recommended values is shown in Fig. 6-3.

The material presented in this section indicates that we need to double our intake of complex carbohydrates, reduce our intake of simple refined sugar by almost 50%, and significantly increase our fiber intake.

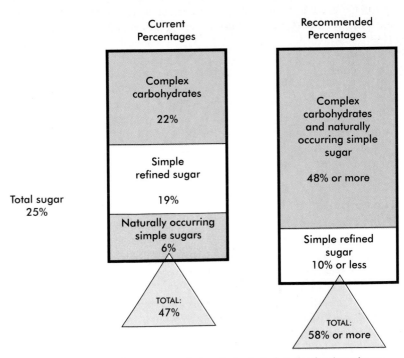

Fig. 6-3 Actual and recommended carbohydrate intakes for Americans.

FATS

Fats (often referred to as lipids or oils) are a secondary source of energy and currently make up approximately 37% of the calories consumed in the average American diet. They appear in a variety of ways in various foods. They may appear as visible fats and oils in the form of butter or oil; they may also occur in the form of fat attached to a steak, ham, or bacon. They may also be less obvious in food such as nuts, cheese, and avocados.

In recent years, fats have fallen into disrepute. The federal government, the American Heart Association, the American Cancer Society, and the National Academy of Sciences are all urging us *to eat less fat*. There are several reasons for this recommendation:

- Each gram of fat provides you with more than twice as many calories as each gram of carbohydrate or protein.
- Excess fat is easily stored in the body, whereas excess proteins and carbohydrates must be converted to fat to be stored. For this reason, excess calories from protein and carbohydrates will affect your metabolism differently from excess calories obtained from fat. It has been shown that the "metabolic cost" associated with 100 excess calories of fat is only 3%; thus 97% of these calories will be stored as fat. With 100 excess calories of carbohydrates, the "metabolic cost" is 23%, and only 77% of these calories will be stored as fat.
- Excess calories from fat can be used as energy or else stored as fat. These are the only options. However, we have seen that excess calories from carbohydrates can be stored as glycogen in the body and can be used to replace the glucose in the blood that constantly must be replenished. Only after the body has made these adjustments will the excess carbohydrates be stored as fat. Fat calories are thus more fattening.
- Dietary fat is thought to be a contributing factor in the development of certain diseases, including cardiovascular disease, diabetes, and certain forms of cancer.

Functions of fats

It should be stressed that fat is an important dietary component and that the problems associated with dietary fats are related to excessive fat intake. In addition to providing energy, fat enhances the flavor of food, and—because it takes twice as long to digest—fat makes a meal seem more filling. Fat also contains two fatty acids that are essential, and it provides transportation for certain fat-soluble vitamins. Moderate deposits of fat serve as support and protection for several of the vital organs and aid in the regulation of body temperature. However, excessive fat deposits create serious health problems.

Saturated and unsaturated fat

Fats contained in food are primarily in the form of triglycerides. Triglycerides are made up of a simple three-carbon alcohol—glycerol—which serves as a backbone to which three fatty acids attach. This is demonstrated in Fig. 6-4.

A fatty acid is basically a chain of carbon atoms linked to hydrogen atoms. If the hydrogen atoms fill each available spot on the chain, then the fatty acid is said to be **saturated.** An **unsaturated** fatty acid contains two or more "empty" spots on the carbon chain. This concept is illustrated in Fig. 6-5.

Each food that contains fat basically has a certain amount of saturated and unsaturated fat. The saturated and unsaturated fat content for select foods is presented in Table 6-7. By dividing the saturated-fat grams by the total-fat grams, the percentage of saturated fat in a particular food can easily be determined. For example, with olive oil,

1.9 of the 14 g of fat come from saturated fat. This represents 14% of the total fat.

In general, fats found in animal foods tend to be high in saturated fat, whereas those found in plant foods tend to be low in saturated fat. Exceptions are the tropical oils—palm oil and coconut oil—which are predominantly saturated. It should be noted that all fats, whether they contain mainly saturated or unsaturated fat, provide the same number of calories—9 calories per gram.

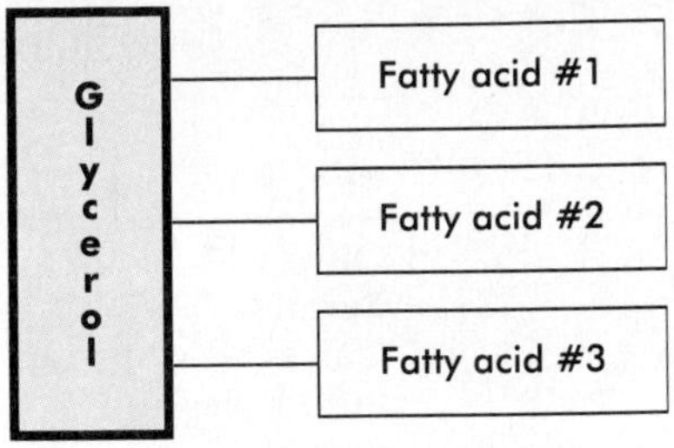

From a health standpoint, it is good to reduce your intake of saturated fat. It is now well established that increased levels of saturated fats in your diet will increase your blood cholesterol level, which increases the incidence of atherosclerosis, and this increases your risk of other cardiovascular diseases. There is also some evidence that polyunsaturated fats may lower your blood cholesterol level. Information relating to this is presented in Chapter 10.

Classification of some of the common sources of fat, according to whether they are predominantly saturated or unsaturated, is presented in the box on p. 198.

Fig. 6-4 **The structure of a triglyceride.**

Essential fatty acids

There are two polyunsaturated fatty acids that the body cannot produce that perform important functions in the body and that therefore are considered as essential. These are **linoleic acid** and **linolenic acid.** These fatty acids play an important role in the immune system, they help form cell membranes, and they aid in the production of certain hormones. In addition, linolenic acid has been shown to play an important role in reducing the incidence of certain forms of cardiovascular disease.

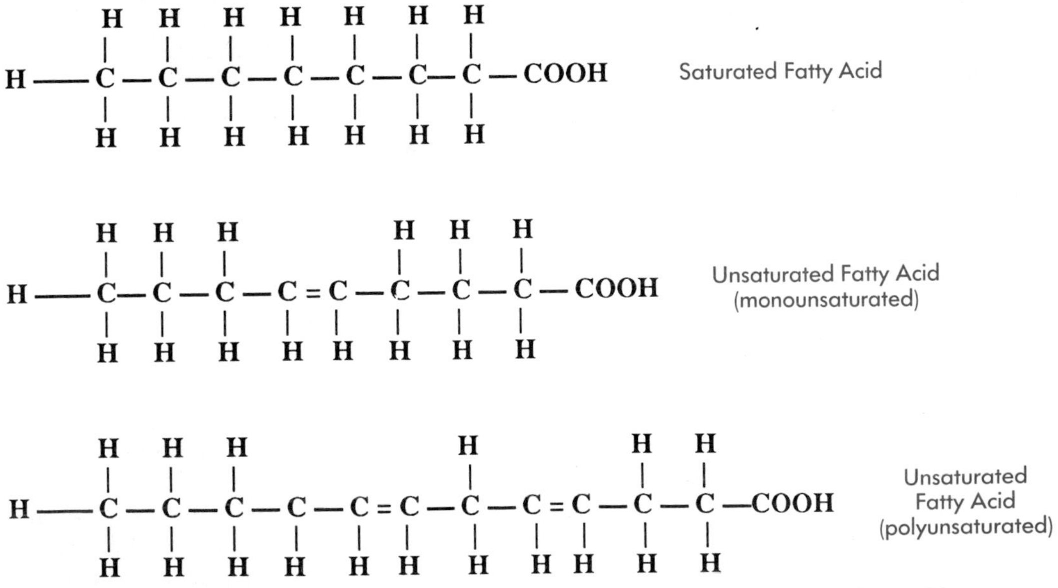

Fig. 6-5 **An example of the differences between saturated and unsaturated fatty acids.**

TABLE 6-7 Saturated fat and unsaturated fat in select foods

Food	Serving size	Calories	Total fat (g)	Saturated fat (g)	Saturated fat (%)
Olive oil	1 tbsp	125	14.0	1.9	14
Peanuts	3 oz	495	42.0	5.7	14
Chicken—white meat	3.5 oz	133	4.5	1.4	30
Sirloin steak	3.5 oz	280	17.5	7.4	42
Butter	1 tbsp	100	11.0	7.0	65

CLASSIFICATION OF SOME COMMON SOURCES OF FAT

SATURATED	MONOUNSATURATED	POLYUNSATURATED
Beef	Almonds	Corn oil
Butter	Avocadoes	Cottonseed oil
Cheese	Olives	Mayonnaise
Chocolate	Olive oil	Safflower oil
Coconut	Peanuts	Soybeans
Coconut oil	Peanut butter	Soybean oil
Cream	Peanut oil	Sunflower oil
Ice cream		Vegetable oil
Lamb		
Milk		
Palm oil		
Veal		

Linoleic acid is readily available in large quantities in nearly all the vegetable oils. Most of us can get all the linoleic acid we need each day in 1 to 2 tsp of practically any vegetable oil.

Linolenic acid, however, is much less readily available. It occurs in significant amounts only in canola oil and soybean oil. If these oils are not consumed regularly, a related form of this can be obtained in large quantities in most of the fatty cold-water fish such as salmon and tuna and in smaller quantities in most other fish. Because of the relationship of this fatty acid to cardiovascular disease, the American Heart Association recommends that we eat at least two servings of fish each week.

Recommendations for fat intake

The actual and recommended fat intakes for Americans are presented in Fig. 6-6. The average American now gets approximately 37% of his or her calories from fat, compared with 42% in 1988. However, this figure is still considerably higher than the recommended 30%.

The recommended percentage is now much easier to achieve than it was several years ago, because there are now so many fat-free products available. We now have fat-free salad dressings, ice cream, yogurt, cheese, tortilla chips, cookies, and so on. In addition, many of the other products are much lower in fat than they were several years ago. For example, Healthy Choice now has a very lean ground beef that has less fat than does chicken (4 g of fat per 4 oz). Also, the fat content of most cuts of pork in 1992 is now 35% less than it was in 1985.

Fat Intake

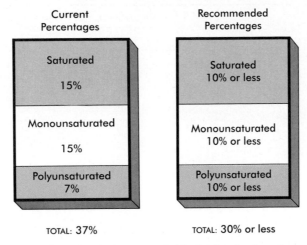

Fig. 6-6 Actual and recommended fat intakes for Americans.

There are many successful weight-loss programs that no longer focus on total calories consumed, but instead concentrate on the number of fat grams consumed. Certainly there is a growing body of research to support this concept.

If you are overweight and have fat to lose, you will probably be more successful in losing this weight and fat if you try to lower your total fat intake to 20% or less, rather than the recommended 30%. Table 6-8 contains information that will help you determine how much fat you should be eating. Table 6-8 shows the grams of fat you can eat each day for a wide range of calories, where 20%, 25%, and 30% of these calories are obtained from fat.

Fat content of foods

Most people are confused when it comes to reading labels, particularly information pertaining to fat. One of the problems is that many labels contain numbers or percentages with little or no explanation as to what these numbers represent. Consider the following three examples:

Extra-lean ham—96% fat-free
Milk—2% fat
Extra-lean ground beef—16% fat

The average person would assume that the ham contain 4% fat, the milk 2%, and the extra-lean ground beef 16%. You will see that this is not so if you are considering calories

Figures such as these, which usually appear in large print on the labels, in most cases refer to the *fat content by weight*. For example, with the extra-lean ham the serving size is 1 oz (28 g), and only 1 of the 28 g comes from fat. This means that ¹/₂₈, or 4%, of the product by weight comes from fat; hence the term 96% fat-free.

TABLE 6-8 Desired caloric intake: fat grams

Daily caloric intake (calories)	Fat grams for selected percentages of calories from fat		
	20%	25%	30%
1200	27	33	40
1300	29	36	43
1400	31	39	47
1500	33	42	50
1600	36	44	53
1700	38	47	57
1800	40	50	60
1900	42	53	63
2000	44	56	67
2100	47	58	70
2200	49	61	73
2300	51	64	77
2400	53	67	80
2500	56	69	83
2600	58	72	87
2700	60	75	90
2800	62	78	93
2900	64	81	97
3000	67	83	100

Example:

If you are trying to limit your caloric intake for the day to 2000 and you are trying to limit your fat intake to 25% of these calories, then you can see that you can consume 56 g of fat for the day.

You need to be more concerned with the percentage of calories in food that comes from fat. To determine this, you need to look at the nutritional information for the product—usually given in small print—and figure this out as follows:

1. Each gram of fat contains 9 calories, so you need to multiply the number of grams of fat by 9 to determine the number of calories coming from fat.
2. Divide this number by the total number of calories from the food to determine the percentage of the calories from fat.

The calculations for the three food items listed previously are as follows:

Extra-lean ham

   Serving size—1 oz
   Calories—30
   Fat—1 g
   Protein—5 g
   Calories from fat $= 1 \times 9$
                                             $= 9$
                                             $= 9/30$
   Percentage of calories from fat $= 30\%$

2% milk
     Serving size—1 cup
     Calories—121
     Protein—8 g
     Fat—5 g
     Carbohydrates—12 g
Calories from fat   = 5 × 9
                              = 45
                              = 45/121
Percentage of calories from fat = 37%

Ground beef—extra-lean—16% fat
     Serving size—3 oz
     Calories—225
     Protein—24 g
     Fat—13 g
     Carbohydrates—0 g
Calories from fat   = 13 × 9
                      = 117
                      = 117/225
Percentage of calories from fat = 52%

Note that these figures are much higher than the figures listed on the label referring to fat by weight. The following box will help you to evaluate foods according to the percentage of their calories coming from fat.

THE PERCENTAGE OF FAT CALORIES FOR COMMON FOODS

>90%	Bacon, butter, cooking oils, margarine, mayonnaise, salad oils, sour cream, tartar sauce, vegetable shortening
80%-89%	Avocadoes, bologna, frankfurters, olives
60%-79%	Beef, ham, cheese, enchiladas, nuts, peanut butter, pork, potato chips, salami, veal
40%-59%	Beef (lean), brownies, bread stuffing, chicken (fried), cookies, corn chips, croissants, doughnuts (cake), fish (fried), French fried potatoes, ice cream, milk (whole), popcorn (with oil), potato salad, scallops (breaded)
20%-39%	Bran muffins, cakes, dinner rolls, cereal (granola), ground beef (extra-lean), ham (lean), lamb (lean—roasted), pancakes (made from mix), tuna (oil packed), waffles (made from mix), yogurt (low-fat)
<20%	Bagels, baked potatoes, breakfast cereal (except granola), chicken (broiled or baked), crackers (low-fat), fish (broiled or baked), fruits, legumes, lentils, muffins (English), pasta, popcorn (air popped), tortillas, tuna (water packed), vegetables

Reducing your fat intake

A large percentage of people fail to realize how much fat they eat. They are constantly making poor choices. The Case Study below will emphasize this point.

CASE STUDY: JOHN AND JOE

John and Joe are both overweight and trying to lose fat. They often go out to eat lunch together. John has learned the importance of reducing the amount of fat that he eats and has become knowledgeable concerning the foods that are high in fat. A typical lunch for John is as follows:

ITEM	SERVING SIZE	CALORIES
Wholewheat bread	2 slices	130
Chicken—white meat, no skin	3 oz	120
Mustard	1 tbsp	0
Lettuce	2 slices	5
Tomato	2 slices	10
Cantaloupe	1/4 small	50
Strawberries	1/2 cup	20
TOTAL CALORIES		335

NUTRITIONAL ANALYSIS	GRAMS	PERCENT OF TOTAL CALORIES
Protein	34	41
Carbohydrate	36	43
Fat	6	16

The nutritional analysis shows that this is a good lunch, providing only 335 calories with less than 20% of these calories coming from fat.

Joe, on the other hand, is not as knowledgeable concerning calories and fat, but he thinks he is also eating well. He makes just three changes in the way he orders his sandwich. He substitutes mayonnaise for mustard and adds two small strips of bacon and $1\frac{1}{2}$ oz of cheddar cheese to the above sandwich.

Following is a summary of the nutritional analysis of Joe's lunch:

TOTAL CALORIES 700

NUTRITIONAL ANALYSIS	GRAMS	PERCENT OF TOTAL CALORIES
Protein	47	27
Carbohydrate	44	25
Fat	37	48

Joe simply can't believe it when he finds out that by making these "insignificant" changes, he has increased the calories from 335 to 700 and he has increased his fat grams from 6 to 37. If Joe was also to eat 2 oz of potato chips with this lunch the total calories would now be 941, with the total fat grams 53.

The following comparison may help you make some changes in the foods you select. These changes could result in a significant reduction in the amount of fat that you eat. Check to see if you generally select the foods that Fat Freddie eats or those of Lean Larry.

Fat Freddie				Lean Larry		
FOOD	PORTION SIZE	FAT (g)		FOOD	PORTION SIZE	FAT (g)
Whole milk	8 oz	8		Skim milk	8 oz	0
Sour cream	3 tbsp	7.5		Nonfat yogurt	8 oz	0
Tuna in oil	3 oz	10.3		Tuna in water	3 oz	1.1
Granola cereal (Nature Valley)	1 oz	5		Bran flakes (Post)	1 oz	0
Quaker— 100% natural cereal (plain)	1 oz	6		Product 19	1 oz	0
Croissant	1 medium	12		Bagel	1 medium	2
Corn chips	1 oz	9		Pretzels	1 oz	0
Hash browns	1 cup	18		Baked potato	1 medium	0
T-bone steak	8 oz	56		Chicken breast	8 oz	8
Fried shrimp	3 oz	10		Broiled shrimp	3 oz	1
Bologna	2 oz	16		Extra-lean ham	2 oz	2
Mayonnaise	1 tbsp	11		Mayonnaise— nonfat	1 tbsp	0
Danish— fruit filled	1 medium	13		English muffin —with jam	1 medium	1
Peanuts—roasted	¼ cup	18		Raisins	¼ cup	0
Cream cheese	1 oz	10		Cottage cheese 1%	1 oz	1

Fat Freddie

Lean Larry

PROTEIN

The most important of the energy nutrients is **protein.** It is appropriate that this word is derived from the Greek word "protos," which means "in first place" or "of prime importance." If you mention the word protein to the average person, he or she will usually associate the word with animal products and will usually relate it to meat, fish, poultry, milk, or eggs. It should be remembered, however, that there are both plant and animal proteins.

Proteins are large complex molecules consisting of anywhere from 24 to as many as 300 **amino acids** joined together in a particular sequence. A great variety of proteins exist because different amino acids combine in unique sequences to form individual proteins. For example, some are flexible and elastic—such as the protein of hair, whereas others are firm and rigid—such as the protein of fingernails.

There are 22 different amino acids that are found in foods, and all but 9 of these are also made by the body. The 9 that cannot be made by the body are called **essential amino acids,** and they must be obtained regularly and in sufficient quantities from the foods that we eat. The 9 essential amino acids are as follows:

Histidine	Methionine	Tryptophan
Isoleucine	Phenylalanine	Valine
Leucine	Threonine	Lysine

Functions of protein in the body

Proteins perform a variety of important functions in the body. They are crucial to the minute-by-minute functioning of our bodies.

- For growth and repair of body tissues

    Muscles, hair, skin, bones, teeth, tendons, ligaments, and so on, are made from protein.

- To regulate body functions

    Enzymes—These are specific proteins that speed up nearly every chemical reaction in the body. There are over 1000 enzymes in the human body. Lactase is an example—it is the enzyme necessary to break down the lactose found in milk.

    Hormones—These are specific proteins that are internal chemical messengers. Insulin is an example. When your blood glucose level is too high, your body produces insulin. This signals the cells to remove insulin from the bloodstream.

    Antibodies—These are blood proteins that attack foreign proteins found in the body, such as bacteria and viruses.

- To transport nutrients

    Hemoglobin is a protein that transports oxygen. Fats also need protein to be transported in the bloodstream.

- To maintain the salt and fluid balance

    Proteins push potassium in and force sodium out of nerve cells to maintain the salt balance. This is also important in maintaining the fluid balance.

- For blood clotting

    Fibrin is a protein and plays an important part in blood clotting.

- To provide energy

    This is not what protein is designed to do. It will occur only if your carbohydrate and fat intake is inadequate.

- To provide glucose

    This will occur only in the absence of sufficient carbohydrates.

Protein requirements

As indicated previously, both the *quantity* and the *quality* of your protein intake are important.

Quantity of protein

There is a Recommended Dietary Allowance (RDA) for protein. It is based on your body weight and is calculated as follows:

1. Calculate your body weight in kilograms

    Body Weight (lb)/2.2 = Body weight (kg)

2. Multiply your body weight in kilograms by 0.8. This will give you your protein requirement in grams.

Example:

Body weight = 154 lb
Step 1. 154/2.2 = 70 kg
Step 2. Protein requirement = 70 × 0.8 = 56 g

CALCULATE YOUR PROTEIN REQUIREMENT:

Record your body weight _____ lb
Step 1. Divide body weight (lb) by 2.2
= _____ / 2.2
= _____ kg
Step 2. Protein requirement = _____ kg × .8
= _____ g

This protein requirement should be considered the minimum amount needed by an inactive person. If you exercise regularly for 45 minutes or more and you want to be sure that you are getting a sufficient amount of protein, you probably should multiply your body weight (kg) by 1.2 rather than 0.8.

Example:

Body weight = 70 kg
Protein requirement = 70 × 1.2
= 84 g

CALCULATE YOUR PROTEIN REQUIREMENT:

Body weight = _____ kg
Protein requirement = _____ kg × 1.2
= _____ g

Quality of protein

Complete protein. Any food containing all 9 of the essential amino acids is classified as a **complete protein.** All animal products are complete proteins; these include meat, fish, poultry, eggs, and dairy products. The amount of protein available from the complete protein sources is given in Table 6-9.

Incomplete protein sources. All other proteins are called **incomplete proteins.** They contain insufficient amounts of one or more of the essential amino acids. The incomplete protein sources can basically be divided into four groups—grain products, green leafy vegetables, seeds and nuts, and legumes. Information concerning the amount of protein available in each of these groups is presented in Table 6-10 for select foods.

TABLE 6-9 Comparison of protein and fat content for complete protein sources

Food	Serving size	Protein (g)	Fat (g)	Calories
Meat (lean)	1 oz	7	3	55
Fish	1 oz	7	3	55
Poultry (lean)	1 oz	7	1-3	40-55
Milk (low-fat)	8 oz	8	1	80
Milk (whole)	8 oz	8	8	150
Cheese	1 oz	6-8	6-9	100-120
Yogurt	8 oz	8	8	140
Egg	1 large	7	6	80

TABLE 6-10 Protein and fat content from incomplete protein sources

Food	Serving size	Protein (g)	Fat (g)	Calories
Grain products (includes starchy vegetables)				
Bran cereal	$\frac{1}{2}$ cup	3-5	0-2	90
Breads	1 slice	2-3	0-2	60-80
Oatmeal (cooked)	1 cup	5	2	130
Rice (cooked)	1 cup	4-5	2	150-200
Potato (baked)	1 medium	5	0	220
Green leafy vegetables (raw)				
Broccoli	1 cup	5	0	45
Brussels sprouts	1 cup	6	0	55
Most other green vegetables	1 cup	2-5	0	50
Seeds and nuts				
Sesame seeds	$\frac{1}{4}$ cup	10	21	221
Sunflower seeds	$\frac{1}{4}$ cup	7	19	208
Walnuts	1 cup	30	71	759
Cashews	1 cup	21	63	787
Peanut butter	1 tbsp	5	8	95
Dry roasted peanuts	1 cup	39	71	840
Legumes				
Peas—green	$\frac{1}{2}$ cup	4	0	70
Beans—navy	1 cup	16	1	259
Beans—lima	1 cup	15	1	217
Beans—pinto	1 cup	14	1	235
Beans—garbanzo	1 cup	15	4	269

Selecting incomplete proteins. In selecting incomplete proteins, it is important to consider which amino acid(s) are missing with each of the groups of foods. These are presented below (the *X*'s indicate that the designated amino acid is missing from that particular food group):

Food group	Lysine	Methionine	Threonine	Tryptophan
Grain products	X		X	
Green leafy vegetables		X		
Nuts and seeds	X			
Legumes		X		X

Different incomplete proteins can be combined to complement one another and provide all the amino acids that are needed by the body. It is important to consume foods from two of these groups so that the same essential amino acid is not lacking in each group. The following combinations will give you all the essential amino acids:

- A grain product with a green leafy vegetable—*Example:* Potato with broccoli
- A grain product with a legume—*Example:* Rice with beans
- A green leafy vegetable with nuts or seeds—*Example:* Brussels sprouts and cashews
- A legume with nuts or seeds—*Example:* Garbanzo beans with dry roasted peanuts

Note that two of the four combinations involve "nuts and seeds." These are not good choices if you are trying to limit your fat intake.

Regardless of the source of the protein, to be used in the body the protein in the food must be broken down by digestion into amino acids, absorbed into the blood, and transported to the cells of the body, where they are used to build the different proteins that are needed by the body. The formation of proteins is summarized in Fig. 6-7 on p. 208.

Note what happens if the body does not get a sufficient amount of all the necessary amino acids at the same time. It cannot use any of them unless it has all of them, and because it has no place to store them—like it does for carbohydrates and fat—the only other option your body has is to convert them to fat and store them as fat. This explains why many vegetarians, even though they do not usually have a weight problem, tend to accumulate excess fat. The reason is that because of what they eat and do not eat, they have difficulty getting a sufficient amount of all the essential amino acids.

Protein intake

Until recently it was not difficult for the average American to take in an adequate amount of protein. In fact, many consumed about double the amount of protein that they needed. However, in recent years we have seen a significant reduction in the amount of fat consumed. Because many of the foods that are high in fat are also high in protein, this has also reduced the total amount of protein that many people get. Those who limit their intake of meat and milk are frequently lacking in protein.

A listing of foods that are high in protein and relatively low in fat appears in Table 6-11. If you need to increase your protein intake these will be good choices for you. A listing of several of the foods that are high in protein and also contain significant

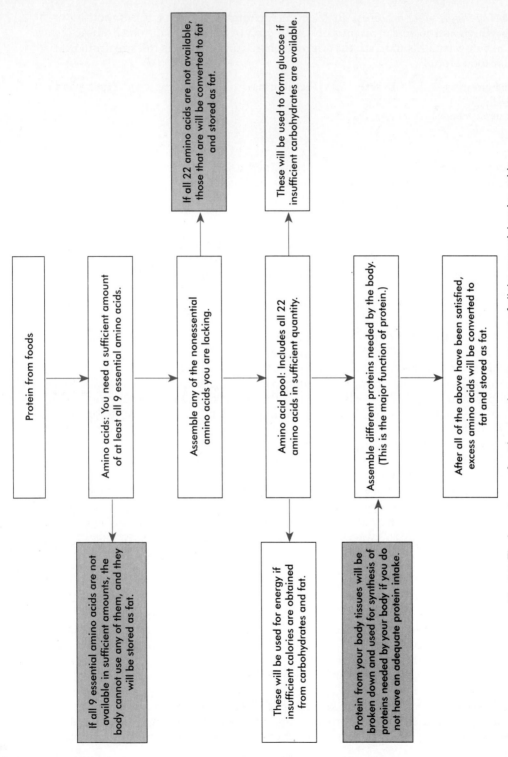

Fig. 6-7 The importance of getting an adequate amount of all the essential amino acids.

TABLE 6-11 Comparison of protein and fat content for selected food items relatively high in protein and low in fat

Food	Amount	Protein (g)	Fat (g)
Breakfast cereals			
Most breakfast cereals—except granola	1 oz	3-5	0-1
Milk and milk products			
Skim milk	1 cup (8 oz)	8	0
Nonfat yogurt (Dannon)	1 cup (8 oz)	9	0
Grain products			
Macaroni	1 cup	6	1
Spaghetti	1 cup	6	1
Meat and fish			
Crab meat	1 cup	23	3
Flounder/sole—baked	3 oz	17	1
Halibut—baked with butter	3 oz	20	6
Oysters	1 cup	20	4
Salmon—baked	3 oz	21	5
—canned	3 oz	17	5
Shrimp—broiled	3 oz	21	1
Tuna—water-packed	3 oz	30	1
Chicken/turkey—white meat, no skin	3 oz	21	4

amounts of fat is presented in Table 6-12. Where possible you should limit your intake of foods from this list.

VITAMINS

Vitamins are organic compounds needed in small quantities by the body to perform specific functions important to growth and development and to the work of nerves and muscles. Although vitamins do not provide energy, they play an important role in releasing energy from the foods that we eat.

Vitamins cannot be manufactured within the body and therefore must be supplied from the foods that we eat. The best method of ensuring an adequate supply of vitamins is to have a well-balanced diet from a variety of foods.

There are presently 13 vitamins that are known to be required by the body and that must be consumed. They can be classified into two groups—fat-soluble vitamins and water-soluble vitamins. The most important difference between the two groups is that the fat-soluble vitamins can be stored in fat in the body, and it is therefore not necessary to eat them each day. There is some danger in consuming extremely large amounts of these vitamins. Water-soluble vitamins cannot be stored in large amounts in the body and must therefore be consumed on a daily basis. Each of the vitamins is identified in Table 6-13. Information is provided for each of them relative to their recommended dietary allowance, the food sources, and their basic functions in the body.

TABLE 6-12 Comparison of protein and fat content for selected food items relatively high in fat

Food	Amount	Protein (g)	Fat (g)
Breakfast cereals			
Granola (Nature Valley)	1 oz	3	5
Quaker—100% natural cereal	1 oz	3	6
Milk and milk products			
Milk—whole	1 cup	8	8
Ice cream—vanilla	1 cup	5	14
Peanut butter	1 tbsp	5	8
Chocolate milkshake	10 oz	9	8
Cheese			
Cheddar	1 oz	7	9
American	1 oz	6	9
Meats			
Bacon	3 slices	6	9
Ground beef—regular	3 oz	20	18
—lean	3 oz	21	16
—extra-lean	3 oz	24	13
Shrimp—fried	3 oz	21	10
Tuna—oil-packed	3 oz	24	7
Scallops	6	15	10
Chicken—dark meat			
without skin	3 oz	21	14
with skin	3 oz	21	18
Leg of lamb—roasted	3 oz	22	13
Miscellaneous foods			
Avocado—raw	1	4	30
Bread stuffing	1 cup	3	5
Cheesecake	1 piece	5	18
Brownie	1	1	4
Croissant	1	5	12
Doughnut—cake	1 large	3	12
Bran muffin	1 small	3	6
Waffle	1	7	10
Nuts—mixed	1 oz	5	15
Egg	1 large	7	6

MINERALS

Minerals are inorganic substances needed by the body in small amounts. They serve a variety of functions within the body, such as maintaining the water balance and the acid-base balance. In addition, they assist in blood clotting, absorption of nutrients, oxygen transportation, and nerve transmission.

TABLE 6-13 **Nutrient needs of the body: vitamins**

Vitamin	Adult RDA		Food sources	Functions
	Men	Women		
Fat-soluble vitamins				
A	1000 μg	8000 μg	Most dark-green leafy vegetables—carrots, pumpkins, sweet potatoes, peaches, apricots, cantaloupes, eggs, milk, fish, butter, and margarine	Promotes good vision; helps keep skin and mucous membrane linings healthy; resistance to certain infectious diseases
D	5 μg	5 μg	Fortified milk, fish-liver oils; some may be produced in the body in response to sunlight; small amounts also contained in butter, liver, egg yolk, salmon, and sardines	Promotes strong bones and teeth and regulates calcium and phosphorus absorption
E	10 μg	8 μg	Plant sources include nuts, vegetable oils, green leafy vegetables, and whole grains	Assists body to use vitamin K; important for formation of red blood cells
K	No specific RDA (70-140 micrograms may be adequate)		Cauliflower, cabbage, spinach, broccoli, and cereals	Assists in formation of blood clots
Water-soluble vitamins				
B₁ (Thiamine)	1.4 mg	1.0 mg	Bran and whole-wheat bread, dried beans, pork, fish, liver, and lean meats	Assists in energy release from carbohydrates; necessary for efficient functioning of heart and nervous system
B₂ (Riboflavin)	1.6 mg	1.2 mg	Cheese, milk, green vegetables, ice cream, enriched bread, and cereals	Assists in the release of energy from food; assists in respiration

Continued.

TABLE 6-13 **Nutrient needs of the body: vitamins—cont'd**

Vitamin	Adult RDA		Food sources	Functions
	Men	**Women**		
B$_3$ (Niacin)	18 mg	13 mg	Meat, poultry, fish, peanuts, whole grain, or enriched cereals and breads	Needed for carbohydrate metabolism and fat synthesis; promotes normal appetite
B$_6$ (Pyridoxine)	2.2 mg	2.0 mg	Meat, poultry, fish, sweet potatoes, vegetables, and whole grains	Aids in absorption of protein; helps convert complex carbohydrates to simple carbohydrates; assists in production in red blood cells
B$_{12}$	3.0 mg	3.0 mg	Animal foods only, such as meat, fish, eggs, cheese, and chicken	Necessary for development of red blood cells; maintainence of normal functioning of nervous system
Folacin (folic acid)	400 μg	400 μg	Whole-wheat products, green vegetables, organ meats, fish, poultry, and eggs	Acts together with vitamin B$_{12}$ to produce hemoglobin
Pantothenic acid	No specific RDA (safe range may be 4-7 mg)		Whole grains, dried beans, eggs, nuts, lean meats, and spinach	Assists in release of energy from foods; assists in hormone synthesis
Biotin	No specific RDA (safe range may be 100-200 mg)		Yeast, liver, egg yolks, and milk	Assists in metabolism of amino acids and carbohydrates; important in formation of fatty acids
C (ascorbic acid)	60 mg	60 mg	All citrus fruits and juices, cabbage, broccoli, green and red peppers, sweet potatoes, and spinach	Tooth and bone formation; promotes iron absorption; necessary for the healing of wounds

Minerals are classified into two categories—macrominerals and microminerals—depending on the amount needed by the body. You need 100 milligrams or more of macrominerals. These include calcium, phosphorus, sulfur, sodium, potassium, chlorine, and magnesium. Microminerals are needed in extremely small amounts. These include iron, copper, zinc, fluorine, iodine, chromium, selenium, and manganese. Specific information relating to the most important minerals is contained in Table 6-14.

TABLE 6-14 **Nutrient needs of the body: minerals**

Vitamin	Adult RDA		Food sources	Functions
	Men	Women		
Calcium	800 mg	800 mg	Milk and milk products, dark green vegetables, and shellfish	To build bones and teeth and maintain bone density and strength; helps muscles contract and relax normally; delays fatigue
Chromium	No specific RDA (safe range may be 0.05-0.20 mg)		Liver, meat, cheese, whole grain cereals, and yeast	Important for glucose metabolism
Phosphorus	800 mg	800 mg	Fish, poultry, meat, dairy products, soft drinks, and nuts	Necessary for normal muscle metabolism, skeletal growth, and tooth development; controls acid-base balance
Sodium	No specific RDA (safe range may be 2000-3000 mg)		Table salt, and from most packaged goods where it is used as a preservative	Helps regulate the water balance; assists in maintaining blood pressure
Potassium	No specific RDA (safe range may be 1500-6000 mg)		Bananas, orange juice, most fruits, potatoes, peanuts	Promotes regular heart beat; controls water balance; contributes to control of blood pressure
Iron	10 mg	18 mg	Liver, kidney, red meat, poultry, egg yolk, whole grain products, dark green vegetables	Formation of hemoglobin, contributes to energy release during metabolism
Copper	No specific RDA (safe range may be 2-3 mg)		Liver, kidney, shellfish, meats, nuts, whole grain cereals	Aids in formation of red blood cells, assists in production of of certain enzymes

Continued.

TABLE 6-14 **Nutrient needs of the body: minerals—cont'd**

Vitamin	Adult RDA		Food sources	Functions
	Men	**Women**		
Magnesium	350 mg	300 mg	Meat, whole grain cereal, nuts, peas, beans, milk, green leafy vegetables	Bone growth; assists in nerve and muscle functioning; regulation of normal heart rhythm
Zinc	15 mg	15 mg	Seafood, beef, liver, eggs, whole wheat bread, oysters	Maintains normal taste and smell; important in healing
Fluorine (fluoride)	No specific RDA (safe range may be 1.5-4 mg)		Water, fish	Increases resistance of teeth to disease; may help prevent osteoporosis
Manganese	No specific RDA (safe range may be 2.5-5 mg)		Nuts, whole grain cereals, peas, beans, coffee, tea, egg yolk	Normal bone growth; activation of enzymes used in carbohydrates and protein metabolism
Iodine	15 mg	15 mg	Iodized salt, seafood, vegetable oil	Necessary for normal functioning of thyroid gland; essential for normal cell function

WATER

Water is the most important nutrient needed by the body. If you are deprived of food you can live for several weeks, but without water you can live for only a few days. It has been described as an indispensable nutrient on which all forms of life depend. Water is second only to oxygen in its importance for sustaining life.

Importance of water

Water is the most abundant nutrient in the human body, accounting for approximately 60% of your total body weight. Your body uses water for a variety of functions, including the following:

- Water is important for the digestion and metabolism of food, acting as a medium in which various enzymatic and chemical reactions take place.
- Water is an important fluid in your blood that carries various nutrients and oxygen to the cells and is also responsible for transportation of waste products.
- Water helps regulate the body temperature by dissipating heat through the skin.
- Water is necessary for efficient movement at each joint, because it contributes to their lubrication.

- The lungs and respiratory passageways must be kept moistened by water to facilitate the efficient intake of oxygen and excretion of carbon dioxide.
- The efficient removal of waste products from the body depends on an adequate supply of water, because these waste products must be dissolved in water.
- Water is a natural diuretic. Without an adequate intake of water, your body will tend to maintain more water than it should.

It can clearly be seen that if you do not drink sufficient water to maintain a "normal" fluid balance, your body will not be able to function efficiently. It is essential that your body maintain its crucial water balance. When the fluid balance is low, dehydration occurs. Severe dehydration can cause death.

How much water should you drink? Not all the water in the body comes from water that we drink. Many of the foods and other fluids we drink contain large amounts of water. Milk, for example, is made up mainly of water, and most fruits and vegetables have high water content. Also, some water is created in your body as the end product of carbohydrate, fat, and protein metabolism.

On a typical day, your body will normally lose the equivalent of 10 to 12 cups of water in one form or another. The water contained in your food will normally provide the equivalent of only 2 to 4 cups per day. This means that you probably need to drink between six and eight glasses of water per day just to maintain your fluid balance. If you exercise a lot or live in a hot climate or you are trying to lose weight, then you probably need to drink even more.

Water intake and weight loss

Adequate water intake is essential if any weight-loss program is to be effective. There are several reasons for this:
- Water suppresses the appetite. If you drink one or two glasses of water before a meal, you will probably not eat as much as you would have eaten if you had not drunk the water.
- An adequate intake of water is essential if the body is to metabolize fat efficiently. The reason for this is that your kidneys will not function efficiently without sufficient water and the liver will be forced to perform some of their functions. One of the primary functions of the liver is to metabolize fat and, if it is forced to perform additional functions, it will not be as efficient as it should be at metabolizing fat.
- With an insufficient intake of water, your body will actually retain more water than it normally would. When your body gets very little water, it treats this as a threat to survival and tries to hold on to all the water that it has. This often shows up in the form of swelling in the feet, legs, and hands. The best way to alleviate this problem and to make sure that an adequate fluid balance exists is to drink lots of water.

Does it make a difference which beverage you drink?

Obviously you can obtain water by consuming such beverages as fruit juice, soft drinks, beer, wine, coffee, tea, and milk. However, there is a difference in the way your body treats pure water and other beverages that contain water.

Apart from the fact that most of these other beverages contain a significant number of calories, many of them contain substances that are not healthful. Following on p. 216 are some examples:

- Beer and wine contain alcohol, which is a toxic substance. In addition, for every ounce of alcohol consumed you need an additional 8 oz of water to metabolize it. This often seriously distorts your fluid balance.
- Many of these beverages contain caffeine. Caffeine itself is a diuretic, which also has several negative effects on the body.
- Fruit juices and soft drinks contain lots of sugar. Sugar requires extra water for metabolism.
- Most of the soft drinks are high in sodium.
- Many of the diet beverages contain chemicals such as preservatives and colorings. These often irritate the stomach lining, and the liver and kidneys require extra water to dispose of them.
- Many of the alternatives to water contain significant amounts of phosphoric acid. This may inhibit the ability of your body to absorb calcium.

Drinking pure water eliminates all these problems. It contains no extra calories to slow down digestion or add unwanted fat, and it contains no irritants or chemicals to irritate the sensitive linings of the digestive tract.

THE FOUR FOOD GROUP PLAN

A well-balanced diet from a variety of foods is essential if all nutrients required by the body are to be obtained. The four food group plan was developed to categorize foods that are similar in origin and nutrient content. A number of servings is recommended from each group to meet the basic daily nutritional requirements. Basic information on the four food group plan is presented in Table 6-15. In principle, the four food group plan is very simple to use. However, depending on the choices you make within each group, you may finish with a caloric intake that is high in fat, cholesterol, sugar, or salt, and you may eat too many calories.

THE NEW AMERICAN EATING GUIDE

Because of these problems, the Center for Science in the Public Interest has prepared a modified version of the four food group plan that provides additional information so that you can make wise choices concerning the foods you select within each group.

With this plan, foods within each of the four groups are divided into three categories. Those you can eat *anytime* are the ones that are low in fat, sugar, and salt. The grain foods in this category are those which are mostly unrefined and therefore are high in fiber and some of the trace minerals.

The second category comprises those foods you should eat *in moderation*. They may contain moderate amounts of fat and may be high in salt, sugar, sodium, or cholesterol. A coding system is used to indicate why each food is listed in this category.

The third category of foods comprises those you should eat only *now and then* or that you should possibly not eat at all. They are foods that are usually high in fat (particularly saturated fat) or that are very high in sugar, salt, or cholesterol. It is suggested that if these foods are eaten, they are to be eaten less frequently and in small amounts.

This plan is referred to as the New American Eating Guide. Basic information relative to each of the classifications within each of the four groups is summarized in Table 6-16.

TABLE 6-15 Four food group plan			
Food group	Servings per day	Sample foods and serving size	Major nutrient contributions
Milk and milk products	2*	1 cup (8 oz) milk, 1 cup yogurt, 1½ cups cottage cheese, 2 cups ice cream, 1-2 oz cheese, 1 cup milk pudding	Calcium Protein Riboflavin Zinc Vitamin B_{12}
Fruits and vegetables	4†	½ cup fruit, vegetable, or juice, 1 medium apple, orange, banana, or peach	Vitamin A Vitamin C Folacin
Grains (bread and cereal products)	4‡	1 slice bread, ½ cup cooked cereal, or 1 oz ready-to-eat cereal (1 cup); ½ hamburger bun, hot dog bun, or English muffin; ½ cup cooked rice, grits, macaroni, or spaghetti; 2 tbsp flour; 6 saltines; 1 6-inch tortilla	Niacin Iron Thiamine Fiber Zinc
Meat and meat substitutes	2	2 to 3 oz cooked meat, fish, or chicken; ¼ cup tuna; 2 eggs; 4 tbsp peanut butter; 1 cup cooked legumes; ½ cup nuts	Protein Iron Riboflavin Niacin Zinc Vitamin B_{12} Thiamine

*Children, teenagers, pregnant women, and nursing mothers need three to four servings or more.
†One selection should be rich in vitamin C, and one should be rich in vitamin A.
‡Enriched or whole-grain products are the best.

THE FOOD PYRAMID

In 1992, The U.S. Department of Agriculture released new standards for a recommended diet in the form of a food pyramid. With this system, foods are divided into six categories and the recommended number of servings for each of these is given (Fig. 6-8 on p. 220). This plan suggests that we need to eat less fat and sugar and eat more fruits, vegetables, and grains.

THE FOOD EXCHANGE SYSTEM

The best system for planning meals and the only one that allows you to analyze your meals is the food exchange system. With this system, foods are classified into six categories, or lists. Some lists contain subgroups. Each food on any given list contains approximately the same number of calories as any other food on the list and approximately the same amount of the energy nutrients. With some of the lists the portion

TABLE 6-16 New American Eating Guide (modified four group plan)

Anytime	In moderation	Now and then

1. Milk products (three to four servings per day for children, two for adults)

Anytime	In moderation	Now and then
Buttermilk (from skim milk)	Cocoa with skim milk[e]	Cheesecake[d,e]
Low-fat cottage cheese	Cottage cheese, regular[a]	Cheese fondue[d,g]
Low-fat milk (1%)	Frozen yogurt[e]	Cheese souffle[d,g,h]
Low-fat yogurt	Ice milk[e]	Eggnog[a,e,h]
Nonfat dry milk	Low-fat milk (2%)[a]	Hard cheeses: blue, brick, Camambert, cheddar, muenster, Swiss[d,g]
Skim-milk cheeses	Low-fat yogurt, sweetened[e]	
Skim milk	Mozzarella, part-skim[1,g]	Ice cream[d,e]
Skim-milk and banana shake		Processed cheeses[d,f]
		Whole milk[d]
		Whole-milk yogurt[d]

2. Fruits and vegetables (four or more servings per day)

Anytime	In moderation	Now and then
All fruits and vegetables except those at right	Avocado[c]	Coconut[d]
Applesauce (unsweetened)	Cole slaw[c]	Pickles[f]
Unsweetened fruit juices	Cranberry sauce[e]	
Unsalted vegetable juices	Dried fruit	
Potatoes, white or sweet	French fries[a or b]	
	Fried eggplant[b]	
	Fruits canned in syrup[e]	
	Gazpacho[b,g]	
	Glazed carrots[e,g]	
	Guacamole[c]	
	Potatoes au gratin[a,g]	
	Salted vegetable juices[b]	
	Sweetened fruit juices[e]	
	Vegetables canned with salt[f]	

3. Beans, grains, and nuts (four or more servings per day)

Anytime	In moderation	Now and then
Bread and rolls (whole grain)	Cornbread[i]	Croissant[d,i]
Bulgur	Flour tortilla[i]	Doughnut[c or d,e,i]
Dried beans and peas	Granola cereals[a or b]	Presweetened cereals[e,i]
Lentils	Hominy grits[i]	Sticky buns[a or b,e,i]
Oatmeal	Macaroni and cheese[a,g,i]	Stuffing (with butter)[d,g,i]
Pasta, whole-wheat	Matzoh[i]	
Rice, brown	Nuts[c]	
Sprouts	Pasta, refined[i]	

Modified from the Center for Science in the Public Interest, Washington, DC, 1982.

TABLE 6-16 New American Eating Guide (modified four group plan)—cont'd

Anytime	In moderation	Now and then

3. Beans, grains, and nuts (four or more servings per day)—cont'd

Anytime	In moderation	Now and then
Whole-grain hot and cold cereals	Peanut butter[c]	
Whole-wheat matzoh	Pizza[f,i]	
	Refined, unsweetened cereals[i]	
	Refried beans[a or b]	
	Seeds[c]	
	Soybeans[b]	
	Tofu[b]	
	Waffles or pancakes with syrup[e,g,i]	
	White bread and rolls[i]	
	White rice[i]	

4. Poultry, fish, meat, and eggs (two servings per day; vegetarians should add servings from other groups)

Anytime	In moderation	Now and then
Cod	Fried fish[a or b]	Fried chicken, commercial[d]
Flounder	Herring[c,b]	Cheese omclct[d,h]
Gefilte fish[g]	Mackerel, canned[b,g]	Whole egg or yolk (limit to 3 a week)[c,h]
Haddock	Salmon, canned[b,g]	
Halibut	Sardines[b,g]	Bacon[d,f]
Perch	Shrimp[h]	Beef liver, fried[a,h]
Pollock	Tuna, oil packed[b,g]	Bologna[d,f]
Rockfish	Chicken liver[h]	Corned beef[d,f]
Shellfish, except shrimp	Fried chicken in vegetable oil (homemade)[c]	Ground beef[d]
Sole		Ham, trimmed[a,f]
Tuna, water packed[g]	Chicken or turkey, boiled, baked, or roasted (with skin)[b]	Hot dogs[d,f]
Egg whites		Liverwurst[d,f]
Chicken or turkey, boiled, baked, or roasted (no skin)	Flank steak[a]	Pig's feet[d]
	Leg or loin of lamb[a]	Salami[d,f]
	Pork shoulder or loin, lean[a]	Sausage[d,f]
	Round steak or ground round[a]	Spareribs[d]
	Rump roast[a]	Red meats, untrimmed[d]
	Sirloin steak, lean[a]	
	Veal[a]	

[a]Moderate fat, saturated.
[b]Moderate fat, unsaturated.
[c]High fat, unsaturated.
[d]High fat, saturated.
[e]High in added sugar.
[f]High in salt or sodium.
[g]May be high in salt or sodium.
[h]High in cholesterol.
[i]Refined grains.

**Food Guide Pyramid:
a guide to daily food choices**

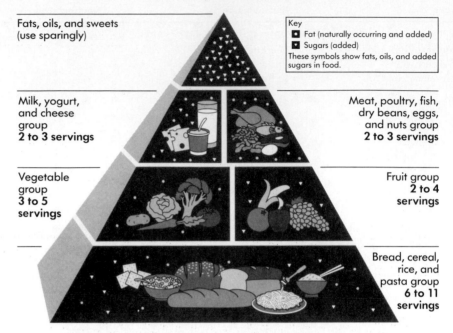

Fats, oils, and sweets
(use sparingly)

Key
◻ Fat (naturally occurring and added)
▾ Sugars (added)
These symbols show fats, oils, and added sugars in food.

Milk, yogurt,
and cheese
group
2 to 3 servings

Meat, poultry, fish,
dry beans, eggs,
and nuts group
2 to 3 servings

Vegetable
group
**3 to 5
servings**

Fruit group
**2 to 4
servings**

Bread, cereal,
rice, and
pasta group
**6 to 11
servings**

Fig. 6-8 The new food pyramid.

size must be adjusted to obtain the desired results. A listing of the six exchange groups and their caloric value together with other nutritional information is presented in Table 6-17.

A listing of the individual foods that make up each of the six exchanges is presented in Appendix C. In addition, Laboratory Experience 6-2 is designed so that you can use the exchange lists to determine the adequacy of your diet.

Planning your food intake

An adequate diet requires more than just sound nutritional knowledge. It may take considerable time and effort to decide what is best for you to eat. This process may be simplified by using the four food group plan together with the exchange system to provide adequacy, balance, calorie control, and variety.

Table 6-18 shows how the four food group plan and the exchange system can be used to get all or most of the major nutrients while consuming less than 1000 calories. The exchange system can be used to estimate the percentage of your calories you get from carbohydrates, fats, and proteins. The example in Table 6-19, based on the foods listed in Table 6-18, shows how easy this is to calculate.

Note that the information relating to your caloric intake is obtained without consulting any tables showing the nutritional values of given foods. It is simply obtained by using information pertaining to the exchange lists as shown in Table 6-17.

TABLE 6-17 Food exchange list (summary)*

List	Approximate portion size	Carbohydrates (g)	Protein (g)	Fat (g)	Calories
Milk	1 cup				
Nonfat		12	8	0	80
Low-fat		12	8	5	125
Whole		12	8	8	150
Vegetable (low-calorie vegetables only)	½ cup	5	2	0	25
Fruit	Varies	15	0	0	60
Bread and starchy vegetables	Varies	15	3	0	70
Meat	1 oz				
Lean		0	7	3	55
Medium-fat		0	7	6	80
High-fat		0	7	8	100
Fat	1 tsp	0	0	5	45

*The exchange lists do not include concentrated sugar. However, concentrated sugar is eaten frequently in the form of sugar, corn syrup, honey, jam, jelly, or candy. A separate list is provided in many nutrition books—a sugar list—where the portion size is 1 tsp. For each of the above forms of concentrated sugar this is approximately 5 g of carbohydrate and equivalent to approximately 20 calories.

TABLE 6-18 Use of the food group plan and the exchange lists

Four food group plan	Conversion to exchange system	Example of food choice	Energy cost (calories)
Milk, 2 cups	Milk list—select two exchanges	1 cup 1% milk 8 oz plain nonfat yogurt	160
Fruits and vegetables, four servings	Fruit and vegetable lists—select four exchanges	½ cup orange juice 1 apple 1 cup broccoli 1 large tomato	130
Grains (bread and cereals), four servings	Bread and starchy vegetable list—select four exchanges	⅓ cup All Bran ½ cup green peas 1 small baked potato 1 slice rye bread	280
Meat, two servings (2-3 oz each)	Meat list—select six exchanges	6 oz fresh fish	330 ———
TOTAL CALORIES			900

TABLE 6-19 Calculating calories and percentages

List	Number	Carbohydrate (g)	Protein (g)	Fat (g)	Calories
Milk	2	24	16	0	160
Fruit	2	20	0	0	80
Vegetables	2	10	4	0	56
Bread	4	60	8	0	272
Meat	6	0	42	18	330
TOTALS		114	70	18	898

Calculation of calories:

Carbohydrates	114×4	$=$	456 calories
Protein	70×4	$=$	280 calories
Fat	18×9	$=$	162 calories

Calculation of percentages:

Carbohydrate	$=$	$\dfrac{456}{898}$	$=$	51%
Protein	$=$	$\dfrac{280}{898}$	$=$	31%
Fat	$=$	$\dfrac{162}{898}$	$=$	18%

Using the exchange lists to plan meals

The food exchange lists can be used to plan meals. Suppose you wanted to eat 1600 calories, with approximately 25% of those calories coming from fat. The sample worksheet in the accompanying box shows how this is done.

Step 1. Calculate the number of calories from fat	$1600 \times .25$
	400 calories
Step 2. Calculate the number of fat grams	400/9
	44 g
Step 3. Select the number of exchanges to supply the 44 grams of fat	You may select:
(Each lean meat exchange = 3 g fat)	8 lean meat = $8 \times 3 = 24$
(Each fat exchange = 5 g fat)	4 fat = $4 \times 5 = 20$
Step 4. Calculate the total number of calories contained in the exchanges selected	8 lean meat = $8 \times 55 = 440$
	4 fat = $4 \times 45 = 180$
(Each lean meat = 55 calories)	
(Each fat = 45 calories)	
TOTAL CALORIES = 440 + 180	
= 620 calories	

Step 5. Calculate the number of calories you have remaining   Calories remaining

(Calories remaining = desired caloric   = 1600 − 620
intake − calories used with fat exchanges)   = 980 calories

Step 6. Determine how these calories are to be used for the following exchanges   You may select the following:

Nonfat milk exchange = 80 calories   2 nonfat milk = 2 × 80 = 160
Vegetable exchange = 25 calories   4 vegetable = 4 × 25 = 100
Fruit exchange = 60 calories   6 fruit = 6 × 60 = 360
Starch/grain exchange = 70 calories   5 starch = 5 × 70 = 350
TOTAL CALORIES = 970

Step 7. List your total plan for the day

2 nonfat milk = 160

4 vegetable = 100
6 fruit = 360
5 starch = 350
8 lean meat = 440
4 fat = 180

TOTAL CALORIES = 1590

Step 8. Select foods from each of the exchange lists (see Appendix A.)

Using the number of exchanges identified in step 9 above, your meal plan for the day may be as follows:

Breakfast

Orange juice	1 cup	2 fruit
Bran cereal	1/3 cup	1 starch
1% Milk	1 cup	1 nonfat milk
Blueberries	3/4 cup	1 fruit

Lunch

Whole-wheat bread	2 slices	2 starch
Sliced chicken	3 oz	3 lean meat
Mayonnaise	1 tbsp	1 fat
Lettuce	2 slices	1/2 vegetable
Tomato	2 slices	1/2 vegetable
Cantaloupe	1/3 small	1 fruit
Strawberries	1 cup	1 fruit
Yogurt (nonfat)	1 cup	1 nonfat milk

Dinner

Lettuce	2 cups	2 vegetable
Baked potato	1 large	2 starch
Broccoli—cooked	1/2 cup	1 vegetable
Tenderloin steak	5 oz	5 lean meat
Salad dressing (nonfat)	3 tbsp	—
Butter	2 tsp	2 fat
Sour cream	2 tbsp	1 fat
Pineapple	3/4 cup	1 fruit

ANALYSIS OF CALORIC INTAKE

The caloric content of food can be measured. To determine the number of calories in any food, the food is dehydrated and burned in a special piece of equipment called a calorimeter. When the food is burned, the increase in temperature is measured, and the caloric content of the food is determined.

Tables have been prepared summarizing the nutritional information for most foods. These tables provide the information that you need so that you can make wise decisions concerning what you eat. You can use these tables to determine your total caloric intake; to determine the percentage of your total calories that you get from carbohydrates, protein, fat, and alcohol; to determine whether you are meeting your Recommended Dietary Allowances for each of the nutrients; and to increase or decrease your intake of a particular nutrient. Nutritional information for many of the common foods is contained in Appendix B in the back of the book.

EXAMPLE: Suppose you wanted to evaluate the following food selections for a particular day:

	Food	Amount
Breakfast	Orange juice	1 cup
	Bran cereal	1 cup
	Skim milk	1 cup
	Banana	1 large
	Blueberries	$^3/_4$ cup
	English muffin	1 large
	Margarine	1 tsp
Lunch	Chicken breast	3 oz
	Whole-wheat bread	2 slices
	Mayonnaise (diet)	1 tbsp
	Tomato	3 slices
	Strawberries	$1^1/_4$ cup
	Shredded wheat	$^1/_2$ cup
	Skim milk	1 cup
Dinner	Mixed green salad	2 cups
	French dressing	2 tbsp
	Carrots (cooked)	$^1/_2$ cup
	Green beans (cooked)	$^1/_2$ cup
	Tenderloin steak (lean)	3 oz
	Potato (baked)	1 small
	Margarine (diet)	1 tbsp
	Whole-wheat bread	2 slices
	Margarine (diet)	2 tbsp

Two options are available to you. You can analyze this diet by using the exchange lists, or you can obtain relevant information for each of the foods from the nutritional tables (see Appendix B).

Analysis using the exchange lists—By consulting the exchange lists (see Appendix A) you can determine how many exchanges you must count for each of the food items. The daily meal plan on p. 225 can be analyzed quickly by adding the number of exchanges and using the information contained in Table 6-17. A summary of this information follows the meal plan.

	Food	Amount	Exchanges
Breakfast	Orange juice	1 cup	2 fruit
	Bran cereal	1 cup	2 starch
	Skim milk	1 cup	1 milk
	Banana	1 large	2 fruit
	Blueberries	³/₄ cup	1 fruit
	English muffin	1 large	2 starch
	Margarine	1 tsp	1 fat
Lunch	Chicken breast	3 oz	3 meat
	Whole-wheat bread	2 slices	2 starch
	Mayonnaise (diet)	1 tbsp	1 fat
	Tomato	3 slices	1 vegetable
	Strawberries	1¹/₄ cup	1 fruit
	Shredded wheat	¹/₂ cup	1 starch
	Skim milk	1 cup	1 milk
Dinner	Mixed green salad	2 cups	2 vegetable
	French dressing	2 tbsp	2 fat
	Carrots (cooked)	¹/₂ cup	1 vegetable
	Green beans (cooked)	¹/₂ cup	1 vegetable
	Tenderloin steak (lean)	3 oz	3 meat
	Potato (baked)	1 small	2 starch
	Margarine (diet)	1 tbsp	1 fat
	Whole-wheat bread	2 slices	2 starch
	Margarine (diet)	2 tbsp	1 fat

EXCHANGE	TOTAL	TOTAL CARBOHYDRATE (GRAMS)	TOTAL FAT (GRAMS)	TOTAL PROTEIN (GRAMS)
Starch	11	165	—	33
Meat	6	—	18	42
Vegetable	5	25	—	10
Fruit	6	90	—	—
Milk	2	24	—	16
Fat	6	—	30	—
TOTALS		304	48	101

Total calories can be estimated as follows:

	GRAMS	×	CALORIES/GRAM	=	CALORIES
Carbohydrates	304	×	4	=	1216
Fats	48	×	9	=	432
Proteins	101	×	4	=	404
TOTAL CALORIES				=	2052

The percentage of the total calories from each of the three nutrients is as follows:

Carbohydrates	=	1216/2052	=	59%
Fats	=	432/2052	=	21%
Proteins	=	404/2052	=	20%

Analysis using the nutritional information tables

A more comprehensive analysis may be obtained by using the information contained in a table of nutritional information for foods (see Appendix B). This is a tedious and time-consuming task. Fortunately, many computer software packages have been developed that will perform most of this busy work for you and will provide you with a large amount of valuable information. The box on p. 227 is part of the analysis for the previously analyzed meal plan using the PRUCAL Computer Software Package. With this program, goals are established based on the specific information for each person relative to age, height, gender, activity level, and frame size. The box on p. 227 shows that the foods consumed provided 2071 calories with 20% from protein, 55% from carbohydrate, and 25% from fat. The actual intakes for each of the 17 important nutrients is given and compared with the RDA values to determine whether the dietary goals are being met.

Several other similar programs are available to assist you in analyzing your caloric intake. The results from these programs can then be used to assist you in making changes in what you eat and how much you eat, so that you can achieve your objectives.

EATING OUT

Eating out has become an important part of the American lifestyle. This is possibly because of the growing number of families in which both the husband and wife work and because of the increase in the number of people living alone who find it easier to eat out rather than cook for themselves. An increase in the number of fast-food outlets available makes it much easier for a person to eat quickly.

However, consumers have become much more concerned about the nutritional content of food, and many restaurants and fast-food chains have been forced to alter their menus to cater to the needs of the consumers. Despite these changes, it is still very difficult to eat well when dining out. Consider, for example, the following "typical" steakhouse meal.

Typical steakhouse meal
Tossed salad with French dressing
Rib-eye steak (8 oz)
Baked potato with butter and sour cream
Coffee with sugar and cream

An analysis shows that this one meal provides over 1600 calories, with 63% of these calories coming from fat and only 24% from carbohydrates. It is no wonder that the typical American diet is so high in fat.

SAMPLE COMPUTER PROGRAM OUTPUT FOR NUTRITIONAL ANALYSIS

PRUCAL

Developed and Copyrighted
by
Colorado State University
Department of Food Science and Human Nutrition

Planning your diet to meet PRUDENT guidelines

Diet Analysis for:	FREDDIE FITNESS
Age:	21
Height:	5 feet 11 inches
Recommended Weight:	158 pounds
Sex:	Male
Frame:	Medium
Activity:	Moderate

This program estimates your individual energy needs (KCALS) based on your sex, the desirable weight for your height and frame size, and your activity level.

The goals are set as follows:

Kilocalories 2686

Calorie distribution

Protein	13%
Total Carbohydrates	57%
Total Sugars	20%
Fat	30%
Saturated Fat	10%
Polyunsaturated Fat	10%

Dietary Fiber	15 grams/1000 KCALS
Cholesterol	300 milligrams/day
Sodium	2000 milligrams/day

Vitamin and mineral goals are set to meet the Recommended Dietary Allowances based on sex and age. The Potassium goal is set at the midpoint of Estimated Safe and Adequate Daily Intake.

FREDDIE FITNESS   DAY ONE   8/17/93

Comparison of Nutrient intake and goals by percentage

Percent of goal

Nutrients	%	0 10 20 30 40 50 60 70 80 90 100 110 120 130+
KCalories	77	**************************************O
Protein	118	***X *****
Total Sugars	85	***********************************O
Dietary Fiber	101	**************************************X
Fat	76	*************************************O
Saturated Fat	50	********************X
Polyunsat Fat	70	****************************X
Cholesterol	62	*************************O
Sodium	121	**************************************O *****
Potassium	127	***************************************: *******
Vitamin A	275	***************************************X ***********
Vitamin C	475	***************************************X ***********
Thiamin	133	***************************************X *****
Riboflavin	161	***************************************X ********
Vitamin B6	152	***************************************X ********
Calcium	127	***************************************X *******
Iron	210	***************************************X ***********
Zinc	96	**************************************X

Goals indicated by a 'O' are maximum goals and should not be exceeded.
Goals indicated by a 'X' are minimum goals and should be met or exceeded.
Goal indicated by a ':' is the midpoint of the Safe and Adequate Range.
The graph lines for Total Sugars, Fat, Saturated Fat and Polyunsaturated Fat should not be longer than the KCalorie line.

Your diet provides 2071 calories, distributed as follows:

Protein	20%	Fat	25%
Total Carbohydrate	55%	Saturated Fat	7%
Total Sugars	22%	Polyunsaturated Fat	9%

Your actual intake per day of the following nutrients is:

Protein	104 gm	Cholesterol	188 mg	Riboflavin	2.7 mg
Total Sugars	115 gm	Sodium	2428 mg	Vitamin B6	3.3 mg
Dietary Fiber . .	41 gm	Potassium	4793 mg	Calcium	1022 mg
Fat	68 gm	Vitamin A	13794 IU	Iron	20.8 mg
Saturated Fat . .	14.9 gm	Vitamin C	14.9 mg	Zinc	14.5 mg
Polyunsat Fat . .	20.9 gm	Thiamin	2.0 mg		

Modified from Colorado State University, Department of Food Science and Human Nutrition, Fort Collins, Colorado.

Eating at fast-food restaurants can be just as bad or worse, depending on the selection of foods. Consider the following selections:

> Bacon cheeseburger
> French fries
> Apple turnover
> Chocolate milkshake

This meal contains approximately 1700 calories, with slightly less than 50% of these calories coming from fat.

Additional information relating to the nutritional content for fast foods is included in Appendix C.

SUMMARY

The following summary will help you to identify some of the important concepts covered in this chapter:

- Most Americans are confused concerning nutrition, and many of them have poor eating habits.
- There are approximately 40 essential nutrients that the body needs. The secret to eating well is to learn how to get adequate amounts of all of these without gaining weight or getting fat.
- Fat is a concentrated source of energy, containing more than twice as many calories as protein and carbohydrates.
- The average American needs to learn how to increase his or her intake of carbohydrates while significantly reducing his or her intake of simple refined sugar.
- Fat, sugar, and alcohol contain "empty" calories and basically contribute very few, if any, of the essential nutrients.
- Complete proteins from animal products contain all nine of the essential amino acids. All other sources of protein are considered incomplete. Incomplete proteins, however, can be combined to complement one another.
- Because many of the foods that are high in fat are also high in protein, by reducing their fat intake, many people now get less than an adequate amount of protein.
- Water is the most important essential nutrient needed by the body. We need to drink at least eight glasses of water each day.
- Various eating plans have been devised to enable you to obtain a well-balanced diet from a variety of foods. The food exchange lists are probably the best available.

KEY TERMS

amino acids   The constituents of protein. An adequate amount of each of these is necessary for the body to make protein.

calorie   A unit for measuring energy—calories in food represent the energy value of foods

carbohydrate   An organic nutrient derived from a plant source, which is the major source of energy in the body.

complete protein   Any food containing all nine of the essential amino acids—includes meats, fish, poultry, eggs, and dairy products.

complex carbohydrate   A compound consisting of many sugar molecules linked together—includes starches and fiber.

energy nutrient   A nutrient that provides energy in the form of calories—carbohydrates, fat, and protein.

essential nutrient   A necessary nutrient that cannot be manufactured by the body and therefore must be obtained from the food you eat.

fat   A nutrient that is a secondary source of energy in the body and that can be stored in the body (also referred to as lipids or oils).

fiber   Any part of a food plant that cannot be broken down and digested by the human body—usually found in the stems, leaves, and seeds of plants.

insoluble fiber   The type of fiber that does not dissolve in water—it is found in the cell walls of many grains, vegetables, and fruits.

incomplete protein   Any food containing protein that does not contain all nine of the essential amino acids—includes grain products, green leafy vegetables, nuts and seeds, and legumes.

minerals   Inorganic substances needed by the body for specific functions.

nutrients   Basic substances needed by the body for a variety of functions.

organic   A nutrient containing carbon that can usually be oxidized or burned to produce energy.

protein   Primary food substance formed from amino acids used by the body primarily to build, repair, regulate, and replace the cells of the body.

Recommended Dietary Allowance (RDA)   The amounts of essential nutrients considered adequate to meet the known nutritional needs of most healthy persons.

refined sugar   A term used to describe sweeteners, such as table sugar, that are created by processing and are added to other foods to sweeten them.

saturated fat   Fat found mainly in animal products that carries the maximum number of hydrogen atoms.

soluble fiber   Fiber that dissolves in water to form a gel—it is the nonstructural material in plant cells, such as pectins and gums.

starch   The most familiar form of carbohydrates found in plants, in seeds, and in the grain from which bread, cereal, spaghetti, and pasta are made.

unsaturated fat   A fat found mainly in plant products that is usually liquid at room temperature. It contains less than the maximum number of hydrogen atoms.

vitamins   Organic compounds needed in small quantities by the body to perform specific functions.

REFERENCES

1. Althoff SA, Svobada M, and Girdano DA: *Choices in health and fitness for life*, ed 2, Scottsdale, Ariz, 1992, Gorsuch Scarisbrick.

2. American Dietetic Association: *Exchange lists*, Chicago, 1986, The Association.

3. Bailey C: *Fit or fat?* Boston, 1978, Houghton Mifflin.

4. Center for Science in Public Interest: *How sweet is it?* Washington, DC, 1985, The Center.

5. Christian JL, Greger JL: *Nutrition for living*, ed 3, Menlo Park, Calif, 1991, Benjamin/Cummings.

6. Church CF, Church HN: *Food values of portions commonly used*, ed 10, Philadelphia, 1985, JB Lippincott.

7. Cottemman SK: *Y's way to weight management*, Champaign, Ill, 1985, Human Kinetics.

8. Crow VCR: *Nutrient needs at a glance*, College Station, Tex, 1985, The Texas Agriculture Extension Service, Texas A & M University System.

9. *Food and your weight*, Washington, DC, 1973, US Department of Agriculture, US Government Printing Office.

10. Hamilton EMN, Whitney EN, and Sizer FS: *Nutrition: concepts and controversies*, ed 4, St Paul, Minn, 1988, West.

11. Hegarty V: *Decisions in nutrition*, St Louis, 1988, Mosby–Year Book.

12. Hurley JS: *Nutrition and health*, Guilford, Conn, 1992, The Dushkin Publishing Group.

13. Katch FI, and McArdle WD: *Nutrition, weight control and exercise*, ed 4, Philadelphia, 1991, Lea & Febiger.

14. Lecos C: Water: the number one nutrient. In *FDA consumer*, US Government Printing Office, October 1984.

15. McLaren M: *Weight loss and nutrition*, San Diego, 1986, Health Media of America.

16. Nutritive value of foods, *Home Garden Bulletin* no. 72, Washington, DC, United States Department of Agriculture, April 1981.

17. Prentice WE: *Fitness for college and life*, ed 3, St Louis, 1991, Mosby–Year Book.

18. PRUCAL: *Prudent diet analysis user's guide*, Fort Collins, Colo, 1986.

19. *Recommended dietary allowances*, ed 9, Washington, DC, 1980, National Academy of Sciences.

20. Rosato FD: *Fitness and wellness—the physical connection*, ed 2, St Paul, Minn, 1990, West.

21. Texas Agriculture and Extension Service: *Hidden sugar in foods*, College Station, Tex, 1985, The Service.

22. Vitamins: fact and fancy, University of California, Berkeley, Calif, *Wellness Letter* 2:1, October 1985.

23. Williams MH: *Nutrition for fitness and sport*, ed 2, Dubuque, Ia, 1988, Wm C Brown.

24. Young EA, Sims O, Bingham C et al: Fast foods 1986: nutrient analyses, *Dietetic Currents* 13:6, 1986.

LABORATORY EXPERIENCE 6–1

Estimating Your Daily Fiber Intake

Following is a listing of many of the foods containing fiber. This list shows the amount of fiber for the designated serving size.

Try to recall the foods that you ate yesterday, and check these off in column 1 on this list.

Next to each item checked off, estimate the grams of fiber you obtained from each item. This will be based on how much of the food you ate in relation to the serving size. Write this value in column 2.

Total up the estimated grams of fiber for the day.

Fiber content of foods

COLUMN 1	COLUMN 2	FOOD	SERVING SIZE	FIBER—GRAMS
		Fruits		
		Apple with skin	1 medium	3.5
		Banana	1 medium	2.4
		Cherries	10	1.2
		Cantaloupe	¼ melon	1.0
		Peach with skin	1	1.9
		Pear with skin	½	3.1
		Prunes	3	3.0
		Raisins	¼ cup	3.1
		Raspberries	½ cup	3.1
		Strawberries	1 cup	3.0
		Orange	1 medium	2.6
		Vegetables—cooked		
		Asparagus	½ cup	1.0
		Beans—green	½ cup	1.6
		Broccoli	½ cup	2.2
		Brussels sprouts	½ cup	2.3
		Cabbage	½ cup	2.0
		Potato—with skin	1 medium	2.5
		Spinach	½ cup	2.5
		Sweet potato	½ medium	1.7
		Zucchini	½ cup	1.8
		Vegetables—raw		
		Lettuce	1 cup	1.0
		Tomato	½ cup	1.1
		Celery	½ cup	1.1
		Cucumber	½ cup	0.4
		Mushrooms	½ cup	0.9
		Legumes		
		Baked beans	½ cup	8.8
		Peas—dried, cooked	½ cup	4.7

		Kidney beans—cooked	½ cup	7.3
		Lima beans—cooked	½ cup	4.5
		Lentils—cooked	½ cup	3.7
		Navy beans—cooked	½ cup	6.0

Nuts and seeds

		Almonds	10 nuts	1.1
		Peanuts	10 nuts	1.4
		Popcorn—air popped	1 cup	1.0

Bread and pasta

		Whole-wheat bread	1 slice	1.4
		Other breads	1 slice	1.0
		Bran muffin	1 medium	2.5
		Bagel	1 medium	0.6
		Rice—cooked	½ cup	1.0
		Pasta—cooked	½ cup	1.1

Breakfast cereals

		All bran with extra fiber (Kellogg's)	1 oz	14.0
		Fiber One (General Mills)	1 oz	12.0
		All Bran (Kellogg's)	1 oz	10.0
		100% Bran with oat bran (Nabisco)	1 oz	8.0
		Uncle Sams (U.S. Mills)	1 oz	8.0
		40% Bran type	1 oz	4.0
		Raisin bran type	1 oz	4.0
		Shredded wheat	1 oz	2.6
		Oatmeal—regular, quick, or instant	1 oz	1.6

Record your total fiber intake for the day, in the space provided below:

Name: _____

Date: _____

Total fiber intake: _____ g

If your total fiber intake is less than 25 g, look carefully at the foods containing fiber and suggest some additional foods you can eat to increase your intake to at least 25 g each day.

Estimation and Analysis of Daily Caloric Intake

The purpose of this Laboratory Experience is to analyze your caloric intake to determine the number of calories and the percentage of these calories that come from fat, carbohydrates, and protein.

Instructions

1. You must record everything that you eat and drink for 2 days—a weekday and a weekend day. Try to select typical days that will reflect your "true" eating habits. Simply fill out the first two columns for each day on each of the prepared sheets that are provided.

2. Consult the Food Exchange Lists (see Appendix A) to estimate how many of the exchanges each food item contains. (An example is given on p. 225 to show you how this is done.)

3. Consult Table 6-17 to determine the number of grams of fat, carbohydrate, and protein in each food. (If the food item does not appear on the exchange list, you may obtain this information from the food label, or you may need to consult Appendix B or a more complete table showing the nutritional content of foods.)

4. Total the values for the day so that you know exactly how many grams of carbohydrates, fat, and protein that you consumed.

5. Perform the calculations as shown on the Summary Sheet (see p. 225 and 226 for an example showing how to do this).

NAME _____

ANALYZING CALORIC INTAKE USING THE FOOD EXCHANGE LISTS _____

FOOD OR BEVERAGE	APPROXIMATE AMOUNT	NUMBER OF EXCHANGES													Carbohydrate* (g)	Protein* (g)	Fat* (g)
		Milk (skim)	Milk (low-fat)	Milk (whole)	Fruit	Vegetable	Starch/grains	Meat (lean)	Meat (medium fat)	Meat (high fat)	Fat	Sugar				
TOTALS																

*Information can be determined from exchange list information or can be obtained directly from food label.

SUMMARY SHEET—ESTIMATION OF CALORIES CONSUMED

	TOTAL GRAMS	×	CALORIES/GRAMS	=	CALORIES
Carbohydrates	_____	×	4	=	_____
Protein	_____	×	4	=	_____
Fat	_____	×	9	=	_____
TOTAL CALORIES					_____

% Carbohydrates $=$ $\dfrac{\text{Calories from carbohydrates}}{\text{Total calories}}$

$=$ _____

$=$ _____ %

% Protein $=$ $\dfrac{\text{Calories from protein}}{\text{Total calories}}$

$=$ _____

$=$ _____ %

% Fat $=$ $\dfrac{\text{Calories from fat}}{\text{Total calories}}$

$=$ _____

$=$ _____ %

ANALYZING CALORIC INTAKE USING THE FOOD EXCHANGE LISTS

NAME _____

FOOD OR BEVERAGE	APPROXIMATE AMOUNT	NUMBER OF EXCHANGES											Carbohydrate* (g)	Protein* (g)	Fat* (g)
		Milk (skim)	Milk (low-fat)	Milk (whole)	Fruit	Vegetable	Starch/grains	Meat (lean)	Meat (medium fat)	Meat (high fat)	Fat	Sugar			
TOTALS															

*Information can be determined from exchange list information or can be obtained directly from food label.

SUMMARY SHEET—ESTIMATION OF CALORIES CONSUMED _____

	TOTAL GRAMS	×	CALORIES/GRAMS	=	CALORIES
Carbohydrates	_____	×	4	=	_____
Protein	_____	×	4	=	_____
Fat	_____	×	9	=	_____
TOTAL CALORIES					_____

% Carbohydrates $\quad = \quad \dfrac{\text{Calories from carbohydrates}}{\text{Total calories}}$

$\qquad\qquad\qquad = \quad$ _____

$\qquad\qquad\qquad = \quad$ _____ %

% Protein $\quad = \quad \dfrac{\text{Calories from protein}}{\text{Total calories}}$

$\qquad\qquad = \quad$ _____

$\qquad\qquad = \quad$ _____ %

% Fat $\quad = \quad \dfrac{\text{Calories from fat}}{\text{Total calories}}$

$\qquad = \quad$ _____

$\qquad = \quad$ _____ %

Interpretation of results

You can now compare your total calories for each day to your RDA value (see Table 6-4). Remember the RDA value for calories is for those trying to maintain their present weight. If you are trying to lose weight you will need to subtract either 500 or 1000 calories from this value, depending on how much weight you are trying to lose. Record your scores in the spaces provided below.

Name: _____
Date: _____
Recommended daily caloric intake: _____ calories
Caloric intake day 1: _____ calories
Caloric intake day 2: _____ calories

Record the percentages of calories from carbohydrates, fats, and protein in the spaces provided below.

PERCENTAGE OF CALORIES	DAY 1	DAY 2	RECOMMENDED PERCENTAGE
Carbohydrates	_____	_____	>58%
Fats	_____	_____	<30%
Protein	_____	_____	>12%

You can also determine whether your total protein intake is adequate. Record the total number of grams of protein consumed each day in the space provided below and also record your calculated RDA values for protein (see p. 205).

Name: _____
Date: _____
Total protein intake:
    Day 1: _____ g
    Day 2: _____ g
RDA value for protein:
  RDA value is 0.8 g for each kg of body weight:
    = _____ g
If you exercise regularly for at least 30 minutes three times a week, you should probably multiply by 1.2 rather than 0.8.
    = _____ g

If your protein intake is more than or less than the appropriate value, you should suggest some additions, deletions, or substitutions you can make to your food intake.

Exercise and Body Composition

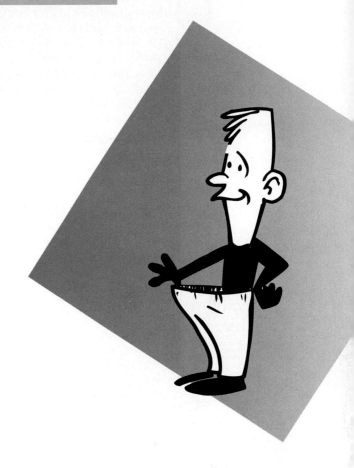

CHAPTER OBJECTIVES

When you understand the material in this chapter, you will be able to:

- Define the terms "obese" and "overweight," and know how to determine each of them
- Evaluate your body composition, and determine your ideal weight
- Discuss the disadvantages associated with excess body fat
- Determine your daily caloric expenditure, and be able to plan a weight-loss or weight-management program based on these results

- Explain the importance of exercise in a weight-loss program and determine how much exercise is necessary and at what intensity you must exercise if you are to be successful at losing weight
- Implement a successful exercise program for weight loss or weight management

239

One of the major health problems in the United States today relates to controlling body weight and/or body fat. A 1991 survey showed that only 22% of the American adult population considered their weight to be within an acceptable range; 64% indicated that they would like to weigh less, while 14% indicated that they would like to weigh more.

Each year billions of dollars are spent on diets, workshops, diet books, diet foods, and special weight-reduction programs. Despite all of this, it is interesting to note that in 1980 the average weight of the American adult was 14 pounds heavier than it was in 1970. Most people who try to control their weight fail because they are unable to incorporate a good exercise and a good nutritional program into their lifestyle.

Even though there is more leisure time available, many individuals are actually less active now than they were in previous years. This is partly because of the introduction of the home computer and video games and the expansion of cable television, which now features special channels for sports, music, and first-run movies. If the time now spent on these activities was previously spent on some form of active recreation, then there is a significant decrease in daily caloric expenditure.

The start of obesity or overweight problems for many people is associated with a decrease in physical activity. Professional or college athletes during training usually have very little trouble maintaining their weight, even though they eat all the food that they want to. Yet many athletes do not maintain their activity level or decrease their food intake when they retire and therefore experience a problem controlling their weight. This is a problem also encountered by many individuals when they finish college and go to work. If their job is sedentary or inactive, these people tend to be less active but usually continue to eat as much as ever. The result, of course, is that their weight increases very rapidly.

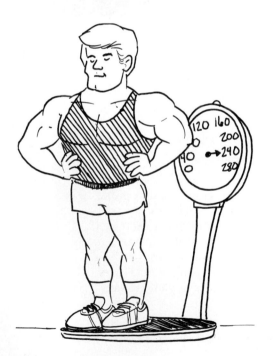

DEFINITION OF TERMS

It is important to differentiate clearly between the terms **overweight** and **obese.**

Overweight

An overweight person is one who weighs more than his or her **desirable weight.** A person's desirable weight has been defined as one at which he or she looks good, feels good, and can function efficiently. Originally, simple tables based on a person's height, age, and sex were used to determine desirable weight. In 1963 the Metropolitan Life Insurance Company introduced a new standard table based on different principles. The company recognized the undesirability of a continued increase in weight during adulthood past the termination of growth and realized at least in theory that people vary according to body build. Weight ranges were then presented for three classes of frame size—small, medium, and large. However, determination of the category in which each individual was to be classified was apparently left to the subjective judgment of the examiner; no criteria were presented for classification purposes.

The present method recommended for determination of frame size involves the measurement of elbow breadth (Fig. 7-1). To measure your elbow breadth, flex your forearm so that there is approximately a 90-degree angle at the elbow joint. Use a pair of calipers to measure the exact distance between the most prominent projection on either side of your elbow.

Elbow breadth: _____ inches

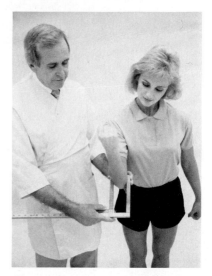

Fig. 7-1 Measurement of elbow breadth for determination of frame size.

The range of values presented in Table 7-1 can be used to determine your frame size. The values presented are for *medium* frame size for men and women. Note that they vary according to your height. If your score is within this range, you would be considered to be a medium frame size. If your score is greater than the score for your height and sex, you would be considered to have a large frame; if your score is lower, you would be considered to have a small frame size. The most recent tables available for determination of desirable weight are Tables 7-2 (men) and 7-3 (women).

Even though these height/weight tables are used extensively, they have some serious limitations.

- The method used for determination of frame size appears to be inadequate.
- The desirable range of weight for a particular height is very large. For example, the recommended weight for a 6-foot man ranges from 149-188 lb. Even for a particular frame size the range is very large (164 to 188 lb for this 6-foot man).
- These tables make no allowances for differences in the development of musculature among individuals. Most highly trained athletes, particularly football players, would be considerably overweight by these standards. However, if these athletes are examined more closely, this excess weight is seen to be caused by muscular development and their percentage of body fat is usually quite low. It is not uncommon to find professional football players who weigh 250 lb or more, with 12% body fat or less. It is not how heavy a person is that is important, but how much fat he or she has.

TABLE 7-1 **Determination of frame size**

Height (women)	Elbow breadth	Height (men)	Elbow breadth
<4'11"	2¼"-2½"	<5'3"	2½"-2⅞"
4'11"-5'2"	2¼"-2½"	5'3"-5'6"	2⅝"-2⅞"
5'3"-5'6"	2⅜"-2⅝"	5'7"-5'10"	2¾"-3"
5'7"-5'10"	2½"-2¾"	5'11"-6'6"	2¾"-3⅛"
<5'10"	2½"-2¾"	>6'2"	2⅞"-3¼"

TABLE 7-2 Metropolitan Life Insurance height/weight tables for men*

Height	Small frame	Medium frame	Large frame
5'2"	128-134	131-141	138-150
5'3"	130-136	133-143	140-153
5'4"	132-138	135-145	142-156
5'5"	134-140	137-148	144-160
5'6"	136-142	139-151	146-164
5'7"	138-145	142-154	149-168
5'8"	140-148	145-157	152-172
5'9"	142-151	148-160	155-176
5'10"	144-154	151-163	158-180
5'11"	146-157	154-166	161-184
6'0"	149-160	157-170	164-188
6'1"	152-164	160-174	168-192
6'2"	155-168	164-178	172-197
6'3"	158-172	167-182	176-202
6'4"	162-176	171-187	181-207

Data from Metropolitan Life Insurance Co.
*Weight is in pounds, with clothing weighing 5 lb; height is with shoes with 1-inch heels.

TABLE 7-3 Metropolitan Life Insurance height/weight tables for women*

Height	Small frame	Medium frame	Large frame
4'10"	102-111	109-121	118-131
4'11"	103-113	111-123	120-134
5'0"	104-115	113-126	122-137
5'1"	106-118	115-129	125-140
5'2"	108-121	118-132	128-143
5'3"	111-124	121-135	131-147
5'4"	114-127	124-138	134-151
5'5"	117-130	127-141	137-155
5'6"	120-133	130-144	140-159
5'7"	123-136	133-147	143-163
5'8"	126-139	136-150	146-167
5'9"	129-142	139-153	149-170
5'10"	132-145	142-156	152-173
5'11"	135-148	145-159	155-176
6'0"	138-151	148-162	158-179

Data from Metropolitan Life Insurance Co.
*Weight is in pounds, with clothing weighing 3 lb; height is with shoes with 1-inch heels.

Despite these disadvantages, these tables are still used frequently. The most frequently used standard to determine whether you are classified as overweight is 10%. If you weigh 10% or more above your desirable weight, you are considered to be overweight. The procedures that are used to determine this are included in Laboratory Experience 7-1.

Body mass index

The body mass index is another method that is widely used to evaluate your weight. It is based only on your height and weight, so it has the same limitations as the height/weight tables. The procedures to follow to determine your body mass index are given in Laboratory Experience 7-2.

Obese

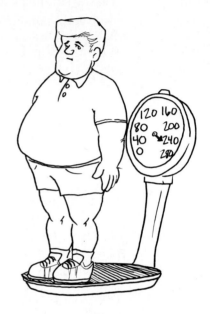

An obese person is one who has an excessive accumulation of *body fat.* This raises the question relating to how much fat you need to have to be considered obese. Unfortunately, there is no clear-cut answer. Instead, fatness should be considered to exist on a continuum, just like your level of aerobic fitness. Based on norms that are available, arbitrary standards are established to evaluate your scores. These norms for both males and females are included in Laboratory Experience 7-3.

Scores for **percentage of body fat** have continued to rise in recent years. In 1968 the average percentage of body fat for college-age students was 12% for men and 20% for women. By 1980 these figures had increased to 15% for men and 22% for women, and by 1990 these scores were 18% for men and 23% for women.

The terms "desirable" and "normal" should not be confused. Men wishing to attain a desirable amount of body fat for optimal health and fitness should probably strive for 12% or less; women should strive to be between 18% and 14%.

BODY COMPOSITION

The term ***body composition*** refers to the percentage of your body weight that is composed of fat in relation to that composed of fat-free tissue. Your fat-free weight is also referred to as your ***lean body weight***. It has been established that the real threat to good health is not total weight, but excess body fat.

Determination of percentage of body fat

It is important to be able to determine your body composition so that you can ascertain how much fat you have and what proportion of your body weight can be attributed to this. By knowing this, you will be able to determine more exactly how much you should weigh. Certainly, this procedure is much better than simply consulting the standard height/weight charts that have previously been discussed.

Your percentage of body fat may be determined by a variety of techniques. Perhaps the best method is to use the underwater weighing technique to determine body density and then use this figure to calculate your percentage of body fat and lean body weight. However, this technique is not practical for use with large groups of people and requires expensive equipment.

Several other approaches have been developed that attempt to estimate a person's percentage of body fat. The most common and possibly the most accurate method involves the use of **skinfold measurements,** provided the person who is taking the measurements is experienced and is able to take each measurement accurately.

Taking skinfold measurements

Taking skinfold measurements requires practice to obtain consistent results. The following are suggestions for measuring skinfold thickness:

- Firmly grasp the fold of the skin between the left thumb and forefinger, and pull the fold away from the body.
- Place the contact surfaces of the calipers approximately ½ inch from the tips of the fingers.
- The caliper should be held perpendicular to the skinfold by the right hand, with the skinfold dial up so that it can be read.
- Wait for approximately 2 seconds until the needle becomes relatively stable.
- Read the measurement to the nearest 0.5 mm.
- Three measurements should be taken at each site, with at least two of these measurements equal. If not, additional measurements must be made until consistency is obtained.
- All measurements should be made on the right side of the body.
- Marking each anatomical site with a black felt pen will enhance consistency.
- Measurements should not be taken when the skin is moist or through leotards or tights.
- Measurements should not be taken immediately after exercise or when the subject is overheated, because the shift in body fluid to the skin may increase the skinfold size.

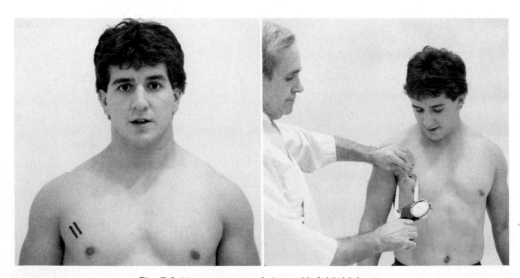

Fig. 7-2 Measurement of chest skinfold thickness.

- Practice is necessary to be able to grasp the same size skinfold consistently at the same location each time.

Skinfold sites

The following are descriptions of the locations for skinfold measurements:

1. *Chest.* Take a diagonal fold on the front of the chest. For *men* this should be midway between the right nipple and the front border of the armpit. For *women* this should be two thirds of the way from the right nipple to the front border of the armpit (Fig. 7-2).
2. *Subscapular.* Take a diagonal fold immediately below the interior angle of the scapula. The natural fold is away from the midline of the body downward (Fig. 7-3 on p. 247).
3. *Triceps.* Take a vertical fold at the back of the right arm, running parallel to the length of the arm, midway between the shoulder and the elbow joints. The arm should be hanging naturally at the side in a relaxed position (Fig. 7-4 on p. 248).
4. *Thigh.* Take a vertical fold on the front of the right thigh midway between the hip and knee joints. NOTE: It is often easier to take this measurement if the subject is seated with the knee slightly flexed, with weight not supported on that leg (Fig. 7-5 on p. 248).
5. *Abdominal.* Take a vertical fold approximately 1 inch to the right of the umbilicus (Fig. 7-6 on p. 249).
6. *Suprailiac.* Take a vertical fold at the front of the hips immediately above the crest of the ilium (Fig. 7-7 on p. 249).
7. *Midaxillary.* Take a vertical fold at the side of the body on the midaxillary line, level with the lower part of the sternum (Fig. 7-8 on p. 250).

There are many different regression equations available that use various combinations of these measurements. The most recent trend has been to use generalized equations that have been developed using large heterogenous samples and that include age as a variable. Five different formulas for men and five for women are summarized:

GENERALIZED BODY COMPOSITION EQUATIONS

Males

Seven-site formula

Body density = 1.11200000 − 0.00043499 (sum of seven skinfolds) + 0.00000055 (sum of seven skinfolds)^2 − 0.00028826 (age)

Measurements used—chest, midaxillary, triceps, subscapular, abdominal, suprailiac, thigh

Six-site formula

Percent body fat = 0.21661 (sum of six skinfolds) − 0.00029 (sum of six skinfolds)^2 + 0.13341 (age) − 5.72888

Measurements used—chest, thigh, suprailiac, abdominal, tricep, subscapular

---

Continued.

GENERALIZED BODY COMPOSITION EQUATIONS—cont'd

Four-site formula

Percent body fat = 0.27784 (sum of four skinfolds) − 0.00053 (sum of four skinfolds)^2 + 0.12437 (age) − 3.28791

Measurements used—chest, suprailiac, abdominal, madaxillary
Three-site formula

Body density = 1.1093800 − 0.0008267 (sum of three skinfolds) + 0.0000016 (sum of three skinfolds)^2 − 0.0002574 (age)

Measurements used—chest, abdominal, thigh
Three-site formula

Body density = 1.1125025 − 0.0013125 (sum of three skinfolds) + 0.0000055 × (sum of three skinfolds)^2 − 0.0002440 (age)

Measurements used—triceps, chest, subscapular

Females
Seven-site formula

Body density = 1.0970 - 0.00046971 (sum of seven skinfolds) + 0.00000056 (sum of seven skinfolds)^2 + 0.00012828 (age)

Measurements used—chest, thigh, triceps, subscapular, abdominal, suprailiac, midaxillary
Five-site formula

Percent body fat = 0.29731 (sum of five skinfolds) − 0.00053 (sum of five skinfolds)^2 + 0.03037 (age) − 0.63054

Measurements used—thigh, suprailiac, abdominal, triceps, subscapular
Three-site formula

Percent body fat = 0.41563 (sum of three skinfolds) − 0.00112 (sum of three skinfolds)^2 + 0.03661 (age) + 4.03653

Measurements used—triceps, abdominal, suprailiac
Three-site formula

Body density = 1.0994921 − 0.0009929 (sum of three skinfolds) + 0.0000023 (sum of three skinfolds)^2 − 0.0001392 (age)

Measurements used—triceps, suprailiac, thigh
Three-site formula

Body density = 1.089733 − 0.0009245 (sum of three skinfolds) + 0.0000025 (sum of three skinfolds)^2 − 0.0000979 (age)

Measurements used—triceps, suprailiac, abdominal

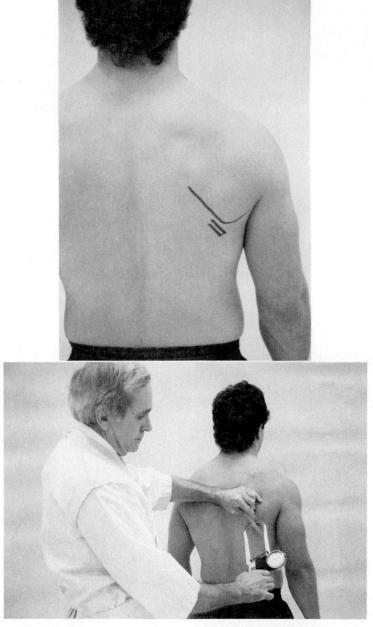

Fig. 7-3 Measurement of subscapular skinfold thickness.

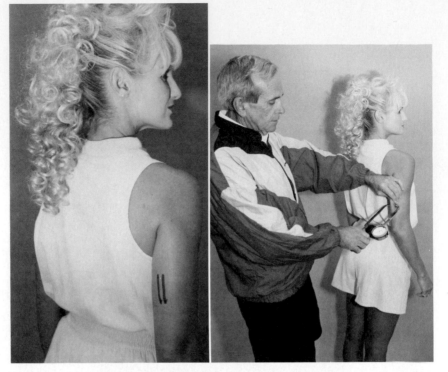

Fig. 7-4 Measurement of triceps skinfold thickness.

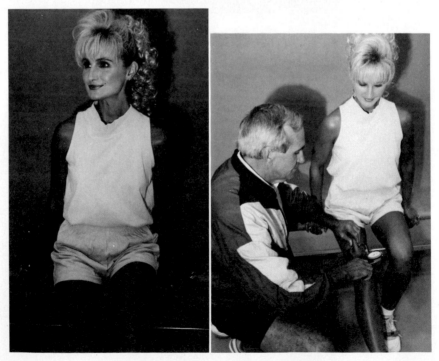

Fig. 7-5 Measurement of thigh skinfold thickness.

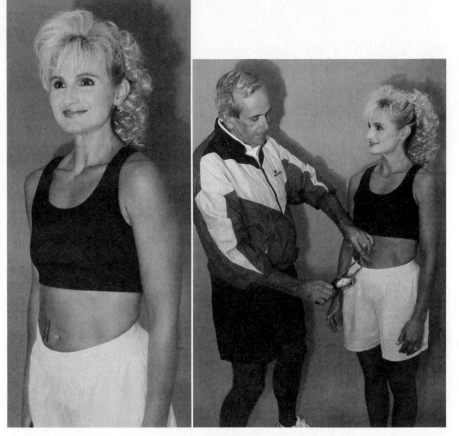

Fig. 7-6 **Measurement of abdominal skinfold thickness.**

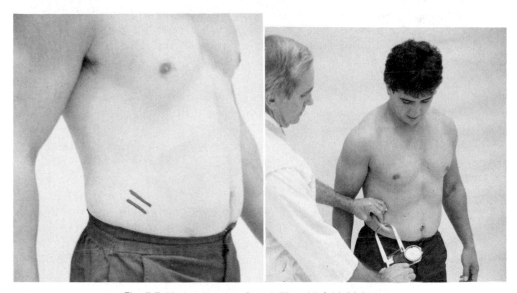

Fig. 7-7 **Measurement of suprailiac skinfold thickness.**

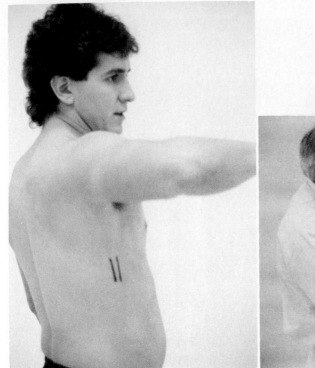
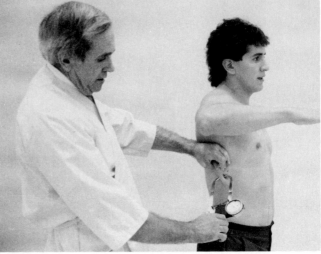

Fig. 7-8 Measurement of midaxillary skinfold thickness.

Note that some of the equations predict *percent body fat* directly, whereas others predict *body density*. With those which predict body density, either of the following equations can then be used to predict percent body fat from body density:

$$\text{Percent body fat} = [(4.57/\text{body density}) - 4.142] \times 100$$
$$\text{Percent body fat} = [(4.95/\text{body density}) - 4.50] \times 100$$

You can determine your percentage of body fat by completing Laboratory Experience 7-3.

DETERMINATION OF DESIRABLE WEIGHT

It is now possible to determine your desirable weight using your body weight and your existing percentage of body fat. This is probably the most accurate method available to determine what you should weigh.

The example given in the box on p. 251 is for a person weighing 180 lb with 21% body fat who wants to reduce his or her percentage of body fat to 12%.

DETERMINATION OF DESIRABLE WEIGHT

Step 1. Determine your body weight and percentage of body fat

Body weight	= 180 lb
Body fat	= 21%

Step 2. Calculate the weight attributable to fat

Fat weight	= 180×0.21
	= 37.8 lb

Step 3. Determine the existing lean body weight

Lean body weight	= Body weight − fat weight
	= 180 − 37.8
	= 142.2 lb

Step 4. Arbitrarily determine the desired percentage of body fat

Ideal percentage of body fat selected is 12%

Step 5. Calculate the desired body weight for 12% body fat

Desired weight	= Lean body weight/1 − desired % body fat
	= 142.2/1 − 0.12
	= 142.2/0.88
	= 162 lb (to the nearest pound)

This is what this 180-lb person should weigh if he or she is to decrease his or her percentage of body fat from 21% to 12%. This would be a realistic goal for this person. For those who have a very high percentage of body fat, a goal more realistic than 12% for men or 18% for women should be selected initially. For these people, a more realistic goal might be to reach the "average" percentage of body fat. These figures are 18% for men and 23% for women. You can determine your desirable weight by completing Laboratory Experience 7-4.

DISADVANTAGES OF EXCESS WEIGHT OR FAT

Many disadvantages are associated with an excess accumulation of weight or fat, including the following:

- There is an increased incidence of cardiovascular disease. Results from the Framingham study showed that obesity is independently related to an increased risk of coronary artery disease. The excess weight places additional stress on the heart, which now must work harder to perform the same amount of work. In addition, obesity is associated with other cardiovascular risk factors. For example, hypertension is found twice as frequently in those considered to be obese, and atherosclerosis is three times more prevalent in those who are overweight than in those whose weight is normal.
- Mortality at a younger age is higher in those who are obese or overweight, resulting in a decrease in life expectancy.

- An excess accumulation of fat, particularly in the legs, can impede the return of blood to the heart and can contribute to an increase in the incidence of varicose veins.
- Overweight and obese persons experience more problems with muscles and joints because the extra weight places additional stress on their joints. This is particularly evident in areas such as the knees, hips, and lower back. The incidence of low back pain is much higher in those who are obese.
- Obesity is associated with increased incidence of diabetes. The incidence of diabetes is three times higher in obese subjects compared with nonobese subjects.
- Blood cholesterol levels are much higher in obese subjects compared with subjects who are at their desirable weight.
- Obesity is associated with an increased incidence of other health problems, such as cirrhosis of the liver and various respiratory problems.
- It has been shown that those who are obese or overweight have more accidents, surgical complications, and complications during pregnancy. In addition, their exercise tolerance is reduced considerably.
- People who are overweight or obese are also at a social and economic disadvantage. Because of their reduced life expectancy, they must pay higher insurance premiums. They are also often discriminated against when applying for a job.

ENERGY BALANCE

Regardless of whether a person tries to control weight by diet or by exercise, the balance between food intake and energy expenditure is very important.

Neutral energy balance

A neutral energy balance exists when the caloric intake is equal to the caloric expenditure. Under these conditions the body weight should remain constant and should neither increase nor decrease by any appreciable amount.

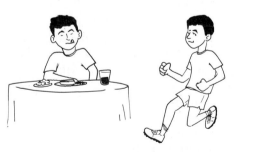

A neutral energy balance.

Positive energy balance

A positive energy balance exists when the caloric intake is greater than the caloric expenditure. The excess food is stored in the form of fat, and the body weight will increase.

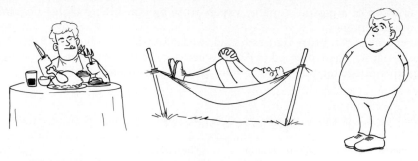

A positive energy balance.

Negative energy balance

With a negative energy balance, the number of calories used will be greater than the number of calories consumed. Stored fat will be used for energy, and the body fat and body weight should be reduced. It is obvious that exercise can make a significant contribution to weight loss if it is performed regularly and if it burns a significant number of calories.

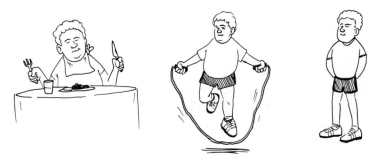

A negative energy balance.

EXERCISE AND ENERGY EXPENDITURE

The energy expenditure of each activity may be calculated by measuring the amount of oxygen used while performing the activity. There is a direct relationship between energy expenditure and oxygen consumption. It takes approximately 1 liter of oxygen to burn 5 calories. The amount of oxygen used by the body is obviously an important measurement, because it can be used to accurately determine your exact rate of caloric expenditure.

For example, if you exercise so that you use 4 L of oxygen per minute, you will use 4×5 — or 20 — calories for each minute of exercise. This is the equivalent of 1200 calories per hour, which is a very high rate of energy expenditure. Note that a 170-lb person would have to run at approximately 9 miles per hour to burn calories at this rate.

It is possible to determine the caloric expenditure for any activity by having a subject perform an activity for a given time and then measure the amount of oxygen used. This value can then be used to accurately determine the exact number of calories used in performing the task.

The energy expenditure for different tasks may vary according to the person's skill level, body weight, and other factors. However, it is possible to obtain a good approximation of a person's energy expenditure by consulting tables prepared from actual measurements.

The energy expenditure figures for selected activities are given in Table 7-4. Note that these figures are expressed in calories per minute per pound of body weight. The caloric expenditure for selected everyday tasks is presented in Table 7-5.

TABLE 7-4 **Energy expenditure for selected physical activities**

Physical activity	Calories/min/lb	Physical activity	Calories/min/lb
Aerobic dance		Racquetball	
Low	0.050	Beginner	0.050
Medium	0.060	Intermediate	0.065
High	0.070	Advanced	0.080
Archery	0.032	Running	
Badminton		Speed: Min/mile:	
Average skill	0.038	5 mph 12.0	0.070
High skill	0.065	6 mph 10.0	0.080
Baseball	0.032	7 mph 8.6	0.090
Basketball		8 mph 7.5	0.100
Half court	0.028	9 mph 6.7	0.110
Full court	0.060	10 mph 6	0.115
Bicycling		11 mph 5.5	0.131
Slow (5.5 mph)	0.025	Sailing	0.020
Moderate (10 mph)	0.050	Skating	
Fast (13 mph)	0.071	Moderate	0.040
Bowling	0.030	Vigorous	0.065
Calisthenics	0.033	Skiing	
Canoeing		Downhill	0.060
Slow (2.5 mph)	0.023	Snowshoeing (2.5 mph)	0.067
Fast (4.5 mph)	0.047	Soccer	0.063
Circuit training		Swimming (crawl stroke)	
Without weights	0.040	30 yards/min	0.045
With weights	0.053	50 yards/min	0.076
Cross-country skiing		Table tennis	0.030
Slow (3 mph)	0.055	Tennis	0.045
Medium (5 mph)	0.075	Touch football	0.060
Fast (7 mph)	0.095	Volleyball	0.030
Field hockey	0.060	Walking	
Fishing	0.016	2 mph	0.020
Golf	0.036	3 mph	0.028
Gymnastics		4 mph	0.042
Light	0.022	Water skiing	0.053
Heavy	0.056	Wrestling	0.060
Hill climbing	0.055		
Judo and karate	0.087		
Jumping rope			
Slow	0.068		
Medium	0.078		
Fast	0.088		

TABLE 7-5 Caloric expenditure for selected everyday tasks

Everyday tasks	Calories/min/lb
Sleeping	0.008
Lying quietly	0.009
Sitting eating, reading, mental work	0.011
Standing	0.012
Sitting, writing	0.012
Washing dishes	0.012
Cooking	0.013
Lecturing	0.014
Driving a car	0.015
Office work	0.016
Light housework	0.016
House painting	0.016
Shopping	0.018
Sweeping floors	0.023
Waiting on tables	0.024
Making a bed	0.027
Cleaning windows	0.028
Mowing lawn	0.028
Ironing	0.028
Gardening	0.032
Shovelling	0.043
Chopping wood	0.049

Caloric expenditure and body weight

The difference in the rate of caloric expenditure that is attributable to weight can be determined by taking the caloric expenditure figure and multiplying it by the body weight and the number of minutes of exercise.

EXAMPLE:

Subject 1. (150 lb) runs 5 miles in 60 minutes

Caloric expenditure $= 0.070 \times 150 \times 60$
$= 630$ calories/hr

Subject 2. (200 lb) runs 5 miles in 60 minutes

Caloric expenditure $= 0.070 \times 200 \times 60$
$= 840$ calories/hr

Note that the 200-lb person uses over 200 calories more than the 150-lb person does in performing the same task.

DAILY ENERGY EXPENDITURE

Your total energy expenditure is defined as the total number of calories you expend in a 24-hour day. To obtain a good estimation of your daily caloric expenditure, you will need to keep an accurate record of everything you do for an entire 24-hour period. Forms for this are included in Laboratory Experience 7-5.

Estimating your daily caloric expenditure

A completed form for recording each of your activities is presented in Table 7-6. Note that you simply record on this form the various activities that make up your day. You start each day at midnight and make your first entry when you wake up in the morning and get out of bed. The most accurate records can be kept if you "fill in" your recording sheet every 2 or 3 hours. At the end of the day, make sure that the total time adds up to 1440 minutes — the number of minutes in 1 day.

After each daily caloric expenditure form has been completed, you need to group some of the activities together and transfer them to the daily caloric expenditure summary form (Table 7-7). NOTE: If you do this for 3 days (2 weekdays and 1 weekend day) and average your figures for the 3 days, you will get a very accurate estimate of your daily caloric expenditure. You can determine your average daily caloric expenditure by completing Laboratory Experience 7-5.

Determining your caloric balance

To determine your caloric balance, you must also determine your caloric intake. To do this, you must keep a record of all the food you eat and everything you drink for a 24-hour period. If a more accurate evaluation is desired, this should be done for 3 days (2 weekdays and 1 weekend day), and the average for these 3 days can then be used. Information concerning this is presented in Chapter 6.

Exercise significantly affects your caloric expenditure

Many persons who are genuinely concerned with losing weight have concentrated only on counting the number of calories in the diet and have completely neglected exercise. Increasing the amount of physical activity can be just as important as decreasing the food intake. Exercise augments dieting in several ways.

- Exercise burns a substantial number of calories. For example, a 180-lb person who walks 5 miles will burn approximately 750 calories. If he or she were to do this five times per week, this would account for more than 1 lb of fat (3500 calories = 1 lb fat).
- Exercise tends to develop muscle tone and thus will contribute to the development of lean body mass while possibly reducing the amount of body fat.
- Exercise may suppress one's appetite, resulting in a reduction in caloric intake.
- Exercise increases the metabolic rate for some time after a vigorous workout, so extra calories continue to be burned during this time. Weight loss will result when a negative caloric balance exists (when the caloric intake is less than the caloric expenditure).

The following example shows the effect that regular exercise can have on the reduction of body weight:

Example:

Initial body weight	= 180 lb
Caloric intake	= 3200 calories/day
Caloric expenditure	= 3000 calories/day

TABLE 7-6 **Daily caloric expenditure form**

Name Freddie Fitness   Date 6/9/93

Starting time	Finishing time	Type of activity or task	Number of minutes
12:00 Midnight	6:30 AM	Sleeping	390
6:30 AM	7:00 AM	Showering, shaving, dressing	30
7:00 AM	7:30 AM	Sitting eating breakfast	30
7:30 AM	8:00 AM	Walking slowly to class	30
8:00 AM	12:00 Noon	Sitting in class	240
12:00 Noon	12:15 PM	Walking to cafeteria (slowly)	15
12:15 PM	12:45 PM	Sitting eating lunch	30
12:45 PM	1:00 PM	Walking to computer lab	15
1:00 PM	3:00 PM	Computer work (sitting)	120
3:00 PM	4:00 PM	Sitting in class	60
4:00 PM	4:15 PM	Walking to gym	15
4:15 PM	4:30 PM	Warming up before activity	15
4:30 PM	5:30 PM	Running (6 miles)	60
5:30 PM	6:00 PM	Showering	30
6:00 PM	6:30 PM	Eating dinner	30
6:30 PM	8:00 PM	Studying	90
8:00 PM	11:00 PM	Watching television	180
11:00 PM	12:00 Midnight	Sleeping	60

TOTAL   1440 minutes

TABLE 7-7 **Daily caloric expenditure summary form**

Name   Freddie Fitness

Date   6/9/93   Body weight   154   lb

Activity	Cal/min/lb	×	Total time (min)	×	Body weight (lb)	=	Calories used
Sleeping and lying quietly	0.008	×	450	×	154	=	554
Sitting (total all your activity you performed while sitting)	0.011	×	780	×	154	=	1321
Standing with little or no movement	0.013	×	60	×	154	=	120
Standing with light activity	0.015	×	0	×	154	=	0
Walking Slow (2 mph)	0.020	×	75	×	154	=	231
Fast (3 mph)	0.030	×	0	×	154	=	0
Other (specify all other activity)							
Running (6 mph)	0.080*	×	60	×	154	=	739
Warming-up	0.033*	×	15	×	154	=	76
(calisthenics)		×		×		=	
		×		×		=	
		×		×		=	
		×		×		=	
	TOTAL TIME		1440		TOTAL CALORIES USED		3041

*These values can be obtained by consulting Table 7-4 or Table 7-5.

This represents an initial positive balance of 200 calories per day. This might seem like an insignificant amount. It is equivalent to 12 French fries, less than 1½ cans of beer or soda, 2 oz of hamburger meat, 1 cup of potato chips, or six strips of bacon. However, in 6 months this small deficit will account for a weight gain of 10 lb, and this person will then weigh approximately 190 lb.

This person has several options to control and/or reduce his or her weight:

- Caloric intake can be reduced by 300 calories per day, while caloric expenditure remains the same. This would result in a weight loss of approximately 5 lb in 6 months, bringing the weight down to approximately 175 lb.
- Caloric intake could remain the same, and a 4-mile walk could be substituted for 1 hour normally spent sleeping 4 days per week. On the days of the walk, an additional 410 calories will be burned. This would account for a weight loss of approximately 6 lb in 6 months and a final weight of approximately 174 lb. Remember that this is actually a weight shift of 16 lb, because if this person does not make any changes, he or she will weigh 190 lb at the end of 6 months. Remember also that this weight change is achieved without reducing caloric intake.
- Caloric intake can be reduced by 200 calories per day while the moderate exercise program of walking 4 miles 4 days each week is incorporated. This program will result in a daily reduction of caloric intake and an increase in caloric expenditure 4 days per week. The net result will be a weight loss of almost 12 lb, bringing the weight down to 168 lb in 6 months.

This example emphasizes the importance of regular exercise in weight control. People must be concerned with the long-term effect of a small daily caloric deficit.

WEIGHT LOSS AND EXERCISE

The maximal rate at which weight should be lost is between 1 and 2 lb per week. To achieve this, you will need a daily caloric deficit of 500 calories for 1 lb per week or 1000 calories for 2 lb per week. Weekly goals need to be set, and if these are not met, then a further adjustment needs to be made in either caloric intake or caloric expenditure. The following example will help to illustrate the "long range" concept of weight control.

Example:

Present body weight	= 180 lb
Desired body weight	= 160 lb
Rate of weight loss	= 2 lb per week for the first 6 weeks, then 1 lb per week

This plan can be summarized as follows:

Week	Date	Target body weight
1	Jan 7	178
2	Jan 14	176
3	Jan 21	174
4	Jan 28	172
5	Feb 3	170
6	Feb 10	168
7	Feb 17	167
8	Feb 24	166

Week	Date	Target body weight
9	Mar 3	165
10	Mar 10	164
11	Mar 17	163
12	Mar 24	162
13	Mar 31	161
14	Apr 7	160

It will take this person 14 weeks to reach the desired goal. If this person were to start on January 1, by April 7 he or she will have achieved the goal, if he or she has the determination to adhere regularly to the program.

Most people have no problem achieving the goals for the first few weeks, and frequently they lose more than they have to during this time. This often tempts them to get off their diet or skip their exercise, and before they know it they are right back where they started. It takes determination, hard work, and discipline to complete a program such as the one illustrated. However, the end results are very rewarding.

How much exercise do you need for weight loss?

If your main objective for exercise is to lose weight, you will probably have to do more than the 20 to 30 minutes that was recommended, 3 to 5 times per week, for the development of aerobic fitness. This is usually insufficient for a person trying to lose weight. The following case study will show you why.

CASE STUDY: JOE

Joe weighed 180 lb and had put on 10 lb during each of the last 2 years. He decided that not only did he not want to gain any more weight, but that he wanted to lose the extra weight that he had accumulated. He decided to start an exercise program where he walked 2 miles, 3 days each week. After 3 months he had lost no weight, and he visited my office to find out what he was doing wrong.

I see a large number of people just like Joe who are unsuccessful because they do not know how to plan their exercise program to achieve their desired results. There is a logical explanation as to why Joe did not lose any weight, despite the fact that he exercised very regularly for 3 months.

To gain 10 lb in a year, you average 100 more calories that you take in, compared with what you use each day. This means that each week Joe had a positive caloric balance of 700 calories. Walking 2 miles burns approximately 240 calories for a person who weighs 180 lb. So, for the 3 days of exercise that Joe decided to do each week, he burned approximately 720 calories more than he would have if he had not exercised. This was only enough exercise to "balance out" the extra 700 calories he was "taking in," and he will see little or no change in his body weight unless he is willing to change his eating habits or else exercise for a longer period of time.

I have found that those who are successful at losing weight and/or body fat are those who make a commitment to exercise continuously for 45 minutes, five times each week.

EXERCISING AT THE RIGHT LEVEL IS IMPORTANT IF YOU ARE TO LOSE FAT

When trying to lose fat, your exercise goal should be to work longer, not harder. It is now well established that low to moderate heart rates are more effective for burning fat than are high heart rates. The reason for this is that carbohydrates—glycogen—can provide energy more efficiently than does fat. When you force your body to work at a high intensity it will use mainly carbohydrates and very little fat. Most of us make a major shift in our metabolism when our exercise intensity is such that our heart rate exceeds 80% of our maximum. Keeping your heart rate below this value will ensure maximum burning of fat.

STARTING A SUCCESSFUL EXERCISE PROGRAM AND STICKING WITH IT

Research shows that over 60% of adults who start an exercise program drop out within the first month. Some of these dropouts try again, but most of them soon quit again. This high drop out rate is unfortunate. There are many who drop out simply because they are misinformed. They think that exercise takes too much time and effort and that it is boring and very inconvenient. This is not necessarily true.

It is important to realize that exercise will take time and effort and will involve discipline and determination. However, it does not mean that it cannot be enjoyable, and you will probably discover that you do not have to work as hard as you thought you would. The old "no pain, no gain" philosophy has been replaced with "gain without pain." Initiating a successful weight-management/exercise program and sticking with it involves several steps. These are as follows:

1. You need to make a commitment to exercise

The first step in beginning an exercise program is to make a commitment that exercise is important to you. Consistency is very important. The most successful participants in our weight-management programs are those who find a way to ensure that they get their 5 days of exercise every week, whereas those who are not as successful come up with excuses as to why they are unable to exercise as frequently as they need to. I see many clients who are frequently out of town on business. Some of them use this as an excuse not to exercise. These people are rarely successful at controlling their weight.

Over 95% of freshmen entering college indicate that exercise is important to them, and yet less than 35% exercise at least three times each week. If exercise is important to you, you will do something about it and find a way to make sure that you exercise regularly.

2. Schedule exercise into your everyday routine

To achieve your specific objectives, you must participate on a regular basis. Those who wait until they "find" time to exercise do not exercise very frequently. If you believe strongly enough in exercise, you will make time available on a regular basis and exercise will become a habit. There is no reason that you cannot schedule exercise each day just like you schedule other activities. What I would suggest is that at the beginning of each week, you look at your schedule for the week. Look carefully at what major commitments you have for the week. You should then tentatively decide which 5 days would be most convenient for you to exercise, and you should mark these days in your schedule book. Each night before you go to bed, look at your schedule for the next day. If it is a day that you had planned to exercise and you now have a very busy schedule, you may have to get up an hour earlier than you normally would if you are to "find" time to exercise.

3. Be patient and start slowly

It is important to start out slowly, to be patient, and not to expect too much too soon. The first few weeks are very important. It is during this time that a large number of people become disheartened and give up. It should be emphasized that you cannot start out at too low a level. It has probably taken you a long time to get out of shape and gain those extra pounds of fat. It will take you more than a few weeks to get back in shape and to lose the extra weight that you have. You need patience and determination.

Moderation is the key as far as how much exercise you need to start with. Too much, too soon may lead to excessive muscle soreness and will increase the chance of musculoskeletal injuries.

4. Determine personal goals

You can waste much time and effort if you do not establish specific goals for your program. These goals should be based on your individual needs. Your goals need to be realistic and you need to allow a reasonable amount of time to achieve them so that you can experience some degree of success. Losing 20 lb in a month or running 10 miles in an hour are unrealistic goals for most people. A realistic goal for you might be to average five exercise sessions for 15 consecutive weeks and accumulate from 12 to 16 miles per week by walking at an intensity sufficient to maintain your heart rate in the desired target zone. Another realistic goal might be to average 20 miles per week walking and to reduce your caloric intake so that in 12 weeks you will lose 15 pounds. You need to determine goals that are important to you, that are realistic, and that will require discipline, determination, and effort.

5. Be willing to work

In any field of endeavor, the people who are the most successful are those who work hard at it. The familiar phrase "I know I should but . . ." is not part of a winner's vocabulary. It has been stated that "man is the architect of his own destiny." You must believe that this is true when it comes to controlling your body weight. Regular exercise is very important if this is to occur.

Many people who do not exercise use the excuse that they just do not have enough energy. You should not let the grind of your daily routine keep you from exercising. Regular exercise will actually increase your energy level and enable you to be more productive in your everyday tasks. You should feel refreshed after a good workout. If you are completely exhausted and have no energy left, in all likelihood you are doing too much or you are working at a higher intensity than what you should be working at.

6. Monitor your progress

It is important to monitor your progress on a regular basis. You can do this by keeping a record of your workouts. This enables you to chart your progress and can be used to establish the success of your program. Keep track of such things as the number of exercise sessions each week, the total miles accumulated, the calories burned, and changes in body weight. Many different computer programs are available that can be used on home computers for this purpose. A sample printout from an exercise logging program is included in Chapter 11 so that you can see samples of the type of information that these programs provide for you.

MISCONCEPTIONS ABOUT WEIGHT CONTROL

Until recent years the role of exercise in weight-control programs has been minimized. The reason for this appears to be that many persons lack sufficient knowledge about the relationship between exercise and weight control. Many of the basic misconceptions that exist are discussed briefly.

Misconception 1: Exercise burns relatively few calories and therefore makes an insignificant contribution to changing the energy balance

Everyone has heard from time to time that it takes several hours of golf or tennis or some other activity to lose 1 lb of fat. The actual figures for several of these activities for a 170-lb person are summarized in Table 7-8.

These figures, although correct, are very misleading. As shown in the previous sections, a difference of only 200 calories per day will make a difference in body weight of 10 lb in 6 months. The activity does not have to be performed continuously nor does the heart rate have to reach the target zone as it does for cardiovascular endurance. The following will help to again emphasize the role that exercise can play in weight control:

Example:

A person who weighs 170 lb decides to substitute 1 hour of tennis for 1 hour of watching television.

Calories burned playing tennis for 1 hour
(tennis requires 0.045 calories/min/lb)

$$= 170 \times 0.045 \times 60$$
$$= 459$$

Calories that would have been spent watching television
(when you sit you burn 0.008 calories/min/lb)

$$= 170 \times 0.008 \times 60$$
$$= 81$$

Extra calories burned

$$= 459 - 81$$
$$= 378$$

If this person were to play tennis four times per week for 6 months, this would account for 39,312 extra calories being burned. This is the equivalent of just over 11 lb of fat. A reduction in body weight of 11 lb in 6 months might seem like an insignificant value; however, it must be remembered that this is obtained without reducing the caloric intake.

TABLE 7-8 Caloric expenditure and weight control for certain activities for a 170-lb man

Activity	Calories/hr	Hours to lose 1 lb of fat
Walking (3 mph)	285	12.28
Basketball	612	5.72
Volleyball	306	11.44
Golf	367	9.54
Tennis	459	7.63

Misconception 2: An increase in physical activity will automatically result in an increase in the amount of food eaten

This statement is definitely false for the average person who exercises up to 1 hour per day. Laboratory tests using rats have shown that when the amount of exercise performed is moderate, from 20 minutes to 1 hour, the food intake does not increase—in fact, it actually decreases. These results are presented in Fig. 7-9. Not only was there a decrease in the daily caloric intake, but there was also a decrease in body weight. With long periods of sustained activity, the food intake did increase; however, the weight remained constant at this optimal level, since the extra activity balanced out the extra caloric intake.

Mayer also was able to obtain similar results working with adults. This study was conducted in India, where it was possible to adequately control many relevant factors. The results of this study are presented in Fig. 7-10. These results indicate that light and medium work result in a decrease in caloric intake and in body weight and that heavy and very heavy work result in an increase in caloric intake but that the body weight remains constant.

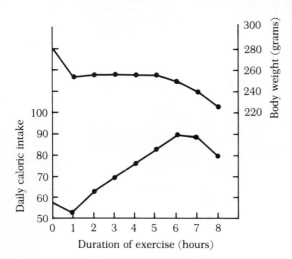

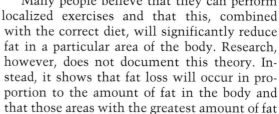

Fig. 7-9 Relationship between food intake, energy expenditure, and body weight. (Modified from Mayer J: *Overweight: causes, cost and control,* Englewood Cliffs, NJ, 1968, Prentice Hall.)

Misconception 3: Exercise can be used to reduce fat from a specific area of the body

Many people believe that they can perform localized exercises and that this, combined with the correct diet, will significantly reduce fat in a particular area of the body. Research, however, does not document this theory. Instead, it shows that fat loss will occur in proportion to the amount of fat in the body and that those areas with the greatest amount of fat will lose more than will the areas where there is less fat.

There appear to be five areas in the body where the majority of the fat accumulates: triceps, subscapular, suprailiac, abdominal, and thigh. These specific areas have been described previously. In women the two most troublesome areas are usually the triceps and the thighs; in men the highest concentration of fat usually occurs in the abdominal area.

Exercise is an important part of weight reduction, because if it is performed regularly, it will use a substantial number of calories and help to prevent loss of lean body weight. However, regardless of the amount or kind of exercise for any specific body part, it will not reduce the fat in that particular area. It should be noted that it may increase muscular development in the specific area and may result in a shift or change in body fluids. These factors may considerably enhance the appearance but will not significantly reduce the amount of fat in that particular area.

Misconception 4: Saunas and steam baths are effective for losing weight

You *do* lose weight through sweating when you take a sauna or steam bath. However, this is only a temporary weight loss; the fluid will quickly be replaced, and your

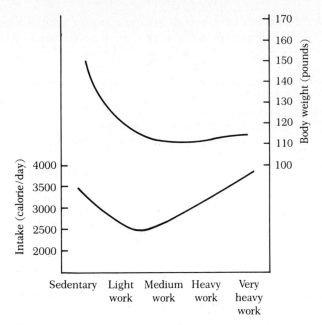

Fig. 7-10 Body weight and caloric intake as related to physical activity in humans. (Modified from Mayer J: *Overweight: causes, cost and control,* Englewood Cliffs, NJ, 1968, Prentice Hall.)

weight will return to its original level. No permanent weight loss results from saunas and steam baths. They are, however, useful for relaxation.

Misconception 5: Passive exercise machines can be used to reduce body weight

Many people think that they can get a machine that will exercise for them and reduce body fat. An example of this type of device is the electrically powered exercycle. You turn it on, and all you have to do is sit on it and let it do all the work. Many health clubs and spas have similar devices, such as vibrators, rollers, and whirlpools. None of these assist in the reduction of body fat or in the shifting of fat deposits from one area to another.

SUMMARY

The following summary will help you to identify some of the important concepts covered in this chapter:

- Obesity is one of the major health problems in America—many people have a hard time achieving and maintaining a desirable body weight and an optimal level of body fat.
- The term "overweight" refers to excess weight, whereas "obese" refers to excess fat.
- To accurately determine your desirable weight, you need to know your percentage of body fat.
- Regular exercise can positively affect your caloric balance, if you exercise for 45 minutes, 5 days each week.
- Exercising at the right intensity is important if you are going to burn fat.
- Exercise of up to an hour per day will not usually result in an increase in the amount of food that you eat.

- Exercises for a specific area of your body are not effective for reducing fat in that particular area. Continuous aerobic exercise at a low intensity must be used to lose fat.

KEY TERMS

body composition   The percentage of your body weight that is composed of fat in relation to that classified as fat free.

caloric expenditure   The total calories for all activities performed over a given time.

caloric intake   The caloric content of all food that is ingested.

desirable weight   The weight at which a person looks good, feels good, and functions efficiently.

lean body weight   The total amount of body weight that is not attributed to body fat.

negative energy balance   The number of calories consumed is less than the number of calories used, resulting in a loss of body weight or body fat.

neutral energy balance   When the caloric intake and caloric expenditure are approximately equal, and body weight remains relatively constant.

obese   An excessive accumulation of body fat.

overweight   When a person weighs 10% or more than his or her desirable weight.

percent body fat   The percentage of the total body weight that is attributable to fat.

positive energy balance   The caloric intake is greater than the caloric expenditure, resulting in an increase in body weight.

skinfold measurement   The measurement of fat at a particular site using skinfold calipers.

REFERENCES

1. Allsen PE, Harrison JM, and Vance B: *Fitness for life: an individualized approach*, ed 3, Dubuque, Ia, 1984, WC Brown.
2. Althoff SA, Svoboda M, and Girdano DA: *Choices in health and fitness for life*, ed 2, Scottsdale, Ariz, 1992, Gorsuch, Scarisbrick.
3. Cooper KH: *The aerobics program for total well being*, New York, 1982, M Evans & Co.
4. Getchell B: *Physical fitness: a way of life*, ed 3, New York, 1983, Macmillan.
5. Golding LA, Myers CR, and Sinning WE: *The Y's way to physical fitness*, ed 2, Chicago, 1982, National Board of YMCA.
6. Hoeger WWK: *Principles and laboratories for physical fitness and wellness*, ed 2, Englewood, Colo, 1991, Morton.
7. Jackson AS, Pollock ML: Practical assessment of body composition, *Physician and Sports Medicine* 13(5):76, 1985.
8. Jackson AS, Pollock ML: Prediction accuracy of body density, lean body weight and total body volume equations, *Medicine and Science in Sports and Exercise* 9(4):197, 1977.
9. Jackson AS, Pollock ML, and Ward A: Generalized equations for predicting body density of women, *Medicine and Science in Sports and Exercise* 12(2):175-182, 1980.
10. Jackson AS, Ross RM: *Understanding exercise for health and fitness*, Houston, Tex, 1986, Mac J-R Publishing CSI Software.
11. Katch FI, McArdle WD: *Nutrition, weight control and exercise*, ed 3, Philadelphia, 1988, Lea & Febiger.
12. Kuntzleman CT: Aerobic shopping, *The Runner*, p. 96, Nov. 1981.
13. McArdle WD, Katch FI, and Katch VL: *Exercise physiology, energy, nutrition and human performance*, ed 3, Philadelphia, 1991, Lea & Febiger.
14. McLarin M: *Weight loss and nutrition*, San Diego, Calif, 1986, Health Media of America.
15. Nieman DC: *Fitness and sports medicine—an introduction*, Palo Alto, Calif, 1990, Bull Publishing.
16. *Physical activity and weight control*, Ottowa, Canada, 1979, Minister of Supply and Services.
17. Prentice WE: *Fitness for college and life*, ed 3, St Louis, 1991, Mosby–Year Book.
18. Sinning W: Use and misuse of anthropometric estimates of body composition, *Journal of Health, Physical Education and Recreation* 51:43, Feb 1980.
19. Svoboda M: Addressing weight management in physical education, *Journal of Health, Physical Education and Recreation*, 51:49, Feb 1980.

Determination of Percentage Overweight

Name _____   Date _____

Complete the following steps to determine what percentage you are overweight or underweight. (Refer to the example at the end of this section if you need help.)

1. Record your actual weight to the nearest pound.
   Weight _____ lb

2. Determine your frame size from your elbow breadth.
   Elbow breadth _____ inches
   Frame size (see Table 7-1) _____

3. Consult Table 7-2 *(men)* or 7-3 *(women)* to determine the range for your desired weight.
   From _____ to _____ lb

4. Determine the midpoint of this range. This figure will be referred to as your desired weight.
   Desired weight _____ lb

5. Determine the difference between your desired weight and your actual weight.
   Difference = Actual weight – desired weight
   = _____ – _____
   = _____ lb

6. Divide this difference by your desired weight to determine the percentage you are overweight or underweight.

   Percentage overweight
   or underweight   = _____ / _____
   = _____
   (indicate + or –)

Interpretation of score

If you are more than 10% above your desirable weight, you would be classified as overweight.

EXAMPLE:

Name: Joe Jock
Height: 70 inches
Weight: 180 lb
Frame Size: Medium
   Desired weight range
   (From Table 7-2)   = 151-163 lb
   Midpoint   = 157 lb
   Difference   = Actual weight – desired weight
   = 180 – 157
   = +23 lb
   Percentage overweight   = 23/157
   = 0.15
   = 15%

Evaluation of Weight Using the Body Mass Index

Your body mass index is calculated as follows (an example is given below if you need help):

1. Record your name, height, and weight in the spaces provided below:
   Name _____
   Height _____ inches
   Weight _____ lb

2. Convert your height to meters by dividing by 39.4 (1 meter = 39.4 inches)
   Height   = Height/39.4
   (meters)   (inches)

                = _____ /39.4
                = _____ meters (correct this to two decimal places)

3. Convert your weight to kilograms by dividing your weight in pounds by 2.2
   Weight (kg)   = Weight (lb)/2.2
                 = _____ /2.2
                 = _____ kg

4. Calculate your body mass index (BMI)
   BMI   = Weight (kg)/Height (meters)^2
                 = _____ / (_____ × _____)
                 = _____ / _____
                 = _____

Interpretation of score

You can interpret your score as follows:
   <20   Below normal weight
   20-25   Normal weight
   25-30   Overweight
   >30   Extremely overweight

EXAMPLE:

   Name: Joe Jock
   Height: 70 inches
   Weight: 180 lb

1. Height (meters) = 70/39.4
                    = 1.78
2. Weight (kg)   = 180/2.2
                    = 81.82 kg
3. BMI   = 81.82/(1.78)^2
                    = 81.82/3.17
                    = 25.81

Determination of Percentage of Body Fat

Name _____

Date _____

Record your skinfold measurements in the spaces provided below:

MEASUREMENT	SCORE (MM)
Chest	_____
Subscapular	_____
Triceps	_____
Thigh	_____
Abdominal	_____
Suprailiac	_____
Midaxillary	_____

You can calculate your percentage of body fat using one of the formulas on pp. 245 and 246, or you can use the nomogram from Fig. 7-11 on p. 270. To use this nomogram you must use the three specific measurements as indicated for males and for females. Take the total of these three measurements, draw a straight line from this value to your age, and read off the percentage from the appropriate place.

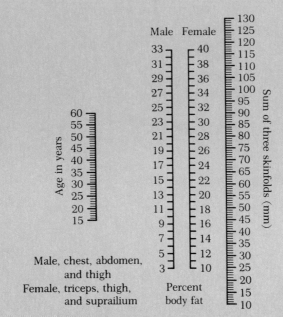

Fig. 7-11 Nomogram for determination of percentage of body fat using age and three designated skinfold measurements.

Record your percentage of body fat in the space provided below:

Name: _____

Date: _____

Percentage of body fat: _____

Interpretation of scores

The norms for percentage of body fat and for each of the skinfold measurements are presented in Table 7-9 (men) and Table 7-10 (women). Circle each of your scores on the appropriate chart. You will be able to evaluate your total percentage of body fat, and you will also be able to see how this fat is distributed.

Ideal percentages are 12% or less for men and 18% to 14% for women. If you achieve these values, all your scores should be in the "good" or "excellent" categories and you should be happy with your distribution of fat.

TABLE 7-9 Norms for percent body fat and for skinfold measurements *(men)*

Category	Percent body fat	Chest	Subscapular	Triceps	Thigh	Abdominal	Suprailiac	Mid-axillary
Excellent	6	2	3	2	4	6	2	5
	7	3	4	3	5	7	3	6
	8	4	5	4	6	8	4	7
	9	5	6	5	7	9	5	8
	10	6	7	6	8	10	6	
		7	8		9	11	7	
		8						
Good	11	9	9	7	10	12	8	9
	12	10	10	8	11	13	9	10
	13	11	11	9	12	14	10	11
	14	12	12	10	13	15	11	12
	15		13			16	12	13
								14
Average	16	13	14	11	14	17	13	15
	17	14	15	12	15	18	14	16
	18	15	16	13	16	19	15	17
	19	16	17	14	17	20	16	18
	20	17	18	15	18	21	17	19
	21	18	19		19	22	18	20
		19			20	23	19	21
						24	20	
						25		
						26		
Fair	22	20	20	16	21	27	21	22
	23	21	21	17	22	28	22	23
	24	22	22	18	23	29	23	24
	25	23	23	19	24	30	24	25
		24			25	31	25	26
						32	26	
						33		
						34		
Poor	26	25	25	20	25	35	27	27
	27	26	26	21	26	36	28	28
	28	27	27	22	27	37	29	29
	29	28	28	23	28	38	30	30
	30	29	29	24	29	39	31	31
	31	30	30	25	30	40	32	32
	32	31	31		31			
		32	32		32			

TABLE 7-10 Norms for percent body fat and for skinfold measurements (women)

Category	Percent body fat	Chest	Subscapular	Triceps	Thigh	Abdominal	Suprailiac	Mid-axillary
Excellent	11	3	3	5	12	6	3	5
	12	4	4	6	13	7	4	6
	13	5	5	7	14	8	5	7
	14	6	6	8	15	9	6	8
	15	7	7	9	16	10	7	
				10		11		
						12		
Good	16	8	8	11	17	13	8	9
	17	9	9	12	18	14	9	10
	18	10	10	13	19	15	10	11
	19	11	11	14	20	16	11	12
	20	12			21	17	12	13
					22	18		
Average	21	13	12	15	23	19	13	14
	22	14	13	16	24	20	14	15
	23	15	14	17	25	21	15	16
	24	16	15	18	26	22	16	17
	25	17	16	19	27	23	17	18
	26	18	17	20	28	24	18	19
		19			29	25	19	
					30	26		
					31			
Fair	27	20	18	21	32	27	20	20
	28	21	19	22	33	28	21	21
	29	22	20	23	34	29	22	22
	30	23	21	24	35	30	23	23
	31		22	25	36	31	24	24
					37	32		
Poor	31	24	22	25	38	33	25	25
	32	25	23	26	39	34	26	26
	33	26	24	27	40	35	27	27
	34	27	25	28	41	36	28	28
	35	28	26	29	42	37	29	29
	36	29	27	30	43	38	30	30
	37	30	28	31	44	39	31	31
	38	31	29			40	32	32

Determination of Desirable Weight

NOTE: Refer to the example given on p. 251.

Name _____

Date _____

Step 1. Determine your body weight and percentage of body fat

Body weight   = _____ lb
Body fat   = _____ %

Step 2. Calculate the weight attributable to fat

Fat weight   = body weight × percentage of body fat
                   = _____ × _____
                   = _____ lb

Step 3. Determine the existing lean body weight

Lean body weight   = Body weight − fat weight
                   = _____ − _____
                   = _____ lb

Step 4. Arbitrarily determine the desired percentage of body fat

Ideal percentage of body fat selected is _____ %

Step 5. Calculate the desired body weight for this percentage of body fat

Desired weight   = Lean body weight/1 − desired % body fat
                   = _____ /1 − _____
                   = _____ / _____
                   = _____ lb (to the nearest pound)

Determination of daily caloric expenditure

Refer to the example given on p. 251 for additional instructions and help. You need to record your activities for 2 days—a weekday and a weekend day. Try to select "typical" days. Start each day at midnight and make sure that the total time for each day adds up to 1440 minutes—the number of minutes in 1 day. Record these activities on Tables 7-11 and 7-12.

After each daily caloric expenditure form has been completed, you need to group some of the activities together and transfer them to the daily caloric expenditure summary forms (Tables 7-13 and 7-14). The example presented previously on p. 258 may help you in calculating your values.

TABLE 7-11 Daily caloric expenditure form

Name _____   Date _____

Starting time	Finishing time	Type of activity or task	Number of minutes

TOTAL   1440 minutes

TABLE 7-12 **Daily caloric expenditure form**

Name _____ Date _____

Starting time	Finishing time	Type of activity or task	Number of minutes

TOTAL 1440 minutes

TABLE 7-13 Daily caloric expenditure summary form

Name _____

Date _____ Body weight _____ lb

Activity	Cal/min/lb	×	Total time (min)	×	Body weight (lb)	=	Calories used
Sleeping and lying quietly	0.008	×	_____	×	_____	=	_____
Sitting (total all your activity you performed while sitting)	0.011	×	_____	×	_____	=	_____
Standing with little or no movement	0.013	×	_____	×	_____	=	_____
Standing with light activity	0.015	×	_____	×	_____	=	_____
Walking Slow (2 mph)	0.020	×	_____	×	_____	=	_____
Fast (3 mph)	0.030	×	_____	×	_____	=	_____
Other (specify all other activity)							
_____	_____	×	_____	×	_____	=	_____
_____	_____	×	_____	×	_____	=	_____
_____	_____	×	_____	×	_____	=	_____
_____	_____	×	_____	×	_____	=	_____
_____	_____	×	_____	×	_____	=	_____
_____	_____	×	_____	×	_____	=	_____
	TOTAL TIME		1440		TOTAL CALORIES USED		[____]

TABLE 7-14 **Daily caloric expenditure summary form**

Name _____

Date _____   Body weight _____ lb

Activity	Cal/min/lb	×	Total time (min)	×	Body weight (lb)	=	Calories used
Sleeping and lying quietly	0.008	×	_____	×	_____	=	_____
Sitting (total all your activity you performed while sitting)	0.011	×	_____	×	_____	=	_____
Standing with little or no movement	0.013	×	_____	×	_____	=	_____
Standing with light activity	0.015	×	_____	×	_____	=	_____
Walking Slow (2 mph)	0.020	×	_____	×	_____	=	_____
Fast (3 mph)	0.030	×	_____	×	_____	=	_____
Other (specify all other activity)							
_____	_____	×	_____	×	_____	=	_____
_____	_____	×	_____	×	_____	=	_____
_____	_____	×	_____	×	_____	=	_____
_____	_____	×	_____	×	_____	=	_____
_____	_____	×	_____	×	_____	=	_____
_____	_____	×	_____	×	_____	=	_____
	TOTAL TIME		1440		TOTAL CALORIES USED		

Weight Management

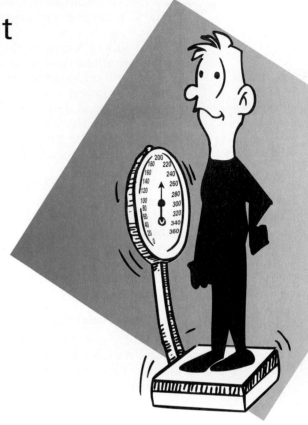

CHAPTER OBJECTIVES

When you understand the material in this chapter, you will be able to:

■ Explain why very few people who use "dieting" as a means to lose weight are successful at losing the weight and keeping it off

■ List the problems associated with very low-calorie diets

■ Identify specific objectives you would like to achieve, and know how to achieve these objectives

■ Identify five positive outcomes associated with eating regularly throughout the day

■ Explain why those people who skip breakfast are more likely to accumulate body fat than those who eat a nutritious breakfast

■ Explain why an adequate amount of both carbohydrates and proteins are an essential part of a good breakfast

■ Evaluate the consistency of your eating and exercise habits, and know what changes you need to make

■ List the 11 guidelines that are essential to any successful weight-management program

L osing weight has become an obsession for a large percentage of the American population. Following is a listing of some statements that have appeared in different books, magazines, and journals during the last several years. Whether they are 100% accurate is not important. They reflect the situation that exists in this country.

- Almost 90% of Americans think that they weigh too much.
- Sixty-five million Americans are presently on one type of diet or another.
- Twenty million Americans are spending an estimated $1 billion annually on liquid diets and programs.
- Americans spend almost $5 billion each year in an attempt to lose weight.
- Each year, Americans spend over $200 million on over-the-counter drugs that contain caffeine and amphetamine-related compounds.
- The sale of low-calorie frozen foods has increased 15% each year for the past several years.
- Of American women, 16% consider themselves to be perpetual dieters.
- From age 25, the average American woman gains almost 1½ lb of fat each year.

It is obvious that despite this obsession, the majority of the people have not been successful at losing the excess weight and/or fat and keeping it off.

WHY DIETS FAIL

It has become clear in recent years that dieting is not the answer. There are several reasons for this.

Most diets restrict your caloric intake so that your metabolism slows down

For many years most people have been told that if they want to lose weight, they must limit the amount of food that they eat and select foods that are low in calories. However, most experts now agree that drastically reducing your calorie intake can significantly slow down your metabolism, which is counterproductive to losing weight.

It is theorized that our bodies have a built-in mechanism—sometimes referred to as your set point—that drives your body to maintain a certain amount of body fat. When you restrict your caloric intake, your body will attempt to compensate by "slowing down" to conserve the amount of body fat that you have. One study showed that when caloric intake was severely restricted, the resting metabolic rate was reduced by almost 45%.

If you are a female and eating less than 1200 calories per day, or a male and eating less than 1500 calories per day, it is likely that such a low caloric intake will have a negative effect on your resting metabolic rate, making continuous weight loss difficult, if not impossible. Most college students can eat a much larger number of calories than this and still be successful at losing weight.

Dieting usually results in depression, which is counterproductive to losing weight

For many people, dieting becomes an antisocial event. People give up friends and meals and, in many cases, give up eating out, because they are afraid that they might eat something that they are not supposed to eat. This usually results in depression and anxiety, which frequently sets the stage for overeating as people turn to food for comfort. Those who diet will be constantly losing weight and gaining it right back again.

Most diets do not encourage permanent lifestyle changes

Good eating habits require a lifetime commitment, otherwise they will result in temporary changes. As your weight goes up and down, this creates definite health problems and may have a negative effect on your metabolism.

There are many weight-loss programs available that involve preplanned "packaged" foods. These programs will usually result in significant weight loss, because the meals are carefully planned and the portion sizes relatively small. However, it does not make sense to eat "packaged" food for the rest of your life, and in many cases when people who have been on these programs start to make their own choices and buy food from the grocery store, they start to regain the lost weight. In many of these programs an attempt is made to "educate" clients while they are in the program about what constitutes good eating. However, it does not make sense to tell people this is how you are supposed to eat and then have them eat preplanned "packaged" foods. One of the major reasons that they do this is that they make most of their money from the sale of their "packaged" food.

With low-calorie diets, weight lost is usually lean body weight

Several studies show that in weight-loss programs where the caloric intake is severely restricted, a large percentage of the weight lost is lean body weight. Many of those who participate in such programs do not have a weight problem, but they have large amounts of excess fat. I frequently evaluate many females who weigh less than 130 lbs and who have over 30% body fat, and I see a significant number of men who weigh less than 180 lbs who have 25% body fat or more. You do not necessarily have to weigh a lot to be obese. In many of these cases the problem is caused by not eating sufficient calories each day.

CRITERIA ASSOCIATED WITH A GOOD WEIGHT-LOSS PROGRAM

With society's current obsession for thinness, together with concerns about the effects of obesity on health, the number of weight-loss programs and associated services has increased tremendously during recent years. Many of these programs are very expensive, and it is often very difficult to evaluate them and decide which program might be best for you. The following criteria might be helpful to you in evaluating your options.

A successful weight-management program should do the following:

- Encourage you to adopt permanent lifestyle habits that you can live with for the rest of your life
- Teach you how to select and prepare the foods that you eat, and how to control the portion sizes
- Teach you how to set reasonable goals, and show you how to achieve these goals
- Not restrict your caloric intake to the extent that you are constantly hungry and/or craving for certain foods
- Not result in your being consistently lacking in energy throughout the day
- Advocate regular aerobic exercise, and teach you how to design a program based on your specific needs

- Promote a realistic weight loss of 1 or 2 lb per week
- Promote eating a variety of foods
- Teach you to identify and modify the behavior patterns that may be contributing to your weight problem
- Encourage you to take personal responsibility for the everyday decisions that you make relative to your exercise and eating habits

GETTING STARTED AND BEING SUCCESSFUL

For you to develop new lifestyle habits relative to exercise and nutrition, you need to learn how to make the right choices each day. These choices relate to when you eat, what you eat, how much you eat, and whether you exercise. You must realize that the choices you make each day relative to each of these will determine how successful you will be at achieving your goals. The following suggestions may be helpful to you in getting started.

Step 1. You must have a positive mental attitude and believe in your ability to succeed

It is extremely important that you believe in yourself. It does not make sense for you not to be able to control your exercise and eating habits. if you believe in yourself, you will be much more likely to try harder and stick with your program. You will handle success and failure much better and should experience less stress. The material in this chapter will show you what you need to do if you are to be successful, but you must believe that this is important and that by implementing these changes each day in your lifestyle you can be successful.

Step 2. You need to learn how to set realistic objectives

You need to learn how to set realistic objectives, making sure that you allow yourself a reasonable amount of time to achieve these objectives. Much time and effort can be wasted unless objectives are established and unless these objectives are organized into specific tangible goals with priorities. These objectives should be based on your individual needs. Do not expect too much too soon.

Many weight-reduction programs concentrate simply on how much weight you need to lose. The material in the previous chapter showed you that losing fat is more important than losing weight. However, because it is much easier to monitor changes in weight, losing weight is usually the most important objective for most participants in a weight-management program. A number of important objectives are identified on the next page.

If one of your objectives is to lose weight, it is very important that you plan to lose this weight slowly and gradually. This is the most effective way to keep it off. Research shows that 95% of all the people who lose weight quickly on low-calorie diets gain most of it, or all of it, back—usually within the first year.

Often when you lose weight rapidly, the majority of the weight loss is caused by a change in your fluid balance or, if you are on a very low-calorie diet, a large percentage of the weight lost will be lean body weight. Most people who weigh more than they would like to are trying to reduce their weight by losing *fat*. With most quick weight-loss programs, this does not occur.

Most experts agree that the maximum rate for weight loss should be 1 to 2 lb each week. A constant 2-lb weight loss each week is very difficult for the majority of those trying to lose weight and is very hard to achieve even for those who are extremely overweight or obese to begin with. It is also important to realize that weight will usually come off faster at first and that you will find it more difficult to lose the closer you get to your goal weight. This is usually because as you weigh less, you use fewer calories performing the same everyday tasks.

POSSIBLE OVERALL OBJECTIVES OF A GOOD WEIGHT-MANAGEMENT PROGRAM

Check off each of the following objectives that you are interested in achieving. I would like to:

- Reduce my body weight
- Have less body fat
- Have more energy throughout the day
- Look and feel better
- Increase my level of aerobic fitness
- Lower my cholesterol level
- Learn how to eat well
- Reduce my chances of cardiovascular disease
- Develop consistent exercise habits
- Reduce my level of stress

Step 3. You need to implement a plan to achieve your objectives

Not only do you need to know where you are going, but you must have a plan as to how to get there. It is important to establish a step-by-step approach that is systematic and carefully designed. It is helpful if it is in writing, so that you can constantly evaluate this plan, update it if necessary, and modify it if it does not work for you. It is important to remember that you must be patient rather than wanting everything at once.

This plan must include specific objectives each week that you will attempt to achieve that will contribute to your being successful at achieving your overall objectives. As these objectives regularly become part of your daily lifestyle, you can add new objectives. You need to work *constantly* at achieving each of these objectives, rather than working with concentrated spurts of energy.

To establish specific objectives, you need first to carefully evaluate your existing eating habits to determine which habits need to be changed and you will then need to develop specific strategies for changing these behaviors. You can evaluate your existing habits by completing Laboratory Experiences 8-1 and 8-2.

At this time, having evaluated your existing habits, you should now attempt to establish some specific objectives relative to your exercise and eating habits. The questions included at the end of Laboratory Experience 8-2 should provide clues to you as to some of the changes you need to make. Use Table 8-1 to list your objectives. Each day that you are successful at achieving each objective on your list, place a check

TABLE 8-1 **Weekly objectives relative to exercise and eating habits**

NAME _____   WEEK COMMENCING _____

List your specific objectives for the week. Place a check next to each objective each day that you successfully achieve it.

    √ = successful at achieving the objective

    x = failed to achieve the objective

Specific objective	Date	Sun	Mon	Tue	Wed	Thu	Fri	Sat
1. _____ _____ _____		—	—	—	—	—	—	—
2. _____ _____ _____		—	—	—	—	—	—	—
3. _____ _____ _____		—	—	—	—	—	—	—
4. _____ _____ _____		—	—	—	—	—	—	—
5. _____ _____ _____		—	—	—	—	—	—	—
6. _____ _____ _____		—	—	—	—	—	—	—
7. _____ _____ _____		—	—	—	—	—	—	—
8. _____ _____ _____		—	—	—	—	—	—	—

mark in the appropriate place. At the end of each day and the end of each week, you can then evaluate how consistent you have been. If your weekly goals have been carefully determined and you meet these consistently, you will be moving in a positive direction toward your overall objectives.

Later in this chapter you will find a weekly self-evaluation form. This includes 11 guidelines that I have found are very important in any weight-management/exercise program. A simple scoring system is included, so that you can evaluate yourself each week and determine more precisely the consistency of your eating and exercise habits.

Step 4. You need to work hard at achieving each of your objectives

In any field of endeavor, those who are the most successful are those who work the hardest. You must be willing to work hard each day at achieving each of your objectives. The familiar phrase "I know I should have, but . . ." is not part of a winner's vocabulary. If you want something bad enough, you will find a way to achieve it. Motivation must come from within.

Step 5. You need to stick with your program

More than 60% of those who start a weight-management/exercise program drop out within the first month. It is important that you learn to be patient. It will take you time to get to where you want to be, and it certainly will involve lots of hard work and discipline. However, the benefits will far outweigh the effort spent. If you implement the steps outlined in this chapter, you will be much more likely to stick with your program.

One way to increase your motivation is to monitor your progress. For some people, changes will show up almost immediately in terms of weight loss. However, simply measuring your body weight may be very misleading, particularly if you are exercising more. If you have not exercised regularly for some time and you become a very consistent exerciser, you are likely to develop muscle tone at the same time that you start to lose fat. This may result in very little, if any, change in your body weight at first, but you should soon begin to notice that your clothes start to fit more loosely. This is a positive sign.

You must also realize that for women during the menstrual cycle, there will be changes in body weight because of excess fluid retention. Also, the amount of carbohydrates and sodium that you eat each day can cause daily fluctuations in your fluid balance that are reflected in your body weight.

The thing to remember is that if you continue to make better choices relative to your eating habits and if you exercise regularly to the extent advocated for weight loss in the previous chapter, your body fat should gradually decrease and these changes will eventually show up on the scales. You should also notice many other positive changes as a result of your new lifestyle. You should have more energy so that you do not become tired so easily, and you should not be constantly hungry throughout the day and be craving for certain foods.

DIETARY GOALS AND GUIDELINES

Three separate publications have been released in recent years in an attempt to encourage good eating habits. These are listed below:
1. Dietary Guidelines for Americans—Published by the U.S. Department of Agriculture and the U.S. Department of Health and Human Services, 1985
2. Dietary Goals for the United States—Published by the Senate Select Committee on Nutrition and Human Needs, U.S. Government Printing Office, Washington, D.C., 1985
3. The Surgeon General's Report on Nutrition and Health—Published by the U.S. Department of Health and Human Services, Washington, D.C., 1989

These provide general guidelines relative to what we should and should not be eating. For example, we now know that if we are to be successful, we need to do the following:
- Avoid too much fat, saturated fat, and cholesterol
- Eat more fruits, vegetables, and grain products

- Limit our intake of sodium and salt
- Reduce our consumption of simple refined sugar

There are two basic problems associated with these guidelines. The average person does not know how much is too much, and he or she does not really know how to implement these recommendations. For example, how do you know how many servings of fruits, vegetables, and grain products you need to eat, and what constitutes a serving? It is also obvious that these guidelines do not focus on the issue of "when to eat." When you eat your meals is probably just as important as what you eat.

THE IMPORTANCE OF EATING REGULARLY

Each day you decide how often you are going to eat and when you will eat. The decisions you make as to what time of the day you eat and in relation to how you space your meals throughout the day can significantly affect how much you will weigh and how much fat you will accumulate.

A large number of people who are overweight or obese suffer from the same problem. It is often referred to as "nighttime eating syndrome." It is defined as an eating pattern where the majority of the calories for the day are eaten in either one or two meals, with a large number of these calories often eaten late in the day.

CASE STUDY: MARY

Mary is a regular exerciser who walks 3 or 4 miles at least 4 days each week. She either skips breakfast each day, or else breakfast consists of coffee and a bran muffin. If she eats lunch, it usually consists of half of a bagel, a small green salad, or a piece of fruit. She usually eats nothing during the afternoon, despite the fact that she feels tired and is usually lacking in energy.

By early evening she is famished and feels that she can reward herself by eating and/or drinking just about anything. Snacking often gets out of control, and she frequently consumes several alcoholic drinks that she feels she deserves, since she has eaten so little during the day. She then eats a large evening meal that is usually high in fat, and she will often continue snacking until late into the evening.

Because she eats so many of her calories late in the day, when she wakes up in the morning she does not feel like eating anything for breakfast and she will repeat the same cycle over and over.

Mary does not have a weight problem, but despite the fact that she has been exercising consistently for several years, she has been unable to reduce the excess fat that she would like to get rid of.

When we eat more frequently, we are more likely to make better choices

In today's world, particularly with all the fast foods readily available, we can get a large number of calories in a small volume of food that can be eaten very quickly. For example, a cheeseburger, French fries, and a chocolate milkshake—which can be eaten in less than 10 minutes—supplies over 1500 calories. A meal such as this is high in fat and sodium and contains very little, if any, fiber.

Because a meal such as this contains so many calories, many of us tend to eat less frequently throughout the day. In fact, a recent national survey showed that only 39% of Americans eat the traditional three meals each day. What many of us need to do is to adopt a more natural eating pattern, where we eat smaller meals more frequently. By doing this, we are more likely to eat more fruits, vegetables, and grain products and fewer animal products, which are usually high in fat.

When you eat only one or two meals each day, snacking often gets out of control and you frequently make poor choices about what you eat.

Eating more frequently reduces the amount of insulin produced by the body

When you eat several small meals throughout the day instead of one or two larger meals, your body will actually produce less insulin. A recent study showed that when two groups followed the exact same diet, those who consumed their calories over several small meals during the day produced significantly less insulin, as compared with those who ate the traditional three meals. Insulin production was 28% lower in those who ate several small meals spaced regularly throughout the day. For those who eat only one or two meals each day, the amount of insulin produced is likely to be even higher. The reason is that insulin is responsible for fat storage and production of fat in the body. The less frequently you eat, the larger the meal is likely to be and the amount of food eaten will usually be greater than what your body can use at that time. When this happens, your body will produce more insulin than normal in an attempt to store the excess calories as fat.

This is nothing new. We have known for some time that those who eat less frequently tend to accumulate more fat. During the last 10 years, over 80% of the people I have tested for body composition who have had a serious fat problem have had poor eating habits relative to when they eat and/or how frequently they eat. Skipping meals is not the answer for those who are trying to reduce their percentage of body fat.

Insulin production affects your appetite

You are much more likely to control your appetite if you eat more frequently, particularly if the meals and snacks are planned in advance. The reason for this again relates to the amount of insulin produced by the body.

Increased levels of insulin production in the body quickly result in a decrease in your blood glucose level. When your blood glucose falls to a low level, you will usually feel tired and hungry and will want to eat again.

Those who eat frequently do a better job maintaining a constant blood glucose level, and by eating before they get too hungry, they will not get to where they are famished and want to eat anything or everything in sight. They will usually be less likely to crave sweets and/or fats. Maintaining a constant blood glucose level within normal limits also allows you to concentrate better, particularly during the late afternoon hours. You should therefore be more productive as a result of this.

Long lapses of time between meals can distort your appetite. You may find that you actually consume more calories in the one or two meals that you eat than you would have had you eaten three or four planned meals.

Skipping meals may also affect your metabolism

Your metabolic rate determines the rate at which your body burns calories. If your metabolism slows down, you will burn calories at a slower rate and a greater amount of the calories consumed will be stored as fat. Increasing the number of meals that you eat each day—particularly if they are high in protein, complex carbohydrates, and fiber—has been shown to increase certain hormones in your body that increase your metabolism. Conversely, we have known for some time that skipping meals is likely to result in a reduction in your metabolic rate.

Eating more frequently can increase your energy level

Skipping meals can significantly reduce your energy level. Including nutritious snacks between meals can increase your energy level. This is extremely important if you exercise late in the day. If you do a good job of scheduling your meals and snacks throughout the day, you should have more energy and not feel as tired at the end of the day.

BREAKFAST: THE MOST IMPORTANT MEAL OF THE DAY

Each day millions of Americans rush out the door without eating breakfast, thinking that by not eating they are saving calories and that this will contribute to weight loss. This is just not so.

It is now well established that breakfast is the most important meal of the day. Despite this, a recent national survey showed that less than 50% of the population reported eating breakfast each day. People who did not eat breakfast were asked why they did not eat breakfast; the following are the three most common responses:
- "I am on a diet and I want to save calories."
- "I just do not have the time."
- "I am not hungry in the morning."

It is now clear that calories eaten during the day are more likely to be used for energy and that those eaten late in the day are more likely to be stored as fat.

Breakfast affects your metabolism

One reason that breakfast is important is that it can positively influence your metabolism. When you wake up in the morning, your body is in a slow fasting state, with your metabolic rate very low. If you do not eat breakfast, your body will not only remain at a low level but will slow down even further. Studies have shown that those who do not eat breakfast have metabolic rates below normal. One reason for this is that each meal that we eat increases the rate at which we burn calories. This is referred to as the *thermic effect of food.* If you eat just one large meal each day, you will actually burn fewer calories than does someone who eats the same amount of food spread over three meals.

Many breakfast foods are low in fat

Those who skip breakfast and eat only one or two meals each day are much more likely to consume a higher percentage of their calories from fat. The reason for this is that there are so many foods that are available for breakfast that contain very little fat, whereas many of the foods that traditionally are eaten later in the day contain large amounts of fat. Cereal, skim milk, and fruit are traditional breakfast foods that contain practically no fat. Of course, if you eat bacon, eggs, and hash browns for break-fast, your fat intake will be extremely high.

Importance of carbohydrates

It is important that your breakfast each day contain an adequate amount of carbo-hydrates. Each day carbohydrates are needed to supply energy. The body can store a limited amount of carbohydrates in the form of glycogen in the muscles and in the liver. You can usually store approximately 1500 calories of carbohydrates in the form of glycogen in your body. If you do not eat breakfast, your carbohydrate stores are likely to be depleted and this will greatly reduce the amount of energy that you will have throughout the day. This is particularly true if you also skip lunch. One of the most frequent comments that I get from the participants in our weight-management classes who start eating breakfast is that "I can't believe how much more energy I now have throughout the day since I have started eating breakfast."

It is also important to keep in mind that you need an adequate intake of carbohy-drates to metabolize fat efficiently. When you skip breakfast, your body will metabo-lize fat less efficiently. This is another reason that those who skip breakfast are much more likely to accumulate more fat, compared with those who eat a nutritious break-fast each day.

Importance of protein

Protein performs a variety of functions in your body, and yet your body does not store protein for use in the body like it stores fats and carbohydrates. For this reason it is important to make sure that you eat foods containing an adequate amount of pro-tein at regular intervals throughout the day.

When you skip breakfast (or one of the other meals), your body will continue to function, but because you get no protein coming into your body, you will force your body to "use" its own protein to perform the important functions that protein per-forms in your body. Your body will usually use protein from your muscle tissue, which is most readily available. This will often then result in an "imbalance" be-tween the amount of fat and muscle in your body. This also explains why very low-calorie diets often result in loss of a significant amount of lean body weight. With a very low caloric intake, it is almost impossible to get the necessary amount of protein that your body needs and your body will use part of its own protein to perform the functions that are necessary in your body. A full glass of milk (preferably skim milk or 1% milk) and a bowl of cereal provide approximately 12 g of protein. This would appear to be an adequate amount of protein for the average person to consume for breakfast. A breakfast containing a piece of fruit, a glass of juice, or a slice of toast with coffee is insufficient in terms of the amount of protein that you need.

Making healthful choices

Making healthful choices is important when deciding what to eat for breakfast. A good breakfast should contain an adequate amount of complex carbohydrates and pro-tein and be very low in fat. Because many of the traditional breakfast foods are very low in fat, your total fat intake for breakfast should be well below the maximum daily recommendation of 30% if you make wise choices.

Four different breakfast plans are included where the total calories are close to 300 and where the percentage of calories from fat is 20% or less.

Breakfast plan #1: Cereal, milk, and fruit

Item	Serving size	Calories
Skim milk	1 cup	90
Cereal		
All Bran	$1/3$ cup ($1/2$ oz)	45
Bran flakes	$1/2$ cup (1 oz)	70
Banana	1 medium	110
TOTAL CALORIES		315

	Grams	Percent of total calories
Protein	15	19
Carbohydrates	59	75
Fat	2	6

Breakfast plan #2: Egg, muffin, and milk

Item	Serving size	Calories
English muffin	1	140
Jelly	1 tbsp	60
Poached egg	1	80
Skim milk	$1/2$ cup	40
TOTAL CALORIES		320

	Grams	Percent of total calories
Protein	15	19
Carbohydrates	49	61
Fat	7	20

Breakfast plan #3: Grapefruit, pancakes, and milk

Item	Serving size	Calories
Grapefruit	$1/2$	30
Pancakes	2	140
Syrup	1 tbsp	50
Skim milk	$1/2$ cup	40
TOTAL CALORIES		260

	Grams	Percent of total calories
Protein	15	15
Carbohydrates	59	75
Fat	2	6

Breakfast plan #4: Bagel, fruit, and milk

Item	Serving size	Calories
Bagel	1	170
Cream cheese	2 tsp	30
Banana	$1/2$ medium	55
Skim milk	$1/2$ cup	40
TOTAL CALORIES		295

	Grams	Percent of total calories
Protein	11	15
Carbohydrates	52	70
Fat	5	15

Because of the importance of protein, each of the four breakfast plans includes milk. Skim milk or 1% milk provides many nutrients and contains very little fat. If you have lactose intolerance or simply do not like milk or yogurt, it is difficult to get the necessary protein for breakfast without getting a lot of fat with it. One solution is to take a protein supplement and mix it with juice and fruit.

If you are not careful, you may find that you are getting as much as half of your calories for the day in one meal, with 50% or more of these calories coming from fat. Following is a typical high-fat breakfast:

Typical high-fat breakfast

Item	Serving size	Calories
Orange juice	1 cup	106
Bacon	3 slices	120
Eggs—fried	2	160
Hash-brown potatoes	1 cup	340
Toast	2 slices	140
Jelly	2 tbsp	120
Butter	2 tbsp	210
Coffee	1 cup	0
Cream—Half & Half	2 tbsp	40
TOTAL CALORIES		1236

	Grams	Percent of total calories
Protein	28	9
Carbohydrates	124	40
Fat	70	51

It may surprise you that this meal contains over 1200 calories, with 51% of these calories coming from fat. It is impossible to be successful with a weight-management program if you are eating this many calories in one meal with such a high percentage of the calories coming from fat.

PUTTING IT ALL TOGETHER: THE 11 GUIDELINES

The importance of the choices that you make each day relative to when you eat, what you eat, how much you eat, and whether to exercise have been discussed previously. The *consistency* with which you make wise choices concerning each of these will basically determine how successful you will be in your weight-management/exercise program.

This weight-management/exercise program is based on 11 specific guidelines that you can use each day to evaluate the consistency of your eating and exercise habits. These guidelines are identified in this chapter, and the importance of each of them is briefly described. Detailed information relative to each of these guidelines has been presented at various places throughout this text.

1. Eat a nutritious breakfast within an hour of waking up

You have probably been told time and time again that "breakfast is the most important meal of the day." This is certainly true if you are trying to lose weight and reduce your body fat. By eating a nutritious breakfast each day, you can positively influence your metabolism, you will have more energy throughout the day, and you will be much more likely to control your snacking throughout the day. A good breakfast must provide an adequate amount of protein and carbohydrates. It is important to eat as soon as you can when you get up in the morning, because your metabolism is low and the food will help to increase your metabolism.

2. Eat at least three planned meals spaced regularly throughout the day

When you eat frequently throughout the day, your metabolism will increase and you will burn more calories than you would have if you had eaten only one or two meals during the day. Skipping meals contributes to an increase in the amount of stored fat in your body. If you plan your meals you will also be much more likely to make better choices about what to eat and will probably find it easier to control how much you eat. Long lapses of time between meals can distort your hunger, and you will often find that when you do eat you will eat more calories in one or two meals than you would if you had eaten three or four planned meals.

3. Eat your evening meal as early as possible

When you eat your evening meal is very important, particularly if it is your biggest meal of the day—which is the case for most people. Eating a large amount of food late in the day is likely to result in more of these calories being stored as fat in your body. The reason for this is that we are usually much less active during the evening hours. There are very few ways you can "use" many of these calories.

4. Drink water frequently throughout the day

This is one concept that just about every weight-loss program agrees on. This is necessary if you are to maintain a normal fluid balance in your body and if your body is to metabolize fat efficiently. By drinking water frequently throughout the day, you will also find it easier to control the amount of calories that you consume. Remember that water is the only fluid that you can drink that contains no calories.

5. If you drink alcoholic beverages, limit your intake

The secret to eating well is to get all the nutrients that you need each day without getting excess calories and without gaining excess weight or fat. Alcohol provides a considerable number of calories with little or no nutritional value. These calories are often referred to as "empty calories." For this reason even moderate drinkers need to drink less if they are overweight or have excess fat. Excessive consumption of alcohol is frequently associated with nutritional deficiencies and may contribute to several serious diseases. It can result in loss of appetite, poor food intake, and impaired absorption of nutrients.

6. Limit your between-meal snacks to low-calorie, nonfat, or low-fat foods

Snacking can be good for you, provided that you plan your snacks and make sensible choices about what you eat. Snacking can be bad if it is not planned and you eat impulsively, because the foods that you will usually choose will be very low in nutritional value and/or very high in fat and/or sugar. You need to learn which foods you can eat regularly and which foods you need to eat sparingly.

7. Limit your intake of simple refined sugars

Similar to alcohol, simple sugars provide calories but few other nutrients. Also, in most cases the more simple sugars you eat, the more you crave. For these reasons it is important that your intake of simple sugars be kept to a minimum.

8. Limit your intake of sodium and salt

Excessive sodium or salt may be hazardous to your health and is likely to create an imbalance in your fluid balance and contribute to an increase in your blood pressure. Since most Americans consume much more sodium than is needed, you should learn how to use less table salt and you need to read food labels carefully, so that you can limit your intake of those foods which contain large amounts of sodium.

9. Limit the amount of fat that you eat each day

If you are to be successful at reducing your body weight and percentage of body fat, you must learn how to limit your fat intake. Not only does fat provide more than twice as many calories as protein or carbohydrate, but we now know that those people who eat more fat accumulate more fat in specific areas of their body. With all the new low-fat and nonfat products now available, it is much easier to reduce the amount of fat that you eat each day.

10. Increase your intake of dietary fiber

Fiber is one of the most neglected nutrients, with the average American consuming less than half the recommended amount of fiber each day. You need to eat lots of fruits, vegetables, and grain products to increase your intake of fiber. If you select a breakfast cereal with lots of fiber, this will help to increase your intake.

11. Exercise regularly

Regular aerobic exercise is important in any weight-management program. If you exercise at the right intensity you will burn fat, which is probably what you are most concerned with. In addition, exercise has a positive effect on your metabolism. After aerobic exercise, your metabolism stays elevated for some time. In addition, exercise can be used to increase your muscle mass. Muscle is more metabolically active than is fat. So by reducing your amount of fat and increasing your lean body tissue, your body will actually burn more calories each day while you are performing your everyday tasks. More fat and less muscle tissue are lost in weight-loss programs that incorporate exercise. The amount of exercise necessary for weight management was discussed in Chapter 7.

THE WEIGHT-MANAGEMENT/EXERCISE PROGRAM
Implementing the guidelines

If you are to be successful, you need to be constantly striving to implement these guidelines into your daily routine. The problem, however, is that most people simply do not know how to do this or else they lack the motivation that is necessary to establish consistent eating and exercise habits.

A simple form has been devised using these guidelines, so that you can evaluate your eating and exercise habits each day and you can then determine how consistent you are. At the same time as you evaluate yourself, you will learn how to make changes relative to each of these guidelines so that you can be successful. This self-evaluation form is presented in Table 8-2.

TABLE 8-2 **Weight-management/Exercise program: weekly evaluation**

Rate yourself on the following 11 guidelines each day, and record your score for each of them. At the end of each day, add up all 11 scores to determine your daily total.

Name:

	Mon	Tue	Wed	Thu	Fri	Sat	Sun
Day: Date:	—	—	—	—	—	—	—

1. Eat a nutritious breakfast within an hour of when you wake up.

    3 points—if your breakfast includes a full glass of either skim milk, 1% milk, low-fat yogurt, or ½ cup low-fat cottage cheese

    2 points—if your breakfast includes cereal or whole-grain toast

    2 points—if your breakfast includes fruit or fruit juice

    2 points—if you eat breakfast and it does not include bacon, eggs, or hash browns

    MAXIMUM 7 points

2. Eat at least 3 planned meals spaced regularly throughout the day.

    0 points—if you eat less than 3 meals a day

    MAXIMUM 3 points

3. Eat your evening meal as early as possible.

    4 points—if you eat before 6 PM

    2 points—if you eat before 7 PM

    0 points—if you eat after 7 PM

    MAXIMUM 4 points

4. Drink water frequently throughout the day (1 glass = 8 oz).

    4 points—if you drink 8 or more glasses

    3 points—if you drink 6 or 7 glasses

    2 points—if you drink 4 or 5 glasses

    1 point—if you drink 2 or 3 glasses

    0 points—if you drink less than 2 glasses

    MAXIMUM 4 points

TABLE 8-2 **Weight-management/Exercise program: weekly evaluation—cont'd**

Rate yourself on the following 11 guidelines each day, and record your score for each of them. At the end of each day, add up all 11 scores to determine your daily total.

Name:	Day: Date:	Mon	Tue	Wed	Thu	Fri	Sat	Sun

5. Limit your alcoholic beverages each day.
  5 points—if you have 0 drinks
  3 points—if you have 1 or 2 drinks
  0 points—if you have 3 drinks
  −2 points—for each drink above 3 (Maximum − 10 points)
	MAXIMUM
	5 points
	MINIMUM
	−10 points
		☐	☐	☐	☐	☐	☐	☐

6. Limit your between-meal snacks to fruit, vegetables, nonfat yogurt, pretzels, or air-popped popcorn (no butter or salt).
  3 points—if you do not snack or limit your snacks to the above foods
  1 point—if you have one snack other than the above (<150 cal)
	MAXIMUM
	3 points
		☐	☐	☐	☐	☐	☐	☐

7. Limit your intake of simple sugars from sources other than fruit.
  2 points—if you do not eat jelly, jam, honey, or candy and you do not drink soda (you may drink <3 diet sodas)
  2 points—if you do not eat baked foods such as cookies, doughnuts, twinkies, cakes, pies, or desserts (you may record 1 point if these foods contain <100 calories)
	MAXIMUM
	4 points
		☐	☐	☐	☐	☐	☐	☐

8. Limit your intake of sodium and salt.
  2 points—if you do not add salt to your food or cook with salt
  1 point—if you consistently select foods low in sodium
	MAXIMUM
	3 points
		☐	☐	☐	☐	☐	☐	☐

TABLE 8-2 Weight-management/Exercise program: weekly evaluation—cont'd

Rate yourself on the following 11 guidelines each day, and record your score for each of them. At the end of each day, add up all 11 scores to determine your daily total.

Name:

	Day: Date:	Mon	Tue	Wed	Thu	Fri	Sat	Sun
9. Limit the amount of fat that you eat each day. 2 points—if you eat no butter or margarine 2 points—if all your dairy products are low in fat 3 points—if you eat no cheese 3 points—if your meat intake consists only of fish, turkey, chicken without skin, or 4 oz or less of lean red meat 2 points—if you eat no food cooked in oil, no fried food, and no products with tropical oils	MAXIMUM 12 points							
10. Increase your intake of dietary fiber. 1 point—for each serving of fruit and vegetables (maximum 5 pts) 1 point—for each serving from grain products and legumes (maximum 5 pts) 1 point—for each 4 g of fiber from breakfast cereals (maximum 3 pts)	MAXIMUM 10 points							
11. Exercise regularly. 1 point—for each minute of organized continuous aerobic exercise where you are on your feet and supporting your body weight and moving ½ point—for each minute of organized continuous exercise that does not meet the above criteria.	MAXIMUM 45 points							
TOTAL POINTS PER DAY	MAXIMUM 100 points							

TOTAL POINTS FOR THE WEEK (add total points for all 7 days) _____

AVERAGE POINTS/DAY (divide the total points for the week by 7) _____

How to use the self-evaluation form

Following are the instructions for using the self-evaluation form:

- You simply rate yourself each day on each of these guidelines using the specific scoring system identified on the form.
- For each guideline there is a maximum number of points that you may record. For example, with the first guideline there are 9 possible points you can earn if you score the maximum number of points possible for each of the criteria pertaining to breakfast. However, you can record only 7 points because this is the maximum number of points you can record for this guideline.
- At the end of each day, add up all 11 scores for the day and record your total points for the day in the appropriate place. There is a maximum of 100 points each day.
- At the end of each week, add up your 7 daily totals and record this total in the appropriate place.
- Determine your average points per day for the week by dividing the total points for the week by 7. Record this value in the appropriate place.

Your average points per day for the week is the score that will indicate how consistent you have been for the week.

What does it take to be successful?

If you are trying to lose weight and/or body fat, we have found that to be successful at losing gradually, you need to achieve the following three criteria each week:

- You need to eat a nutritious breakfast all 7 days each week. (You will need to score 7 points for guideline 1 each day.)
- You need to make a commitment to exercise continuously for at least 45 minutes for a minimum of 5 days each week in any type of weight-bearing activity such as walking, jogging, basketball, racquetball, aerobics, or stair-climbing. If you have not been exercising regularly when you start this program, it may take you 2 or 3 weeks to gradually increase the length of each exercise session until you can participate continuously for 45 minutes. Start out at a very low level until 45 minutes of continuous work feels comfortable and then gradually increase the intensity. (You will need to score 45 points for Guideline 11, 5 days each week.)
- You need to average 70 or more points per day for each week. This total is based on 5 days of exercise. If you exercise 6 days then you will need to average 75 points, and if you exercise all 7 days then this total needs to be 80 or more points.

Does the program work?

It has taken over 3 years to develop the scoring system for the weekly self-evaluation form and to determine the criteria that you need to meet to be successful. Over 80% of the clients enrolled in our weight-management/exercise programs who meet the above three criteria each week and who have weight and/or body fat to lose are successful at gradually losing this weight and/or fat. Some lose only $1/2$ to 1 lb of weight per week, whereas others lose up to 2 lb. Some lose very little weight initially but significantly reduce their percentage of body fat. The following case study is one of hundreds of successful participants in this weight-management program. It shows how successful you can be if you decide to take charge of your eating and exercise habits.

CASE STUDY: LYLIAN

Lylian was a non-exerciser who enrolled in our weight-management/exercise program in September 1990. She had extremely poor eating habits, was overweight, and had an excessive amount of fat. She decided that it was time to make a commitment and to take charge of her eating and exercise habits.

During the 10 weeks she was in this program, there was not one morning that she did not eat breakfast and there was not one week that she did not exercise at least 5 times for 45 minutes. Her average points per day for each of the 10 weeks ranged from 72 to 96. Her average for the 10 weeks was 81. Before the program started, she was averaging less than 40 points per day. These scores reflect a major change in her eating and exercise habits.

She was very consistent during the program, and because of this she was very successful. Following is a comparison between her initial and final test results.

MEASUREMENT	SEPTEMBER 1990	DECEMBER 1990
Body weight (lb)	170	148
Percent body fat	41	30
Body fat measurement (mm)		
Subscapular	28	19
Triceps	32	24
Thigh	46	33
Abdominal	48	33
Suprailiac	41	24
Midaxillary	40	24
Cholesterol (mg/dl)	186	139
Aerobic fitness level		
(ml/kgbw/min)	19	28

Not everyone is alike, and it may be necessary to "fine-tune" this program so that you determine the amount of exercise you need to do each week to "balance out" the eating habits that you have established. Do not be discouraged if you do not see a change in your body weight initially. The reason for this has been explained previously. A number of clients who go through our weight-management/exercise program see only minimal changes in their body weight; however, when their body fat is measured again at the end of the program they are surprised by the amount of fat that they have lost.

If you initially have extremely poor eating habits and have not been regularly exercising for some time, do not expect to immediately achieve all three criteria that you need to meet to be successful. It is unlikely that you will be able to make all the necessary changes at once. Work on them one at a time. As specific objectives regularly become part of your lifestyle, you can concentrate on becoming more consistent with each of the other objectives. You should see an increase each week in the average number of points for the week.

Evaluating your exercise and eating habits

Use the self-evaluation form—Table 8-2—to evaluate a "typical" day for you. By doing this, you will see which of these guidelines are already part of your lifestyle and you should be able to identify changes that you can make immediately. In Laboratory Experience 8-3, you will evaluate yourself for an entire week. This will give you a much better idea of the consistency of your eating and exercise habits.

Make 10 copies of Table 8-2 so that you can use these for 10 consecutive weeks. We have found that most people will take more than a week or so to change some of their habits. By working each week at getting more consistent with each of these and recording your score each week, you will be more motivated to stick with your program. You will be able to see progress in your weekly scores if you are more consistent.

SUMMARY

The following summary will help you to identify some of the important concepts covered in this chapter:

- Despite the fact that weight loss has become an obsession in America, very few people have been successful at losing excess weight and keeping it off.
- Most diets fail because they restrict your food intake and do not encourage permanent lifestyle changes.
- For permanent weight loss, you should lose weight slowly by making changes in your lifestyle that you can live with for the rest of your life.
- Initially in a weight-loss program, you can lose fat but you may not lose any weight.
- You need to eat at regular intervals throughout the day. Skipping meals is counterproductive to losing body fat.
- Eating a nutritious breakfast is essential if you are to be successful at controlling the amount of body fat that you have.
- The day-to-day consistency of your exercise and eating habits will determine how successful you will be.

REFERENCES

1. Boyle MA, Zyla G: *Personal nutrition*, ed 2, St Paul, Minn, 1992, West.
2. Christian JL, Greger JL: *Nutrition for living*, ed 3, Redwood City, Calif, 1992, Benjamin/Cummings.
3. Coats C, Smith P: *Alive and well in the fast food lane*, Orlando, Fla, 1987, Carolyn Coats Bestsellers.
4. Cottrell RR: *Wellness—weight control*, Guilford, Conn, 1991, Dushkin.
5. *Dietary Guidelines for Americans*, US Department of Agriculture and Department of Health and Human Services, Washington, DC, 1985.
6. *Dietary Guidelines for the United States*, Senate Select Committee on Nutrition and Human Needs, US Government Printing Office, Washington, DC, 1985.
7. Nash JD: Weight control programs—what's the best choice? *Healthline* 7:1-4, Jan 1988.
8. Pritikin: Is snacking good for you? *Vantage Point* 1:6, April 1991.
9. Shapiro L: Feeding frenzy, *Newsweek*, pp. 46-53, May 27, 1991.
10. The Surgeon General's Report on Nutrition Health, US Department of Health and Human Services, Washington, DC, 1989.
11. Wardlaw GM, Insel PM, and Seyler MF: *Contemporary nutrition*, St Louis, 1992, Mosby–Year Book.

Do Your Daily Habits Encourage Weight Management?

To determine whether your daily habits encourage weight management and to help you identify changes that you need to make, simply circle the appropriate number in response to each question.

HOW OFTEN DO YOU:	RARELY	SOMETIMES	OFTEN
1. Eat fried foods rather than foods that are baked, broiled, or boiled?	3	2	1
2. Eat a nutritious breakfast?	1	2	3
3. Choose low-fat or nonfat foods?	1	2	3
4. Plan ahead of time the foods that you eat?	1	2	3
5. Skip meals?	3	2	1
6. Overeat and wish that you had not eaten so much?	3	2	1
7. Eat at fast-food restaurants because you do not have time to sit down and relax and enjoy a quiet, leisurely meal?	3	2	1
8. Get up in time so that you can eat breakfast at home?	1	2	3
9. Crave for a dessert after eating an adequate meal?	3	2	1
10. Buy troublesome foods such as chips, ice cream, cookies, etc.?	3	2	1
11. Eat in one main place when eating at home?	1	2	3
12. Engage in other activities, such as reading or watching television, while eating?	3	2	1
13. Avoid the negative influence of friends and peers on your eating habits?	1	2	3
14. Take 20 minutes or longer to eat your meals?	1	2	3
15. Exercise regularly?	1	2	3
16. Leave food on your plate?	1	2	3
17. Drink at least 6 glasses of water in a day?	1	2	3
18. Drink more than 2 alcoholic drinks in a day?	3	2	1
19. Drink at least 1 glass of water or other low-calorie fluid before each meal?	1	2	3
20. Eat in response to something other than hunger?	3	2	1

Add the numbers together that you circled.

Enter your score here _____

Interpretation

Interpret your score this way:

20-36	Very poor—Your eating habits need a lot of attention.
37-47	Average—You are doing all right, but there is room for improvement.
48-60	Very good—You have developed good consistent habits; however, do not reward yourself by overeating.

LABORATORY EXPERIENCE 8–2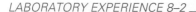

Learning About Your Eating Habits

To learn more about your eating habits, you need to keep a food diary for at least 2 days—a weekday and a weekend day (see Tables 8-3 and 8-4). Following are the instructions you will need to complete these food diary forms:

Time of eating

For every meal or snack, record the time when you begin eating or drinking and when you finish.

Meal or snack

Indicate whether it is a meal or a snack. Be sure to remember that everything you drink between meals is considered a snack. If it is a meal, indicate whether it is breakfast, lunch, or dinner.

Place of eating

Record where you are when you eat that meal or snack or have that drink. If you are at home, record the room of the house you are in; otherwise, record whether you are in a restaurant, car, office, bar, etc.

Food and amount

Indicate what you eat and the approximate amount. If you eat at home and you have a small scale, you will find it beneficial to measure the amount of the food that you eat so that you become more aware of portion sizes. If you do not know the exact amount, you will need to estimate this amount. If you estimate the amount of food, keep in mind that most people usually underestimate this amount.

Posture

Indicate your physical position while you are eating or drinking—lying down? sitting? standing? walking? etc.

Associated activity

Record what else you are doing while you are eating or drinking. For example, preparing dinner, watching television, reading, driving a car, talking on the telephone, etc.

Social situation

Indicate whether you are alone, with someone, or with a group of people each time you eat.

Mood

Record how you feel before you start to eat. Were you content? happy? sad? depressed? angry? bored? tired? rushed? lonely? tense? etc.

Hunger level

Record how hungry you are before you start to eat. Rate your hunger level on a 10-point scale ranging from a score of 1, which would indicate that you were not hungry, to a score of 10, which would indicate that you were very hungry.

Evaluating your daily food recall diary

By carefully evaluating your 3-day food diary, you will become more aware of what you eat and how much you eat. You may find out that you are one of those people who do not realize how much they eat until they write everything down. You will also be able to see patterns as to when and why you eat.

Your food recall forms may also show you that you eat too quickly without paying attention to your food or taking the time to enjoy it. If you eat frequently while standing up or while you are engaging in other activities, this is a good indication that you need to slow down and take the time to enjoy your food.

Analysis of the three food recall forms

By answering the following questions you may be able to identify some of these patterns:

- How many days did you skip at least one meal? _____
- How many times did you eat when you were not really hungry? _____
- How many times did you eat because you were bored? _____
- How many times did you eat because you were angry and/or depressed? _____
- How many days did you snack on foods that you know you should not have eaten? _____
- How many days did you drink more than one alcoholic beverage? _____
- How many days did you eat at least one dessert? _____
- How many times did other people trigger unwanted eating behavior? _____
- How many times did you eat a meal and when you were finished, you wished that you had not eaten so much? _____

TABLE 8-3 Daily food recall diary #1

Complete this form for at least 1 weekday and 1 weekend day. Try to select typical days.

Time start-end	Meal or snack	Place	Food	Amount	Posture	Associated activity	Social situation	Mood	Hunger level

Name _____

Date _____

TABLE 8-4 Daily food recall diary #2

Complete this form for at least 1 weekday and 1 weekend day. Try to select typical days.

Time start-end	Meal or snack	Place	Food	Amount	Posture	Associated activity	Social situation	Mood	Hunger level

Name _____

Date _____

Evaluating the Consistency of Your Eating and Exercise Habits

To determine the consistency of your exercise and eating habits, it may be beneficial for you to evaluate your eating and exercise habits for a complete week. Simply use the weekly self-evaluation form in Table 8-5 and score yourself each day. The procedures to follow have been given previously.

Calculating your score

To calculate your score for the week, simply total your score for each day. You then add the 7 daily totals and divide by 7 to determine your average score for the week.

Interpretation of score

To have the consistency you need to be successful at losing weight or simply to have good consistent eating and exercise habits, you need to average 70 or more points. This score is based on the premise that you exercise no more than 5 times each week. If you exercise 6 times, you need to average 75 points, or if you exercise all 7 days, your average needs to be 80 points.

TABLE 8-5 Weight-management/Exercise program: weekly evaluation

Rate yourself on the following 11 guidelines each day, and record your score for each of them. At the end of each day, add up all 11 scores to determine your daily total.

Name:

	Mon	Tue	Wed	Thu	Fri	Sat	Sun
Day: Date:	—	—	—	—	—	—	—

1. Eat a nutritious breakfast within an hour of when you wake up.
   3 points—if your breakfast includes a full glass of either skim milk, 1% milk, low-fat yogurt, or ½ cup low-fat cottage cheese
   2 points—if your breakfast includes cereal or whole-grain toast
   2 points—if your breakfast includes fruit or fruit juice
   2 points—if you eat breakfast and it does not include bacon, eggs, or hash browns

   MAXIMUM 7 points

2. Eat at least 3 planned meals spaced regularly throughout the day.
   0 points—if you eat less than 3 meals a day

   MAXIMUM 3 points

3. Eat your evening meal as early as possible.
   4 points—if you eat before 6 PM
   2 points—if you eat before 7 PM
   0 points—if you eat after 7 PM

   MAXIMUM 4 points

4. Drink water frequently throughout the day (1 glass = 8 oz).
   4 points—if you drink 8 or more glasses
   3 points—if you drink 6 or 7 glasses
   2 points—if you drink 4 or 5 glasses
   1 point—if you drink 2 or 3 glasses
   0 points—if you drink less than 2 glasses

   MAXIMUM 4 points

5. Limit your alcoholic beverages each day.
   5 points—if you have 0 drinks
   3 points—if you have 1 or 2 drinks
   0 points—if you have 3 drinks
   −2 points—for each drink above 3 (Maximum −10 points)

   MAXIMUM
   5 points
   MINIMUM
   −10 points

6. Limit your between-meal snacks to fruit, vegetables, nonfat yogurt, pretzels, or air-popped popcorn (no butter or salt).
   3 points—if you do not snack or limit your snacks to the above foods
   1 point—if you have one snack other than the above (<150 cal)

   MAXIMUM
   3 points

7. Limit your intake of simple sugars from sources other than fruit.
   2 points—if you do not eat jelly, jam, honey, or candy and you do not drink soda (you may drink <3 diet sodas)
   2 points—if you do not eat baked foods such as cookies, doughnuts, twinkies, cakes, pies, or desserts (you may record 1 point if these foods contain <100 calories)

   MAXIMUM
   4 points

8. Limit your intake of sodium and salt.
   2 points—if you do not add salt to your food or cook with salt
   1 point—if you consistently select foods low in sodium

   MAXIMUM
   3 points

9. Limit the amount of fat that you eat each day.
   2 points—if you eat no butter or margarine
   2 points—if all your dairy products are low in fat
   3 points—if you eat no cheese
   3 points—if your meat intake consists only of fish, turkey, chicken without skin or 4 oz or less of lean red meat
   2 points—if you eat no food cooked in oil, no fried food, and no products with tropical oils

   MAXIMUM
   12 points

Continued.

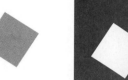

TABLE 8-5 **Weight-management/Exercise program: weekly evaluation—cont'd**

Rate yourself on the following 11 guidelines each day, and record your score for each of them. At the end of each day, add up all 11 scores to determine your daily total.

Name:

	Day: Date:	Mon	Tue	Wed	Thu	Fri	Sat	Sun

10. Increase your intake of dietary fiber.
  1 point—for each serving of fruit and vegetables (maximum 5 pts)
  1 point—for each serving from grain products and legumes (maximum 5 pts)
  1 point—for each 4 g of fiber from breakfast cereals (maximum 3 pts)
	MAXIMUM
	10 points
		☐	☐	☐	☐	☐	☐	☐

11. Exercise regularly.
  1 point—for each minute of organized continuous aerobic exercise where you are on your feet and supporting your body weight and moving
  ½ point—for each minute of organized continuous exercise that does not meet the above criteria.
	MAXIMUM
	45 points
		☐	☐	☐	☐	☐	☐	☐

TOTAL POINTS PER DAY	MAXIMUM 100 points	☐	☐	☐	☐	☐	☐	☐

TOTAL POINTS FOR THE WEEK (add total points for all 7 days) _____

AVERAGE POINTS/DAY (divide the total points for the week by 7) _____

Stress Management

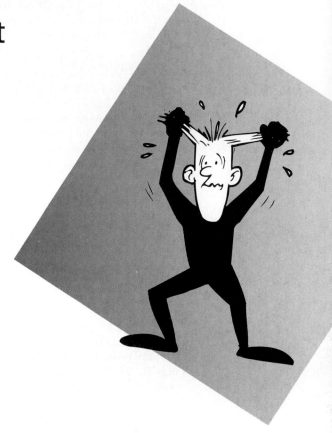

CHAPTER OBJECTIVES

When you understand the material in this chapter, you will be able to:

- Define stress, and know the difference between too much stress, too little stress, and optimal stress
- Discuss the way in which your body reacts to stress, and identify the three stages of stress
- Discuss the problems associated with too much stress
- Identify stressful situations, and determine how much stress is too much

- Differentiate clearly between Type A and Type B behaviors
- Discuss the role of exercise in stress reduction
- Identify strategies you can use to effectively deal with stress
- Determine your level of stress

S tress is a normal part of everyday living—something we cannot avoid. It is necessary if we are to be productive, but it can be harmful if it occurs too frequently, is too intense, or lasts too long. Stress may be defined simply as our reaction to a specific situation or event. It is not the event that causes the stress but the reaction to it. The following case study will illustrate this.

CASE STUDY: ANNEMARIE

Annemarie is an 18-year-old who has just graduated from high school in a small rural community where she has many friends. She has lived at home with her parents all her life and has been "going steady" with the same boy for nearly 2 years. She is preparing to leave this environment to attend college in a large city 700 miles away.

She is very happy to be the first person in her family to attend college, but she is very apprehensive about some of the adjustments she now must make. Some of her "anxiety" is caused by the following:

- Her parents want her to do well in college.
- Her boyfriend does not want her to leave.
- She has to live on campus and share a room, and she is worried about whether she will "get along" with her roommate.
- She is concerned about having to eat on campus and is afraid she will gain weight like most other freshmen.
- She does not know which classes she should take.
- She has never had to worry about grades in high school, but now she knows that she will have to "compete" for good grades.

This is a typical college situation that many freshmen face, and it is obvious that such situations cause different reactions from different people. It would appear to be important to learn to balance stress with the demands placed on you with everyday living. To do this you will need to do the following:

- Become more knowledgeable about stress
- Determine the amount of stress in your life
- Learn to identify the specific situations that cause stress for you
- Develop effective ways of dealing with stress and reducing your stress level

DEFINITION OF BASIC TERMS

Stress has been defined as your reaction to a specific situation or event. This reaction can be either positive or negative and would include such responses as anger, joy, rejection, frustration, and happiness. It is obvious that stress is associated with both unpleasant and pleasant situations.

Distress is a term used to refer to high level of stress resulting in negative responses such as tension and frustration. Constant distress can negatively affect your health and performance.

Eustress is a term used to refer to a "good" stress that results in what is perceived as a positive reaction such as joy and happiness. It is usually associated with pleasurable situations such as getting married, graduation, promotion, and successfully completing a difficult task. Despite the fact that these types of events are viewed as "positive," they can also negatively influence your level of stress.

For example, getting married means that you must often make some major lifestyle adjustments. These may include buying or renting a house or apartment, buying furniture, moving, and having added financial responsibilities. These can all cause distress.

A **stressor** is any situation or event that initiates the stress response. The same stressor may result in two entirely different responses. For example, many people play golf for the enjoyment and relaxation that they get from playing. With others, who are usually very competitive, it creates so much frustration that they have a hard time controlling the stress that it creates for them.

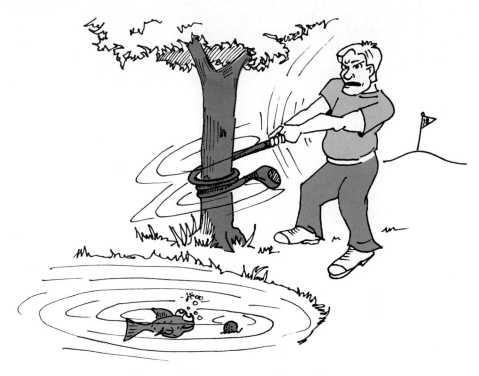

Some activities create stress for participants.

QUANTIFYING STRESS

It may be beneficial to find a way to *quantify* stress. A logical approach might be to consider stress as existing on a scale or continuum (Fig. 9-1).

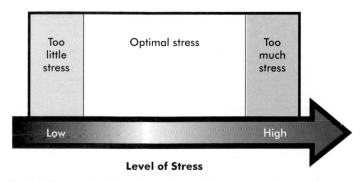

Fig. 9-1 Stress should be viewed as existing on a continuum or scale.

An optimal level of stress is defined as the level at which you perform most efficiently without encountering any harmful side effects. An optimal level of stress can help you concentrate better on the job at hand and reach peak efficiency. You are likely to be able to think more clearly, your motivation level will be higher, and you will be in total control of the situation.

An extremely high level of stress is often referred to as negative stress. There are many people who perform their best work under extreme pressure. However, if high stress levels cannot be relieved by relaxation, you will not be able to function efficiently. Negative stress has also been associated with increased risk of coronary heart disease, hypertension, diabetes, and many other physical ailments.

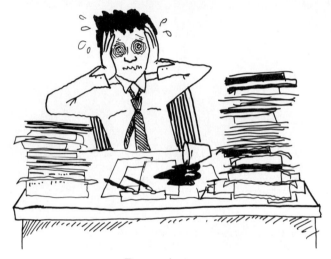

Too much stress.

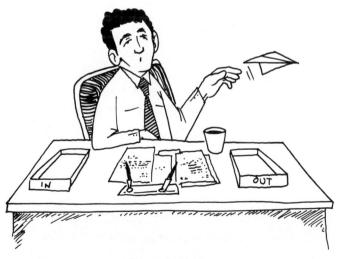

Too little stress.

A low level of stress is usually detrimental also. It may result in decreased motivation and performance, irritability, and boredom. We need a certain level of stress to be productive.

THE NATURE OF STRESS

Your body has a built-in response to stress that occurs automatically, without conscious thought. Your natural reaction in response to a stressor is to prepare for physical activity.

Our bodies react the same way as in ancient times, when people had two choices on finding themselves face-to-face with physical stress: either they could fight or they could try to run away from it. This is referred to as the "fight or flight" response. Both of these responses require the body to quickly perform more physical work than normal.

Your physiological response to stressors may occur in three stages.

Stage I: These are immediate physiological changes that occur within the body to prepare for high-intensity physical activity. These include the following:

> Your heart rate increases to circulate more blood to the muscles.
> Your blood pressure rises.
> Your breathing rate increases to provide more oxygen to the blood.
> Your muscles tense in anticipation of increased activity.
> Additional energy is automatically made available from stored carbohydrates.
> Perspiration increases in an attempt to control your body temperature.

Stage II: The second stage is often referred to as the resistance stage. In this stage the body reacts to the stressor, and most functions within the body return to normal. The body adjusts to the increased level of stress by secreting various hormones that have a calming effect on the body and that help you to adjust to the stressful situation.

Stage III: If the stress continues over an extended period or is extremely intense, the body may enter the third stage, where exhaustion and disease may occur.

The problem is that the majority of today's stressors are not physical in nature but are primarily emotional. Rarely is it appropriate to "attack" our problems or to "run away from them." However, our bodies still react in the same way. They are primed for action, and this just does not occur. The result is a prolonged state of tension that often results in irritability, depression, anger, anxiety, hostility, apathy, and fatigue.

In an attempt to cope with this prolonged state of tension, many people turn to such things as alcohol, drugs, smoking, overeating, or some other unhealthful practice. These do not relieve stress; in fact, in most cases they add to the problem. When your level of stress becomes extremely high and ongoing, your physical and emotional health are adversely affected. The more intense the stress or the longer it lasts, the more serious the consequences.

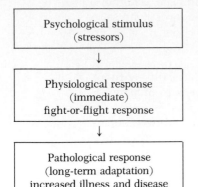

Fig. 9-2 Short-term and long-term effects of stress. (Modified from Dehn MM: *Well on the way to optimal health and fitness,* Irving, Tex, 1987, Health Management Consultants.)

PROBLEMS ASSOCIATED WITH TOO MUCH STRESS

It has been estimated that more than 50% of all diseases in the United States have a stress-related origin. The diseases most frequently mentioned include cardiovascular disease, cancer, **hypertension, migraine headaches,** ulcers, allergies, and asthma.

- The incidence of cardiovascular disease is much higher in those who are classified as having a high stress level, as compared with those who experience very little stress.
- The hormones secreted in the body in abundance as part of the "fight or flight" response tend to remain in the body and may lessen the body's ability to fight infection.
- Stress is the cause of certain muscular problems. For example, many headaches are caused by continued contraction of certain muscles in the head and neck.
- Stress can contribute to high blood pressure, which is a risk factor associated with cardiovascular disease. It can also contribute to problems with the liver and kidneys.
- Constant levels of high stress can make you confused and may make it difficult for you to concentrate. This may make you more accident prone.

The relationship between stress and illness is summarized in Fig. 9-2.

> Nearly one third of all Americans feel under "great stress" just about every day or several days per week.

IDENTIFYING STRESSFUL SITUATIONS

It is important to be able to recognize and identify the situations in your life that cause stress.

Stress may be caused by minor day-to-day events

Each day we encounter a variety of situations that in themselves are insignificant but that collectively can accumulate to negatively affect your level of stress. Following are some examples of day-to-day events that may increase your level of stress:

- Waiting in line
- Misplacing your keys or glasses
- Hosting a party
- Being late for an appointment
- Being caught in a traffic jam
- Not hearing your alarm and sleeping in
- Having a disagreement with a friend

Note that it is not the event that causes stress but your response to the specific situation. If you become impatient, irritated, frustrated, or apprehensive in response to any of these situations, or situations similar to these, your stress level will increase.

When you experience situations such as those mentioned previously, before you react negatively and let them bother you, you need to ask yourself, "Will this situation have an effect on my life tomorrow or next week?" In most cases it will not. Despite this, it is still often difficult to change the way you react to "minor" everyday stressors such as these.

Stress may be caused by lifestyle changes

Both positive and negative lifestyle changes require you to adjust to a new or different situation and can therefore be stressful. Following are some examples of lifestyle changes:

- Getting married
- Taking a vacation
- Starting a family
- Buying a new house
- Getting fired
- Relocating in a different city
- Experiencing the death of a close friend
- Getting promoted

Some lifestyle changes are completely out of your control, but many are controllable. If you are adjusting to many changes within a short period, you are much more likely to have a high level of stress. You should take your time and plan your changes gradually. It would not make sense to graduate from college, start a career, get married, buy a house, and start a family within the first year of graduation.

Many people tend to overreact to change. For example, some people worry so much about what appears to be an unpleasant event that this causes as much stress or even more than actually experiencing the event. In coping with this type of stress, you should try to focus on those factors which you can control, rather than on those over which you have no control.

Stress may be caused by overload

Overload occurs when you find yourself faced with demands that have accumulated to an unmanageable level and that exceed your capacity to meet them. These demands may be related to work, school, or home.

When you become overloaded, you try to do too many things at the same time, with the result that you have too many deadlines to meet and not enough hours in the day to accomplish all that needs to be done. When this occurs, you often have trouble deciding which task to attempt first.

Some people become totally involved in their work and thrive on overload. They are usually remarkably satisfied with their lives and are willing to make sacrifices in other areas so that they have time to complete their work. These people are often referred to as "workaholics."

This situation is far too stressful for most people, and it often results in the following:

- Lack of motivation, despite the fact that they are overloaded
- A feeling of frustration and helplessness
- Decreased productivity
- Inability to think clearly
- Inability to sleep soundly

- Chronic fatigue
- Reduced judgment and recall

When this situation occurs, it is important to sit down, try to relax, and get things in perspective. You need to decide on priorities and then complete one step at a time. Added stress associated with work can also result from the following:

- Having to meet deadlines
- Being forced to make important decisions
- Having high levels of expectation relating to job performance
- Lacking confidence in your ability
- Having too much responsibility

Being aware of what causes your stress is the first step involved in finding a solution to the problem.

HOW MUCH STRESS IS TOO MUCH?

People react differently to potentially stressful situations. However, there are certain signs and symptoms that could indicate that you are under too much stress. Your first step in trying to cope with stress is to learn to recognize some of these early signs and symptoms. Those which relate to your mood or disposition are identified below.

Check off those responses that apply to you.

HOW FREQUENTLY DO YOU FEEL:	RARELY	SOMETIMES	OFTEN
Insecure. You frequently think the worst possible outcome.	____	____	____
Irritable. You may be short-tempered or impatient.	____	____	____
Depressed. You are easily upset—you may eat or drink in response to how you feel.	____	____	____
Angry. You may be hostile, violent, or irrational.	____	____	____
Overly aggressive. You may be demanding, selfish, or insensitive.	____	____	____
Easily distracted. You find it difficult to concentrate—you may be preoccupied or may experience decreased productivity.	____	____	____
Forgetful. You may be absentminded or suffer from insomnia.	____	____	____
Anxious. You may be frequently worried or nervous.	____	____	____
Reckless. You may act violently, or you may be careless or self-destructive.	____	____	____

There are also other internal signs and symptoms or particular responses that may indicate a potential high stress level. These are as follows:

Check the frequency with which the following responses apply to you.

	RARELY	SOMETIMES	OFTEN
Pain or tension in your back or neck	_____	_____	_____
Increased frequency of eating	_____	_____	_____
Increased smoking	_____	_____	_____
Tension headaches	_____	_____	_____
Easily startled by unexpected sounds	_____	_____	_____
Profuse sweating	_____	_____	_____
Pounding of heart or irregular heart beat	_____	_____	_____
Hands feel moist and/or cold	_____	_____	_____
Upset stomach	_____	_____	_____
Increased blood pressure	_____	_____	_____
Difficulty standing still	_____	_____	_____
Difficulty sitting quietly	_____	_____	_____
Reduced attention span	_____	_____	_____

By evaluating your response to these early signs of excess stress, you should be able to identify situations that may create problems for you. With regard to the two sets of signs and symptoms, if several of your responses are "often" or "sometimes," then you could be considered as either having a high level of stress, or else you are a high-risk candidate for developing a high level of stress. You need to avoid or confront the specific stressors that create problems for you.

The following case study will show you how to do the following:
- Confront a specific problem
- Identify the causes
- Plan so that you can avoid such a problem in the future

CASE STUDY: SCOTT

Scott is a very "competitive" college student who likes to excel. He never seems to have enough time and is constantly rushing to meet specific guidelines. Today he has an exam at 9:30 AM. He "overslept" and missed his first class because he stayed up until 5:00 AM studying for the exam. Not only did he miss his first class, but he did not have time to eat breakfast or to "review" his notes for the test. His stress level is extremely high as he rushes out the door and barely makes it in time for his examination.

By analyzing the events that happen in a stressful situation such as this, you should be able to come up with a plan in an attempt to avoid this situation in the future. Scott could have begun studying for the test several days in advance, so that he did not have to "cram" everything into 1 night. He could have then gotten a good night's rest, had a leisurely breakfast while he reviewed his notes, attended his first class, and made it to the examination refreshed without the extra stress caused by rushing, missing a class, and not eating breakfast.

You need to analyze specific events such as these that create high levels of stress for you, and plan how you can modify your behavior and reduce your level of stress.

PERSONALITY FACTORS

Your attitude and your perception of the stressor will determine your reaction to each specific stressful situation. Those who see problems as worse than they really are will be likely to reach a higher level of stress and maintain this level for a longer period. Basically, people can be classified into two groups according to how they perceive specific situations.

The first class, **Type A,** is associated with a high level of stress. Type A personalities rate high on the following criteria:

Ambition—an intense, sustained drive to achieve self-selected but usually poorly defined goals
Competitiveness—a profound inclination and eagerness to compete
Aggressiveness—persistent desire for recognition and advancement
Chronic sense of time urgency—continuous involvement in multiple functions, while constantly subject to restrictions
Drive—persistent efforts to accelerate the rate of execution of many physical and mental functions

These traits are normally present in most individuals, but the Type A person possesses them to an excessive degree. Individuals in this group include those who cannot stand to have unscheduled time on their hands, who are impatient with the world, who become very upset when they are kept waiting, and who always walk, talk, and eat rapidly.

Those who rate low on these traits are classified as **Type B.** These people usually are able to relax easily. Very seldom do they let outside factors adversely influence their emotional state. The level of anxiety and tension of a Type B person is therefore very low.

There are some short-term benefits associated with being a Type A person. However, more often than not, in the long run it impairs efficiency and creates definite health problems. It is also interesting to note that Type A people have a lower than average self-esteem. This may explain why they feel that they must attempt to do more and to work at a faster pace.

If you have a Type A personality, it is very difficult to change. You will need to work hard at learning to adjust differently to given situations. You need to become less competitive, to concentrate on one task at a time, and to slow down. Specific lifestyle changes that may be beneficial to you are found in the following section on stress management.

STRESS MANAGEMENT

The first step in coping with stress is to be aware that stress exists and that, if it persists, its effects can be detrimental to your health and wellness. Some people simply refuse to accept the fact that they are under too much stress and fail to recognize the signs and symptoms associated with excess stress.

The next step is to identify the environmental situations that cause your stress. We have seen that much of our stress is caused by the following:

- Minor day-to-day hassles
- Significant lifestyle changes
- Too many responsibilities and deadlines

In many cases we cannot change the nature of the stressors, but we can learn new skills so that we can control the effects that stressors have on us.

Lifestyle changes

By intentionally changing those aspects of your lifestyle and environment that create stress, you can reduce your level of frustration, anxiety, hostility, and irritability. Making these changes may not be as difficult as it may at first appear. Following are some suggestions that may be helpful:

- When a major change occurs in your life, you can minimize the amount of stress by reducing the number of other changes made. Continue to engage in familiar and enjoyable activities that help you to relax.
- Try to slow down and allow yourself more time to do the things that need to be done. If you are always rushed in the morning, get up earlier so that you have more time. Establish a routine that becomes automatic and that allows plenty of time. When traveling, try to leave 10 to 20 minutes earlier than normal so that you do not have to rush from one place to the next. Try to eliminate the things you do hurriedly that don't save you much time, such as changing lanes on the freeway or running a red light because you are in a hurry.
- Plan each day by listing the tasks that need to be accomplished in their order of importance, so that the most important ones can be completed first. If a task appears to be long and complicated and you become frustrated at even getting started, break it down into a series of smaller tasks. Work on each of these,

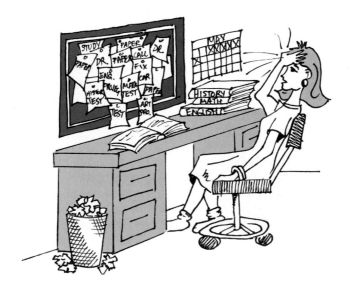

one at a time. As each task is completed, check it off. This will give you a sense of satisfaction and will increase your level of motivation instead of increasing your level of stress.

- Use a good time-management technique by matching things that need to be accomplished with the time you have available. Do not accept additional responsibilities if you do not have time to complete the tasks you are presently working on. Learn to assign work and additional responsibility to others. Do not plan too many things close together or at the same time. Avoid taking work home with you; learn to leave with unfinished work from day to day.
- If you experience a time when you feel unproductive and have difficulty completing a task, take a short break to stretch, walk, relax, or simply get away from it for awhile.
- Make your work environment as relaxing as possible. Such things as soft music, healthy plants, and nice furniture may help.

Personality changes

By intentionally changing the stressful aspects of your personality, you can improve the way you react to stressful situations.

How you react to a given situation is usually a habit that has been learned and developed over a period and possibly maintained in your lifestyle for a number of years. You need to realize that these habits will be extremely difficult to change; it will take time, effort, and discipline. However, keep in mind that with determination it can be done.

If you are to be successful, the following may be important:

- You may need to realize that you will not get the same satisfaction with new experiences as you did with old ones. However, with time, how you feel will fall in line with what you do.
- Evaluate each positive change. Each time you make different choices, old bonds will loosen and new behavior will become easier.
- Be as objective as possible. Do not underestimate what you can achieve.
- Reinforce positive outcomes.

If you are to be successful in changing your habits, the following may be important considerations.

Improving your self-concept. You must believe in your ability to succeed. This is important, because it determines how much effort you will expend in trying to change your habits, how long you will persist, and how much stress you will experience while you are changing your lifestyle. You need to develop a positive attitude by making up your mind that you *can* make specific changes and then by working hard to meet the challenge at hand. You will need to change your negative self-talk and irrational thinking and work on raising your self-esteem.

Improving your relationships with others. When changing your habits, the support and encouragement you get from other people are very important. It will be beneficial to you at this time to try to improve your relationship with your fellow workers, your friends, and your family. You need to be understanding and tolerant toward them, to be willing to understand their viewpoints, and to realize that this may be different from how you feel. Your social life at this time can be extremely important. You need to get together with your friends regularly, keep in touch with your family members, and try to become involved with church, club, or organizational activities or projects.

Taking care of yourself. You can adapt better to changes if you take good care of your body. This can be achieved by simply following a few simple guidelines.

- Get sufficient sleep so that you feel awake and refreshed each morning.
- Participate regularly in an aerobic exercise program.
- Eat regular, healthful meals.
- Maintain normal weight.
- Moderate your use of alcohol and caffeine.
- Refrain from smoking or inhaling the smoke of others.

Relaxation techniques for stress management

Physiologically, relaxation is the opposite response to the stress response and is the key to balancing stress. Several different relaxation techniques are available that allow you to regulate body processes. By using these techniques, you become more aware of your body and how it responds to stress.

Deep breathing technique. One of the "fight or flight" responses to stress is an increased respiration rate—you breathe more rapidly. Deep breathing is simply a technique where you consciously breathe slowly and deeply in an attempt to relieve tension in the body. With this technique you inhale slowly through your nose; your stomach should expand at this time. You then hold your breath for a few seconds before exhaling through your mouth.

Meditation. Meditation is another relaxation technique that can help reduce your stress by "clearing your mind" and blocking out any thoughts that might be responsible for increased tension. When your mind is clear, you then try to concentrate on a pleasant thought or situation.

Progressive muscle relaxation. This relaxation technique consists basically of a series of exercises designed to contract and relax the major muscle groups of the body. The objective is to reduce the tension in the muscles. You begin by tightening the muscle and then releasing the tension while you concentrate on how different the two tension levels feel. This technique can be used with the stretching exercises described in Chapter 5 and can provide an excellent form of relaxation.

Listening to music. Sitting or lying and listening to music can be an excellent way to relax and to cope with stress.

Stretching. If stress persists over an extended period, muscle tension is likely to develop in certain parts of the body. This situation can often be alleviated by simply performing stretching exercises for the part or parts of your body affected.

GUIDELINES FOR REDUCING STRESS*

The following guidelines may be helpful to you in reducing your level of stress:

1. Exercise regularly

We have seen that the natural reaction of the body to stress is the "fight or flight" response, as your body prepares for an increased level of physical activity. However, most of the stressors we encounter in today's world are mental in nature rather than physical. Because of this, a natural reaction would be to undertake some form of phys-

---

*Parts of this section are summarized from *Wellness Newsletter*, Randall Sports/Medical Products, 2:2, Kirkland, Wash, 1990.

ical activity to use this extra energy as you attempt to accelerate the dissipation of the by-products of stress.

It has also clearly been shown that those people who are physically fit and who exercise regularly can handle stress more easily than those who are unfit. Exercise has a "calming" effect on the body. As a result of exercise you will not only look better but you will *feel* better, and you should be more relaxed and better able to deal with the stress in your life.

In addition, if you exercise regularly you are likely to have a lower resting heart rate and lower blood pressure, and you should be able to handle better the negative effects of stress on your body relative to these two responses.

It should be realized, however, that for some people exercise can increase their level of stress. This is particularly true where competition is involved. Those people who have a high level of stress and who are very competitive should not select a competitive form of exercise.

2. Improve your personal appearance

By exercising and eating right, you can often improve your personal appearance. When you look better you usually feel better. By feeling better, you will have a much more positive attitude and outlook and will be in a position to react more favorably in certain stressful situations.

3. Adopt good eating habits

A healthful eating plan can increase your resistance to stress. By eating well you can increase your energy level and help your body to resist illness and infection. Skipping meals and getting too few complex carbohydrates and too much simple refined sugar can trigger a drop in your blood glucose level, resulting in irritability and fatigue.

4. Learn to think clearly

If you are to schedule time effectively, establish realistic goals, and determine priorities, you need to be able to think clearly. To do this you must get a sufficient amount of sleep. Lack of sleep often results in poor decisions, and you will not be able to think clearly.

5. Think positively

No matter what you are trying to achieve, you must believe that you can be successful and you must think positively rather than always coming up with negative thoughts. You need to make up your mind that you *can* do it and then plan how you are going to do it.

6. Learn how to make decisions for yourself

You need to be in control and make sure that *you* decide what you need to do each day. You are going to have to learn how to say "no" to other people when they ask you to do something that you will not have time to do, because you are struggling to complete the tasks and activities that you are already doing.

7. Learn to listen to other people

If you listen more and talk less, you will probably be able to cope with stress better.

8. Schedule time to relax

Try to plan your schedule so that you have time to sit or lie down and relax by listening to music, reading a book, or watching television. Getting outdoors and enjoying nature is also an excellent way to relax. Positive and negative coping skills are included in Laboratory Experience 9-2.

9. Express your feelings openly

Many of the everyday problems that contribute to a high level of stress are caused by lack of communication. People who tend to keep their feelings inside frequently "blow up" and take out their anger and frustration on others. By not discussing problems and resolving them, they often get out of control.

10. Do your best

The adage "Do your best, and leave the rest" is probably the best advice anyone could give you for reducing and coping with stress.

SUMMARY

The following summary may help you to identify some of the important concepts covered in this chapter.

- Stress is something we cannot avoid—a certain level of stress is necessary if we are to be productive.
- Our responses to stressful situations may be either positive or negative.
- The body's natural response to stress is to prepare for physical activity.
- Stress that is prolonged and intense contributes to many physical and mental disorders.
- Stress can be caused by simple everyday events.
- Changes in our lifestyle can significantly affect our level of stress.
- Trying to do too much can negatively affect your level of stress.
- Improving your self-concept and your relationship with others can help you to cope with stress better.
- Exercise can have a very positive effect on stress.
- By eating right you can increase your resistance to stress.

KEY TERMS

distress A high level of stress—associated with negative responses such as anxiety, tension, and frustration.

eustress A positive reaction to stress, resulting in responses such as joy and happiness.

hypertension Consistently elevated blood pressure.

migraine headache Intense pain in the head, usually confined to one side of the head. May be preceded by changes in vision.

stressor Any change that causes a person to react in a stressful manner.

Type A personality A person who is aggressive, anxious, and impatient and who works excessively.

Type B personality A person who is relaxed, not rushed, and not affected by deadlines or demands.

REFERENCES

1. Althoff SA, Svoboda M, and Girdano DA: *Choices in health and fitness for life*, ed 2, Scottsdale, Ariz, 1991, Gorsuch Scarisbrick.
2. Anspaugh DJ, Hamrick MH, and Rosato FD: *Wellness: concepts and applications*, St Louis, 1991, Mosby–Year Book.
3. Cooper KH, Gallman JS, and McDonald JL: Role of aerobic exercise in reduction of stress, *Dental Clinics of North America* 30:4-6, October 1986.
4. Dehn MM: *Well on the way to optimal health and fitness*, Irving, Tex, 1987, Health Management Consultants.
5. *Fit to win: your handbook*, The Army's Health Promotion Program, Washington, DC, 1987, US Government Printing Office.
6. Floyd PA et al: *Wellness: a lifetime commitment*, Winston-Salem, NC, 1991, Hunter Textbooks.
7. Forman JW, Myers D: *The personal stress reduction program*, Englewood Cliffs, NJ, 1987, Prentice Hall.
8. *Interpreting your test results*, Lake Geneva, Wisc, 1985, Fitness Monitoring.
9. Kiesling S: Tension relief, *American Health* March/April 1982.
10. Krames Communications: *A guide to managing stress*, Daly City, Calif, 1985.
11. Kusinitz MI, Fine M: *Your guide to getting fit*, ed 2, Mountain View, Calif, 1991, Mayfield.
12. Miller A: Stress on the job, *Newsweek*, pp. 40-45, April 25, 1988.
13. Murphy P: Stress and the athlete: coping with exercise, *The Physician and Sportsmedicine* 14(4):141-146, April 1986.
14. Nieman DC: *The sports medicine fitness course*, Palo Alto, Calif, 1986, Bull.
15. Prentice WE, Bucher CA: *Fitness for college and life*, ed 3, St Louis, 1991, Mosby–Year Book.
16. Randall Sports/Medical Products, *Wellness Newsletter* 2:2, 1990, Kirkland, Wash.
17. Robbins G, Powers D, and Burgess S: *A wellness way of life*, Dubuque, Ia, 1991, Wm C Brown.
18. Roth DL, Holmes DS: Influence of physical fitness in determining the impact of stressful life events on physical and psychological health, *Psychosomatic Medicine* 47:2, March/April 1985.
19. *Start taking charge: adaptation to stress*, Aetna Life Insurance Co, Seattle, 1984, Bob Hope International Heart Research Institute.
20. Swarth J: *Stress and nutrition*, San Diego, 1986, Health Media of America.

LABORATORY EXPERIENCE 9–1 _____

Determining Your Stress Level

To evelute your level of stress and to help you identify changes that you need to make, circle the number under the appropriate response to each question.
Use the following guidelines in making your decisions:

Rarely—Almost never
Sometimes—Once or twice each week
Often—Four or more times each week

HOW FREQUENTLY DO YOU:	RARELY	SOMETIMES	OFTEN
1. Experience one or more of the symptoms of excess stress such as tension, pain in the neck or shoulders, or headaches?	1	3	5
2. Find it difficult to concentrate on what you are doing because of deadlines or other tasks that must be completed?	1	3	5
3. Become irritable when you have to wait in line or get caught in a traffic jam?	1	3	5
4. Eat, drink, or smoke in an attempt to relax and/or relieve tension?	1	3	5
5. Worry about your work or other deadlines at night and/or on weekends?	1	3	5
6. Wake up in the night thinking about all the things you must do the next day?	1	3	5
7. Feel impatient at the slowness with which many events take place?	1	3	5
8. Find yourself short of time to complete everything that needs to be done?	1	3	5
9. Become upset because things have not gone *your* way?	1	3	5
10. Tend to lose your temper and get irritable?	1	3	5
11. Wake up in the night and have a hard time getting back to sleep?	1	3	5
12. Drive over the speed limit?	1	3	5
13. Interrupt people while they are talking or complete their sentences for them?	1	3	5
14. Forget about appointments and/or lose objects or forget where you put them?	1	3	5
15. Take on too many responsibilities?	1	3	5

Add the numbers together that you circled.

Enter your score here _____

Evaluate your score according to the following criteria:

Potential level of stress

Low	<35
Moderate	35-42
High	43-50
Very high	>50

Positive and Negative Coping Skills

People react differently to stressful situations. Following is a list of what would be considered "positive" responses.
Check off the appropriate response for each of these. If there are other positive ways that you deal with stress, please list them at the bottom of the list.

RESPONSE	NEVER	SOMETIMES	OFTEN
Meditate	____	____	____
Stretch	____	____	____
Engage in progressive muscle relaxation	____	____	____
Listen to music	____	____	____
Exercise aerobically	____	____	____
Watch television	____	____	____
Go to the movies	____	____	____
Read	____	____	____
Work on puzzles or play games	____	____	____
Go for a leisurely walk	____	____	____
Go to a health club	____	____	____
Relax in a steam room or sauna	____	____	____
Spend time alone	____	____	____
Go fishing or hunting	____	____	____
Participate in some form of recreational activity such as golf	____	____	____
Do some work in the yard	____	____	____
Socialize with friends	____	____	____
Sit outside and relax	____	____	____
Engage in a hobby	____	____	____
Other responses—list	____	____	____
_____	____	____	____
_____	____	____	____
_____	____	____	____

Listed below are some negative ways of reacting to stress. Check off the appropriate column for each of these. If there are other negative ways you react to stress, list these at the bottom of the list.

RESPONSE	NEVER	SOMETIMES	OFTEN
Act violently	____	____	____
Yell at someone	____	____	____
Overeat	____	____	____
Do not eat for long periods	____	____	____
Drink an excessive amount of alcohol	____	____	____
Drink lots of coffee	____	____	____
Smoke tobacco	____	____	____
Kick something	____	____	____
Throw something	____	____	____
Drive fast in a car	____	____	____
Swear	____	____	____

Modified from Anspaugh DJ, Hamrick MH, and Rosato FD: *Wellness: concepts and applications*, St Louis, 1991, Mosby–Year Book.

Pace up and down
Bite your fingernails
Take tranquilizers
Take valium or other drugs
Other responses—list

_____

_____

_____

You should compare the number of positive and negative responses. If your negative responses outnumber your positive responses, you have reason to be concerned about your stress level. You will need to try some of the positive responses in an attempt to reduce your level of stress.

Exercise and Cardiovascular Disease

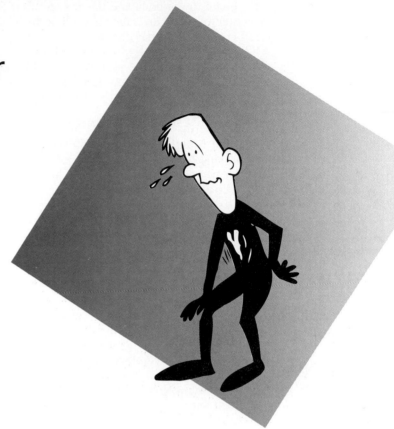

CHAPTER OBJECTIVES

When you understand the material in this chapter, you will be able to:

- Identify the diseases that affect the cardiovascular system
- Define atherosclerosis, and explain why it is the underlying cause of most cardiovascular disease
- Discuss the lifestyle behaviors that contribute to the development of cardiovascular disease
- Identify the primary and contributing risk factors associated with cardiovascular disease
- Explain why the number of deaths from cardiovascular disease has decreased significantly in the last 10 years
- Identify the two important lipoproteins, and differentiate clearly between them
- Explain why the cholesterol/HDL ratio is a better indicator of cardiovascular disease than simply using the total cholesterol level
- Differentiate clearly between type I and type II diabetes
- Explain how exercise can positively influence other cardiovascular risk factors
- Evaluate your lifestyle, and identify changes you can make to reduce your chances of cardiovascular disease
- Determine your risk of cardiovascular disease

The word **cardiovascular** refers to the heart and blood vessels that make up the lifestream of the human body. Basic information about the circulation of the blood in the body and the changes that occur with regular aerobic exercise was presented in Chapter 2. Before reading this chapter, you may want to review the material contained in that chapter.

Although the death rate from cardiovascular disease has declined significantly in the United States in the past 20 years, this group of disorders is still by far the leading cause of death; it accounts for more than 945,000 deaths each year, which is approximately 43% of all deaths. Deaths from cancer total approximately 497,000 each year.

Consider the following facts relative to cardiovascular disease:

- Each American still has a 50% chance of developing some form of cardiovascular disease.
- Nearly one in four Americans has one or more forms of cardiovascular disease.
- Almost one out of two Americans dies of cardiovascular disease.
- Cardiovascular diseases are not just a threat to elderly persons—nearly one fifth of all persons who die from cardiovascular disease are under the age of 65, and 45% of all heart attacks occur to persons in this age-group.

CARDIOVASCULAR DISEASE

Diseases affecting the cardiovascular system may be inherited; they also can be caused by various personal habits or by infection or injury. The major cause of cardiovascular disease is the build-up of fatty substances along the inside walls of blood vessels. These blood vessels then narrow to create a condition known as **atherosclerosis.** Blood may not be supplied in a sufficient quantity to various parts of the body; those areas are thus deprived of a sufficient supply of oxygen.

The heart, which is composed of muscular tissue, also requires its own continuous blood supply. This supply is delivered through a special set of arteries known as the *coronary arteries.*

With cardiovascular disease, damage may occur to the heart itself, in the coronary arteries, or in other blood vessels throughout the body. Thus cardiovascular disease is not a single disorder, but rather comprises several specific diseases.

COMMON CARDIOVASCULAR DISEASES

The estimated number of deaths each year caused by the major types of cardiovascular disease are given below.

Coronary heart disease (heart attack)	497,850
Stroke	147,470
Hypertensive disease	31,630
Rheumatic fever and rheumatic heart disease	6000
All other cardiovascular diseases	262,050
TOTAL	945,000

Atherosclerosis

Atherosclerosis is the underlying cause of more than 95% of all cardiovascular disease. It is the more common form of **arteriosclerosis,** or hardening of the arteries. With atherosclerosis the arterial walls thicken, as well as harden.

The process may start with several lipids present in the bloodstream, including cholesterol, triglycerides, phospholipids, and fatty acids. It is believed that atherosclerosis usually begins with a deposit of some form of fatty material on the inner layer of the arterial wall. Such a deposit is known as a **plaque.** After a time, these deposits may become embedded in the intima, the inner layer of the artery. The lumen—or opening—through which the blood must pass gradually narrows with each deposit, and the blood flow may be seriously impaired. This is illustrated in Fig. 10-1.

Atherosclerosis may begin developing early in life, yet the symptoms may not appear until much later. A person can have the condition for 50 years or more and not

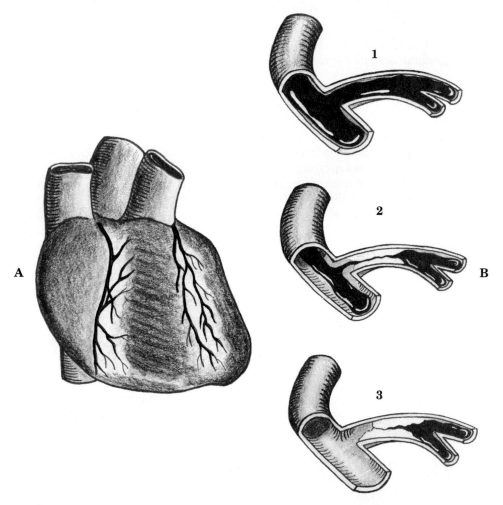

Fig. 10-1 **A,** The heart showing the right and left coronary arteries. **B,** The development of atherosclerosis: *1,* normal blood flow; *2,* restricted blood flow; *3,* completely blocked coronary artery

die from it. However, many people are not so fortunate; each year almost 1 million people in the United States die from diseases caused by atherosclerosis.

Coronary heart disease

Coronary heart disease, often referred to as a heart attack, causes almost 500,000 deaths in the United States each year. A heart attack occurs when a section of the heart muscle is deprived of its blood supply. The gradual narrowing of the coronary arteries sets the stage for this development. Most heart attacks occur when a blood clot (thrombus) lodges in one of the narrowed arteries, cutting off or limiting the blood supply to a particular area of the heart. Although such an attack is usually sudden, it commonly stems from slowly developing atherosclerosis in the coronary arteries.

When part of the heart is deprived of sufficient oxygen, certain damage may occur. This damage is referred to as **myocardial infarction.** *Myocardium* is the Latin name of the heart muscle. The word *infarction* means death to tissue by loss of its normal supply of oxygenated blood. Thus the term *myocardial infarction* means that a small portion of the heart muscle has died, because an artery or branch of an artery that formerly supplied it with oxygenated blood has been closed.

With regular aerobic exercise, not only is the incidence of coronary heart disease much lower, but the survival rate is much higher. This is possibly due to the development of a system of smaller blood vessels that detour the blood around a blockage in a coronary artery. This secondary system is called **collateral circulation,** and these vessels are much more extensively developed in active people than in individuals who are not active.

Signs of a heart attack. A common initial symptom of coronary heart disease is chest pain, called *angina pectoris,* which results when the heart muscle does not receive enough blood. The pain can be described as a pressing or squeezing sensation, and it usually lasts for a few minutes. It is focused in the center of the chest below the sternum, although it may spread to the shoulders and may also be felt in one or both arms. Immediate rest usually provides relief. This condition usually occurs when the heart's need for oxygen increases, such as during physical exertion or as a result of stress.

Angina pectoris may be accompanied by one or more of the following—dizziness, fainting, shortness of breath, and excessive sweating. If you have chest pain and discomfort lasting for more than 2 minutes, you need to seek emergency medical help immediately. It should be noted, however, that sharp, short twinges of pain that last for only a few seconds are not usually signals of a heart attack.

Stroke

A stroke occurs when a part of the brain is deprived of its blood supply, leaving the nerve cells in that part of the brain unable to function properly. When this happens, the parts of the body controlled by these nerve cells also cannot function.

The importance of a regular supply of oxygen to the brain is clearly demonstrated during prolonged vigorous exercise, when the body demands additional oxygen for the working muscles to use. Blood is diverted from various parts of the body to the working musculature. The brain is the only area where the blood supply does not change, which demonstrates the importance of a steady supply of blood to the brain. The blood supply to the brain may be impaired by clotting, compression, or hemorrhage.

The most common cause of a stroke is a thrombus lodged in one of the arteries leading to the brain. If such a blockage occurs, the blood supply to part of the brain is impaired, and the person has suffered from **cerebral thrombosis.** In the case of a stroke, as with a heart attack, atherosclerosis is an important underlying cause. A stroke also can be caused by a brain tumor or by excess pressure on the brain or on an artery supplying blood to the brain. A fourth cause of stroke is bleeding, or hemorrhage, in an artery supplying blood to the brain, which reduces the supply of blood available to the brain.

IDENTIFICATION OF RISK FACTORS ASSOCIATED WITH CARDIOVASCULAR DISEASE

Preventive medicine is the key to reducing the chances of having a heart attack. It is obvious that what we eat and how we live largely determine our susceptibility. In a recent survey in the United States, more than 92% of the participants agreed with the following statement: "If we lived more healthful lives, ate more nutritious foods, smoked less, maintained our proper weight, and exercised regularly, it would do more to improve our health than anything doctors or medicine could do for us."[21]

During the past 30 years, attempts have been made to determine the basic cause or causes of heart disease. Large populations have been observed over long periods and their living habits and medical records carefully analyzed in relation to the incidence of coronary heart disease. The Framingham heart study[21] began in 1949 under the direction of The National Heart, Lung and Blood Institute. Over 5000 participants started in this program, and of these almost 3000 still remain. These subjects are monitored each year, and the information obtained relative to heart disease and lifestyle habits has contributed greatly to our knowledge of cardiovascular disease. Another large study involved over 17,000 Harvard alumni who were studied for more than 20 years. These studies have helped identify several factors associated with an increased risk of cardiovascular disease.[23]

Risk factors that cannot be changed

Four of the risk factors associated with cardiovascular disease cannot be altered by the individual:

1. *Heredity:* Evidence supports the hypothesis that a history of heart disease in the immediate family increases the possibility of cardiovascular illness.
2. *Gender:* Research indicates that the incidence of heart attacks is lower in women under 45 years of age than in men of a comparable age.
3. *Race:* Hypertension, accompanied by a higher incidence of heart attack deaths and stroke, is much more prevalent among black Americans than among whites.
4. *Age:* The incidence of heart attack and the death rates attributable to it increases with age. For example, for those who are 65 years of age or older, 60% of all deaths are caused by cardiovascular disease. This figure is only 11% for those aged 15 to 24 years and 27% for the age-group 35 to 44 years.

Risk factors that can be changed

Fortunately, many of the risk factors associated with premature death from cardiovascular disease can be reduced by an adjustment in living habits. It is interesting to note that the 25% decrease in deaths associated with cardiovascular disease in the past 10 years has coincided with the following:

- A reduction in cigarette smoking
- A decrease in the average serum cholesterol level

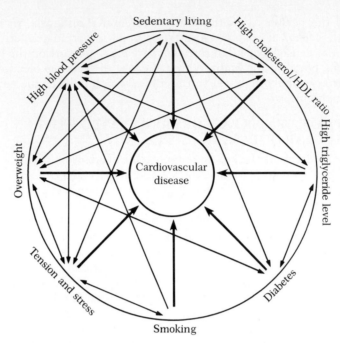

Fig. 10-2 Modifiable risk factors associated with cardiovascular disease.

- A decrease in the consumption of foods high in fat
- An increase in the number of people controlling hypertension
- An increase in the number of people exercising regularly

The risk factors that can be changed are depicted in Fig. 10-2.

Notice that not only do each of these factors contribute directly to cardiovascular disease, but many of them interact to intensify the risk. An arrow pointing from one factor to another indicates that that factor has a negative influence on the one to which it points. Arrows pointing in both directions between two factors (such as with overweight and high blood pressure) indicate that the two factors have a negative influence on each other.

The American Heart Association suggests that the risk factors be grouped into two classifications—major risk factors and contributing risk factors.

Major risk factors are those which the research has shown to be directly associated with an increase in the risk of cardiovascular disease. They are sometimes referred to as primary risk factors. They are identified in the figure to the left:

Contributing risk factors are also associated with an increased risk of cardiovascular disease but not as directly, and their significance has not yet been as clearly determined. They are often referred to as secondary risk factors and are identified in the figure on the next page.

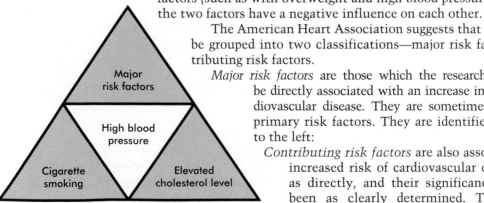

Major risk factors associated with cardiovascular disease.

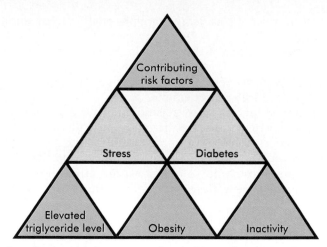

Contributing risk factors associated with cardiovascular disease.

MAJOR RISK FACTORS
Cigarette smoking

It is encouraging to note that in recent years the incidence of smoking has dropped significantly. However, in 1990 more than 50 million Americans continue to smoke and are either unwilling or unable to quit; this represents approximately 26% of the adult population. This number has decreased by 30% in the last 22 years.

Cigarette smoking has many detrimental effects. The World Health Organization states that "the control of cigarette smoking could do more to improve health and prolong life than any other single action in the field of preventive medicine."[8]

Consider the following facts, which have been summarized from material from the American Heart Association and from reports from the Surgeon General of the United States:

- Cigarette smokers have a 70% higher rate of early death from all causes than do nonsmokers.
- Tobacco is associated with an estimated 325,000 premature deaths each year.
- An additional 10 million Americans are currently suffering from chronic diseases caused by smoking.
- The risk of developing lung cancer is 10 times greater for cigarette smokers than for nonsmokers.
- Life expectancy for cigarette smokers has been shown to be greatly reduced. For example, a person between 20 and 35 years of age who smokes two packs of cigarettes per day has a life expectancy 8 to 9 years shorter than that of a nonsmoker of the same age.

It is interesting to note that those who smoke cigarettes also tend to have poorer health habits. When compared with nonsmokers, smokers:

- Exercise less
- Are less likely to check their blood pressure
- See their dentist less frequently
- Are less likely to know their cholesterol level
- Consume more alcohol

In light of these facts, it is not surprising that 90% of all current smokers have experienced a desire to quit.

The following is a summary of the research available on cigarette smoking and cardiovascular disease:

- Those who smoke cigarettes regularly have a much higher incidence of cardiovascular disease than those who do not smoke.
- Those with a history of regular cigarette smoking have a considerably higher early death rate from cardiovascular disease than those who do not smoke.
- The greater the number of cigarettes smoked daily, the higher the incidence of coronary heart disease and the higher the incidence of sudden death after heart disease. For example, those who smoke one pack of cigarettes or more per day are twice as likely to have a heart attack than those who do not smoke (Fig. 10-3).
- Pipe and cigar smokers rate only slightly higher than nonsmokers with regard to the incidence of cardiovascular disease (Fig. 10-3).

Most people who smoke regularly are aware of smoking's detrimental effects on overall health and wellness. In summary, these effects are the following:

- Smoking releases nicotine and other toxic substances into the blood, adversely affecting the inner linings of the blood vessels. This makes it easier for cholesterol and triglycerides to be deposited on the arterial walls and for plaques to form.
- Smoking makes red blood cells more cohesive, thus increasing the formation of blood clots.
- Smoking reduces the body's level of **high-density lipoprotein (HDL)** and increases the **low-density lipoprotein level (LDL).**

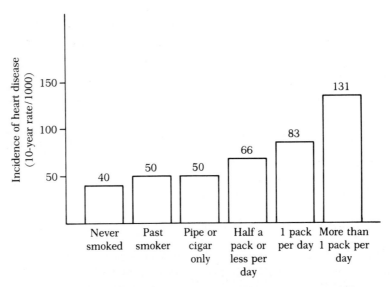

Fig. 10-3 The relationship between smoking and the incidence of the first heart atack in a 10-year period for men aged 30 to 59 years. (Data from *Heart book: a guide to prevention and treatment of cardiovascular disease*, New York, 1980, American Heart Association.)

- Smoking increases the heart rate.
- Smoking constricts blood vessels and may increase blood pressure.

The good news about all this is that a person who quits smoking quickly reduces his or her excess risk of cardiovascular disease. From a health standpoint, the only way to go about it is to QUIT. Of those who successfully quit smoking, 95% do so on their own, and those who quit all at once are more successful than those who try to quit in steps. Successful quitters give the following reasons for stopping:

- Health concerns
- Wanting to set an example for others, particularly family members
- Desire for self-control
- Aesthetic reasons, such as breath odor and loss of taste for food

Even though there is no direct relationship between exercise and smoking, many people try to quit smoking and change their nutritional habits when they start a serious exercise program.

If you quit smoking and you are trying to lose weight, it is important that you make some adjustments in your eating and/or exercise habits. The reason for this is that smoking speeds up your metabolism. Studies show that smoking one pack of cigarettes per day can increase your metabolism by approximately 250 calories. So if you quit smoking, you would have to either eat 250 calories less per day or exercise so that you burn 250 more calories, simply to maintain your pre-sent weight. In terms of exercise, this is equivalent to walking 2 to $2^1/_2$ miles for most people. You can determine the equivalent amount of food by consulting Appendix B.

High blood pressure

Blood pressure is the amount of force that blood exerts against the walls of the arteries. Blood pressure is generated by the heart as it contracts and is maintained by the elasticity of the arterial walls.

Blood pressure changes constantly during each cardiac cycle. Each time the heart contracts, the blood pressure goes up as more blood is forced from the heart into the arterial system. The contraction phase of the cardiac cycle is called systole; thus the upper blood pressure figure is referred to as systolic blood pressure. The relaxation phase of the cardiac cycle is called diastole, hence the lower blood pressure figure is known as diastolic blood pressure. Additional information about blood pressure and the procedures for measuring it are included in Chapter 2.

Consistently high blood pressure is called **hypertension**, one of the risk factors of cardiovascular disease. The higher the blood pressure, the greater the risk. High blood pressure can also contribute to kidney failure.

Although it is difficult to define the limits of "normal" blood pressure, there seems to be general agreement that a reading that is consistently at 140/90 mm Hg or higher indicates a significantly greater risk of cardiovascular disease, and a person with such a reading should initiate serious measures to reduce his or her blood pressure.

It has been estimated that more than 62 million Americans have blood pressure readings higher than 140/90 mm Hg, and that in approximately 35 million of these people, the pressure exceeds 160/95 mm Hg. In only about 10% of the cases is the cause for hypertension known.

If you have high blood pressure, the following recommendations may be of help:

- If you are overweight your primary goal should be weight reduction. Losing as little as 10 lb has been shown to have a significant effect on your blood pressure.

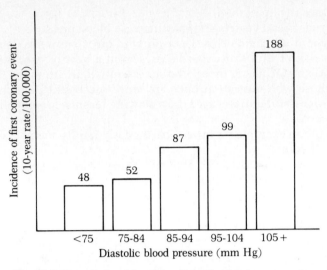

Fig. 10-4 The relationship of the diastolic blood pressure to the incidence of coronary heart disease. (Data from *Heart book: a guide to prevention and treatment of cardiovascular disease*, New York, 1980, American Heart Association.)

- Reduce your sodium intake—excessive sodium intake contributes to approximately 25% of the cases of high blood pressure. You need only approximately 1000 mg of sodium per day. It may be obtained from several sources—small amounts occur naturally in some foods, it is added to foods during processing, or it may be added to foods during cooking or at the table. Most added sodium comes from salt—1 tsp of salt contains over 2000 mg of sodium. The average American gets approximately 7500 mg of sodium per day. The National Research Council recommends between 1100 and 3300 mg/day. Those with high blood pressure or a history of hypertension should try to limit their intake to 2000 mg or less per day.
- Learn to relax so that you can minimize the effects of stress in your life.
- Participate regularly in a good aerobic exercise program.
- Stop smoking (if you are a cigarette smoker).
- Decrease your alcohol intake.
- Be careful about taking high doses of nose drops or over-the-counter sinus medicines. These may raise your blood pressure.

Research has shown that people with consistently high blood pressure have greater risk of coronary heart disease (Fig. 10-4). If diet and exercise do not reduce your blood pressure, medication may be necessary. You should follow your doctor's recommendations.

Elevated cholesterol level

Cholesterol is an odorless, white, fatlike substance found in the body and in all foods of animal origin. It performs several crucial functions:
- It is an important constituent of all cell walls.
- It is important for conducting nerve impulses.

▪ It is used to make various hormones, such as estrogen and testosterone.

▪ It is used to make bile, which aids in the process of breaking up fat.

Research indicates that the amount of cholesterol in the blood (serum cholesterol) is one of the most important risk factors associated with the development of athero-sclerosis. Atherosclerosis occurs when the inner lining of the artery is damaged in some way. Such damage is usually caused by a toxic substance, such as nicotine. Under these conditions, cholesterol can penetrate the inner lining of the artery and a plaque (fatty deposit) can form. Once the arterial lining has been damaged, the extent of the buildup within the artery will depend largely on the amount of cholesterol in the blood stream. That, in turn, will be influenced by three factors:

▪ The amount of cholesterol manufactured by the liver

▪ The amount of cholesterol and saturated fat in the food eaten

▪ The efficiency with which the body breaks down and excretes cholesterol

The production and breaking down of cholesterol occur primarily in the liver, and usually the two are balanced such that the amount of cholesterol in the blood is maintained within safe limits. However, some people have an inherited tendency for a very high cholesterol level, whereas others seem to have a very low level regardless of what they eat. In general, however, a person's cholesterol level apparently is influenced most by how much saturated fat and cholesterol he or she eats. Other contributing factors include excess body fat, high level of stress, and lack of exercise.

Research has shown that people with a high level of serum cholesterol have a greater chance of developing coronary heart disease (Fig. 10-5). Note that with a total blood cholesterol level of less than 200 mg/dl, the incidence of coronary heart disease is relatively low. The risk levels for total blood cholesterol proposed by the National Heart, Lung, and Blood Institute follow on p. 340.

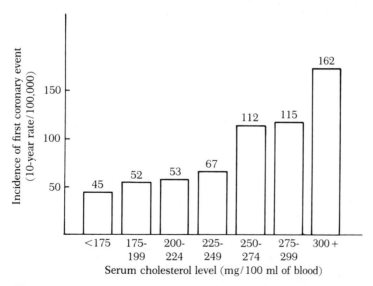

Fig. 10-5 The relationship of the serum cholesterol level to the incidence of the first coronary event. (Data from *Heart book: a guide to prevention and treatment of cardiovascular disease*, New York, 1980, American Heart Association.)

TOTAL BLOOD CHOLESTEROL LEVEL

Desirable	<200 mg/dl
Borderline to high	200–239 mg/dl
High	>240 mg/dl

The ideal values for adults would appear to be somewhere between 120 and 160 mg/dl. The incidence of cardiovascular disease is lowest when the serum cholesterol level is below 160 mg/dl. Table 10-1 on pp. 343-345 compares the fat and cholesterol content of several foods and gives the saturated fat content for each. The information in Table 10-1 can help you identify the total amount of fat in each food listed, as well as the amount of saturated fat in these foods. You should also look closely at the information pertaining to fast foods, which is included in Appendix C. When selecting foods, you should try to pick low-fat items and pay particular attention to the amount of saturated fat.

The following changes are recommended for people whose blood cholesterol is too high:

- Decrease your total fat intake.
- Eat less saturated fat.
- Decrease your dietary cholesterol.
- Increase your intake of water-soluble fiber—found mainly in fruits, vegetables, grains, and legumes.
- Lose weight or fat if you are overweight or obese.
- Participate regularly in aerobic exercise.
- Reduce your stress level.

Cholesterol/HDL ratio

The total amount of cholesterol in the blood is an excellent measurement for predicting your risk of developing coronary heart disease. However, you can get an even better indication of your risk with a more sophisticated measurement of cholesterol.

Lipids (fats) are insoluble in water and cannot be transported in the blood by themselves. They combine with protein to form **lipoproteins.** There are three major lipoproteins:

- High-density lipoproteins (HDLs)
- Low-density lipoproteins (LDLs)
- Very low-density lipoproteins (VLDLs)

The amounts of protein and lipids present in each of these is summarized in Fig. 10-6.

The HDLs are the smallest and most dense—they contain approximately 50% proteins and about 18% cholesterol. HDLs are very stable and tend to attract loose particles of cholesterol in the blood and remove them from the bloodstream. Research has shown that people with a high HDL level have a lower incidence of heart disease. For this reason, these lipoproteins have become known as "good" cholesterol.

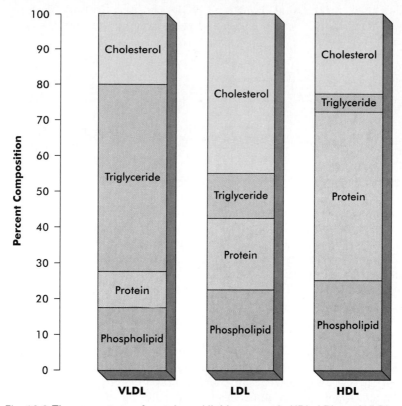

Fig. 10-6 The percentage of protein and lipids present in HDL, LDL, and VLDL.

LDLs, on the other hand, contain large amounts of cholesterol (43%) and relatively small amounts of protein (25%). Their poor stability often allows cholesterol to break away from the protein, making persons more susceptible to coronary heart disease. Increased LDL levels are associated with an increased incidence of cardiovascular disease. For this reason, LDLs are often referred to as "bad" cholesterol. VLDLs contain mainly triglycerides and only very small amounts of cholesterol.

The ratio of total cholesterol to HDL cholesterol is probably the best single measurement for predicting cardiovascular disease. The lower the ratio, the less is your chance of having coronary heart disease. To determine your ratio, simply divide your total cholesterol value by your HDL value.

EXAMPLE:

If your total cholesterol is 200 and your HDL is 50, you can calculate your ratio as follows:

$$\text{Total cholesterol/HDL ratio} = 200/50$$
$$= 4.0$$

The risk levels for the total cholesterol/HDL ratio are as follows. Because the HDL level differs significantly between men and women, a separate set of scores is necessary for each sex.

CHOLESTEROL/HDL RATIO

	MEN	WOMEN
Low risk	<5.0	<4.4
Moderate to high risk	5.0–5.7	4.4–5.1
High risk	>6.7	>5.1

Also of importance are your HDL and LDL levels. Your desirable LDL level is less than 130 mg/dl. Between 130 and 160 mg/dl is borderline, and above 160 mg/dl you are at high risk for cardiovascular disease. With regard to HDL, men whose level is less than 25 mg/dl and women whose level is less than 40 mg/dl are at three times the normal risk for developing cardiovascular disease.

Your total cholesterol/HDL ratio is influenced primarily by what you eat and what you do. To lower this ratio and thereby reduce your chance of coronary heart disease, you must lower your LDL level and increase your HDL level.

To lower your LDL level, you should do the following:
- Reduce your intake of foods high in cholesterol (Table 10-1).
- Reduce your intake of foods high in saturated fat (Table 10-1).
- Exercise regularly in a good aerobic exercise program.
- Maintain a desirable weight and a desirable percentage of body fat.

Aerobic exercise can contribute more to increasing your HDL level than any other single factor. Studies show that people who exercise regularly have a higher HDL level than do people who do not exercise. An extremely high level of exercise is associated with an extremely high level of HDL.

Research also has pinpointed three substances that lower your HDL level. When possible, these should be avoided.

Cigarette smoking: One pack of cigarettes per day will reduce your HDL level by 5 points or more.

Birth control pills: Regular use of birth control pills will also reduce your HDL level by 5 points or more.

Prescription medications: Several medications used for blood pressure and/or heart disease have a detrimental effect on your HDL level.

Amount of exercise necessary to change blood lipids

Considerable research has been done on the effects of exercise on blood lipids. These studies show that men and women who participate regularly in aerobic exercise generally have a slightly lower total cholesterol level and a much higher HDL level.

It appears that the *minimum* amount of exercise needed to precipitate these changes corresponds closely to the amount prescribed for development of aerobic fitness—30 minutes of continuous activity performed three to five times per week with the heart rate sustained in the target zone. In a walking or running program,

TABLE 10-1 Fat and cholesterol content of selected foods*

Food	Serving size	Saturated fat (g)	Total fat (g)	Cholesterol (mg)
Beef				
Top round lean (broiled)	3½ oz	2.2	6.2	84
Ground lean (broiled)	3½ oz	7.3	18.5	87
Prime rib (broiled)	3½ oz	14.9	35.2	86
Processed meats				
Link sausage, smoked (pork and beef)	3½ oz	10.6	30.3	71
Bologna (beef)	3½ oz	11.7	28.4	56
Frankfurter (beef)	3½ oz	12.0	29.4	48
Salami (pork or beef)	3½ oz	12.2	34.4	79
Pork				
Ham (extra lean)	3½ oz	1.4	4.2	45
Pork-center loin (lean)	3½ oz	4.7	13.7	111
Pork spareribs (braised)	3½ oz	11.8	30.3	121
Poultry				
Chicken (roasted)				
White meat without skin	3½ oz	1.3	4.5	85
White meat with skin	3½ oz	3.1	10.9	84
Dark meat without skin	3½ oz	2.7	9.7	93
Dark meat with skin	3½ oz	4.4	15.8	91
Fish				
Cod	3½ oz	0.1	0.7	58
Perch	3½ oz	0.2	1.2	115
Snapper	3½ oz	0.4	1.7	47
Rockfish	3½ oz	1.6	6.3	49
Mackerel	3½ oz	4.2	17.8	75
Crustaceans				
Crab	3½ oz	0.2	1.8	100
Lobster	3½ oz	0.1	0.5	72
Shrimp	3½ oz	0.3	1.1	195
Liver meats				
Chicken	3½ oz	1.8	5.5	631
Beef	3½ oz	1.9	4.9	389
Eggs				
Egg yolk	1	1.7	5.7	272
Egg white	1	0	Trace	0
Whole egg	1	1.7	5.6	272

*From *Facts about blood cholesterol,* US Department of Health and Human Services, 1986, National Institute of Health.

Continued.

TABLE 10-1 Fat and cholesterol content of selected foods*—cont'd

Food	Serving size	Saturated fat (g)	Total fat (g)	Cholesterol (mg)
Nuts				
Almonds (dry roasted)	3½ oz	4.9	51.6	0
Pistachios (dry)	3½ oz	6.1	48.4	0
Peanuts (dried)	3½ oz	6.8	49.2	0
Cashews	3½ oz	9.2	46.4	0
Brazil nuts	3½ oz	16.2	66.2	0
Milk and cream				
Skim milk	1 cup	0.3	0.4	4
Low-fat milk (1% fat)	1 cup	1.6	2.6	10
Whole milk (3.7% fat)	1 cup	5.6	8.9	35
Light cream	1 cup	28.8	46.3	159
Heavy cream	1 cup	54.8	88.1	326
Yogurt and sour cream				
Plain yogurt (skim milk)	1 cup	0.3	0.4	4
Plain yogurt (low-fat)	1 cup	2.3	3.5	14
Plain yogurt (whole milk)	1 cup	4.8	7.4	29
Sour cream	1 cup	30.0	48.2	102
Soft cheeses				
Cottage cheese (low-fat)	1 cup	1.5	2.3	10
American (processed spread)	1 cup	30.2	48.1	125
Cream cheese	1 cup	49.9	79.2	250
Hard cheeses				
Mozzarella (part skim)	8 oz	22.9	36.1	132
Mozzarella (whole)	8 oz	29.7	49.0	177
Provolone	8 oz	38.8	60.4	157
Swiss	8 oz	40.4	62.4	209
Muenster	8 oz	43.4	68.1	218
American (processed)	8 oz	44.7	71.1	213
Cheddar	8 oz	47.9	75.1	238
Vegetable oils and shortening				
Safflower oil	1 cup	19.8	218.0	0
Sunflower oil	1 cup	22.5	218.0	0
Corn oil	1 cup	27.7	218.0	0
Olive oil	1 cup	29.2	216.0	0
Soybean oil	1 cup	31.4	218.0	0
Margarine, soft	1 cup	32.2	182.6	0
Margarine, stick or brick	1 cup	34.2	182.6	0
Peanut oil	1 cup	36.4	216.0	0
Household vegetable shortening	1 cup	51.2	205.0	0
Cottonseed oil	1 cup	56.4	218.0	0
Palm oil	1 cup	107.4	218.0	0
Coconut oil	1 cup	188.5	218.0	0

TABLE 10-1 Fat and cholesterol content of selected foods*—cont'd

Food	Serving size	Saturated fat (g)	Total fat (g)	Cholesterol (mg)
Animal fats				
Chicken fat	1 cup	61.2	205.0	175
Lard	1 cup	80.4	205.0	195
Beef fat	1 cup	102.1	205.0	223
Butter	1 cup	114.4	183.9	496

this would mean approximately 10 to 15 miles per week. Several studies have shown, however, that even greater changes occur in blood lipid levels if the amount of activity is increased substantially above this level.

Benefits of reduced cholesterol

Several recent studies have demonstrated conclusively that lowering the cholesterol level in the blood helps reduce the incidence of coronary heart disease. A 12-year study costing $150 million—performed by The National Heart, Lung and Blood Institute—showed conclusively that reducing the serum cholesterol level results in a decrease in heart disease. The research concluded that for those who reduce their blood cholesterol levels by 25%, there will be a 49% reduction in the incidence of cardiovascular disease. Other research shows the following:

- A diet with moderate fat intake reduced the level of cholesterol by 3% to 4% for all participants. People on a much stricter diet had a decrease of 10% to 15%.
- People who took cholestyramine, a cholesterol-lowering drug, had cholesterol levels reduced by as much as 25%.
- Overall, people whose cholesterol levels were lowered an average of 8% had a 19% lower rate of fatal and nonfatal heart attacks.
- Cholesterol reduction is also associated with lower rates of atherosclerosis and coronary bypass surgery.

Multiple risk factors

With regard to the three primary risk factors, the incidence of heart disease increases in proportion to the number of risk factors present. This is illustrated in Fig. 10-7 on p. 346. Notice that when none of the risk factors are present, the risk of cardiovascular disease is less than that for the average American. A person who smokes and has a high cholesterol level and high blood pressure has a risk of 3.84. This means that he or she is 3.84 times more likely to have a heart attack than is the average American.

INFORMATION ON CONTRIBUTING RISK FACTORS

Even though these risk factors may not have a "direct" relationship to cardiovascular disease, they are still very important factors. Following is information relative to each of these factors.

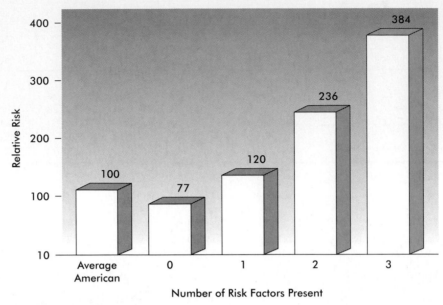

Fig. 10-7 The relative incidence of cardiovascular disease in proportion to the number of risk factors present.

Elevated triglyceride level

Triglycerides are another form of fat circulating in the bloodstream. Most people know quite a bit about cholesterol but very little about triglycerides. High levels of triglycerides also contribute to the high incidence of cardiovascular disease.

Of the fat we eat, 95% is in the form of triglycerides; this is also the type of fat that is stored under the skin in the fat cells. Triglycerides in the blood either come from the food we eat or are manufactured by the liver. A high intake of refined sugar and/or alcohol often causes the liver to overproduce triglycerides. Therefore high sugar and/or alcohol consumption usually raises triglyceride levels significantly.

A high level of triglycerides is also associated with increased development of atherosclerosis and is therefore classified as a risk factor. High triglyceride levels are particularly dangerous for people with a high cholesterol level.

The box below shows the level of risk associated with different triglyceride readings.

TRIGLYCERIDE LEVEL (mg/dl)

Low risk	<140
Borderline to high risk	140-180
High risk	>180

If your triglyceride level is high, the following suggestions may be of value to you:
- Reduce your body weight and/or body fat. If you are overweight or obese, a reduction in weight and/or fat usually results in a decrease in your triglyceride level.

- Reduce your intake of refined sugars and alcohol.
- Participate regularly in a good aerobic exercise program. (A recent study showed that people with a high triglyceride level who exercised for 1 hour three times a week reduced their triglyceride level by 25% over a 4-month period.)
- Reduce your fat intake to less than 30% of your total calories.
- Reduce your intake of saturated fat to less than 10% of your total calories.

Some evidence suggests that oils from fish can be used to lower triglyceride levels. Also, most people whose diets have a high percentage of complex carbohydrates have very low triglyceride levels.

High level of tension or stress

Stress is defined as a physical or emotional factor that causes tension. It is an important part of living, and if you handle it properly, you can learn to relax and cope with your anger, fear, tension, and external pressure.

People react differently to specific situations that occur daily; how a person reacts to a situation will determine his or her stress level. Each person can be classified as one of two types. The first is type A—people exhibiting a high stress level and rating high on the following criteria:

1. *Ambition:* An intense, sustained drive to achieve self-selected but usually poorly defined goals
2. *Competitiveness:* A profound inclination and eagerness to compete
3. *Aggressiveness:* A persistent desire for recognition and advancement
4. *Profound sense of time urgency:* Continuous involvement in multiple functions, while constantly subject to restrictions
5. *Drive:* Persistent efforts to accelerate the rate of execution of many physical and mental functions

These traits are normally present in most individuals, but the type A person possesses them to an excessive degree. People in this group include those who cannot stand to have unscheduled time on their hands and who become very upset when they are kept waiting.

Those who rate low in these traits are classified as type B. This is the type of person who usually is able to relax easily. Very seldom does this individual let outside factors adversely influence his or her emotional state. A type B person's level of anxiety and tension is therefore very low.

The relationship between the level of stress and cardiovascular disease has been evaluated, and research clearly shows the following:

- Cardiovascular disease is much more prevalent in the high-stress group (type A) than in the low-stress group (type B).
- Those with a high stress level also have a higher cholesterol level, compared with those with a low stress level.
- The incidence of cigarette smoking is higher in those with a high stress level than in those with a low stress level.

Many people who have a high stress level and have difficulty coping with this stress turn to drugs, alcohol, smoking, and overeating. These are all unhealthful, and they help increase the incidence of cardiovascular disease. Many people turn to exercise as a means of coping with this stress. Chapter 9 deals with stress, especially the role exercise plays in preventing and controlling it.

Obesity and excess weight

Most people are familiar with the health hazards associated with excess fat and excess weight (these were identified in Chapter 7). The conclusion is that it is clearly more healthful to keep body fat and body weight within acceptable limits.

The procedures for measuring body fat and for determining ideal weight also were clearly identified in Chapter 7. If you do not have the opportunity to conduct these tests, you can probably just think back to the time when you felt that you looked your best, and you can probably recall what your weight was then.

Obesity and/or excess weight are risk factors associated with cardiovascular disease. For example, in the Framingham study, people who were 20 lb or more overweight suffered three times as many heart attacks as those of normal weight. The link between obesity and cardiovascular disease may possibly be caused by the following:

- Extra stress is placed on the heart because of the added workload.
- People who are obese or overweight tend to exercise less.
- Obesity is closely associated with increased blood pressure. (One study showed that successful weight reduction reduced hypertension by 41%.)
- Obesity is usually accompanied by increased levels of cholesterol and triglycerides.
- Diabetes occurs more frequently in people who are overweight and/or obese.

Diabetes

Glucose is a simple sugar we get by digesting carbohydrates. It is transported in the blood throughout the body and serves as the major source of energy for each of the body's cells. A high blood glucose level is the primary characteristic of diabetes.

Insulin, a hormone secreted by the pancreas, is responsible for controlling your blood glucose level. Normally, when the blood glucose level rises, more insulin is secreted and most of the body's cells respond by "taking up" glucose from the blood. This excess glucose is stored as glycogen in the muscles or liver or converted to fat and stored in the body. Usually the blood glucose level then quickly returns to normal. However, this process breaks down in the more than 11 million Americans who have diabetes; their bodies cannot maintain a normal blood glucose level.

There are basically two types of diabetes. **Type I diabetes** accounts for fewer than 10% of the cases. With this type of diabetes, the body cannot produce enough insulin. For this reason this type is often referred to as insulin-dependent diabetes. **Type II diabetes** is known as noninsulin-dependent diabetes. Sufficient insulin is available, but for some reason the body does not react to it and is unable to control the blood glucose level. More than 90% of all diabetics are noninsulin-dependent. This disorder usually occurs in people over the age of 40, and almost 90% of the patients can be classified as obese at the time of onset of the disease.

An elevated fasting blood glucose level may be an early sign of diabetes. The box on p. 349 can help you evaluate your blood glucose level.

It has been shown that many people who have diabetes not only have excess glucose in the blood, they may also have difficulty metabolizing fat. This often causes increased atherosclerosis throughout the body and contributes to a high incidence of cardiovascular disease. More than 80% of all diabetics die from some form of cardiovascular disease.

FASTING BLOOD GLUCOSE LEVEL

CATEGORY	BLOOD GLUCOSE LEVEL (mg/dl)
Normal	<115
Borderline to high	115–140
High	>140

Exercise is the key to controlling diabetes. Research shows that sedentary people have a much higher incidence of diabetes than do active people and that this result occurs independently of the differences in obesity. There appear to be several reasons for this:

- Exercise promotes the use of glucose for energy. Diabetics who exercise regularly thus can control their blood glucose levels better and require less insulin than those who do not exercise.
- Exercise increases the number of insulin receptors in the cells and therefore contributes to insulin's effectiveness in removing glucose from the bloodstream.
- Exercise can contribute to the reduction or prevention of obesity. Regular aerobic activity of the correct intensity and duration can prevent the loss of lean body mass and can reduce the amount of body fat. The role that exercise plays was described in detail in Chapter 7.

There is no known cure for diabetes, so it is extremely important to control this disease. This can be done most effectively through diet and exercise and, in extreme cases, by the administration of insulin.

Lack of activity

A previous discussion emphasized the harmful effects of America's sedentary lifestyle. It was shown that automobiles, elevators, television sets, home computers, and many other mechanical devices have reduced expenditure of physical effort. Indisputably, these changes have had a detrimental effect on the fitness level of Americans.

Numerous studies have shown that physical inactivity and lack of exercise are associated with a significantly higher rate of cardiovascular disease. One such project involved a 16-year study of nearly 17,000 Harvard alumni. Data from that study are summarized in Table 10-2.

TABLE 10-2 **Death rates/10,000 among 16,936 Harvard alumni, 1962-1978, classified according to physical activity**

Causes of death	Physical activity level (calories/week)		
	<500	500-2000	>2000
All causes	84.8	66.0	52.1
Cardiovascular disease	39.5	30.8	21.4

This study clearly shows an inverse relationship between the amount of physical activity and the incidence of death from all causes and death from cardiovascular disease. In this study, as in several others that show similar findings, other potential risk factors—such as smoking, obesity, and hypertension—also were analyzed. They did not appear to account for the relationship between physical inactivity and the risk of coronary heart disease.

Notice in the study cited in Table 10-2 that the amount of exercise associated with the lowest death rate (from cardiovascular disease and from all causes) is the amount required to burn 2000 or more calories per week. This is more exercise than is prescribed for the development of aerobic fitness. For example, a 154-lb person running at a speed of 12 minutes per mile would have to run for approximately 40 minutes five times per week to burn 2000 calories. You can use the caloric expenditure values for selected physical activities in Table 7-4 to determine the calories you burn in your exercise program.

The information in Fig. 10-2 shows that sedentary living contributes to each of the other risk factors except smoking. Regular exercise can positively influence each of these factors and can reduce your risk of cardiovascular disease.

This relationship between aerobic fitness level and selected risk factors can clearly be seen in the data on more than 3000 men from the Aerobics Clinic in Dallas. These data are summarized in Table 10-3.

Notice that an increase in the aerobic fitness level is associated with a positive change in each of the cardiovascular risk factors. The changes include the following:

- Reduced level of cholesterol and triglycerides
- Lower body weight and lower percentage of body fat
- Lower resting blood pressure (both systolic and diastolic)
- Higher level of HDL cholesterol

These factors would explain, at least in part, why several studies have shown that physically active people have a much lower incidence of coronary heart disease than do inactive people.

Many heart attacks occur during sudden bursts of vigorous activity, such as during the first snowstorm of the season, when shoveling is necessary, or during the hunting season, when the body is called on to do more work than it is accustomed to. People who exercise regularly show a lower incidence of cardiovascular disease at these times, and they are much more likely to survive a heart attack if one occurs.

TABLE 10-3 **Aerobic fitness level and selected cardiovascular risk factors**

Aerobic fitness level	Body weight (kg)	Percent body fat	Blood pressure (mm Hg)	Cholesterol (mg/dl)	Triglyceride (mg/dl)	HDL cholesterol (mg/dl)
Poor	90.0	29.3	133/87	238	182	37
Fair	86.3	26.9	127/84	237	172	40
Average	82.8	24.0	125/83	228	140	42
Good	79.4	20.8	123/81	222	114	45
Excellent	76.4	18.2	122/80	217	87	50

There are several possible explanations for this. Regular exercise increases the efficiency of the circulatory system, so the same amount of work can be performed with less stress on the heart. There may also be an increase in the diameter of the coronary arteries, accompanied by the development of additional capillaries (collateral circulation), so that blood may actually be able to bypass a partially obstructed artery. Remember also that exercise places stress on the body, and it is therefore accustomed to working at a higher level than a sedentary person is.

PREVALENCE OF CERTAIN RISK FACTORS

Following is a summary showing the prevalence of several of the risk factors associated with cardiovascular disease.

RISK FACTOR	ESTIMATED NUMBER OF AMERICANS (MILLIONS)
Cigarette smoking	52.9
Elevated cholesterol level	
>240 mg/dl	48.8
>200 mg/dl	102.7
Hypertension	
>140 mm Hg systolic or	
>90 mm Hg diastolic	62.7
Obesity/excess weight	
>20% above desirable weight	46.3
Inactivity*	132.2
Completely sedentary	61.0
Irregular activity	71.2

*Inactivity is defined as exercise of less than three times each week.

In recent years most of these figures have improved, but they are still much higher than they should be. They certainly explain why the number one cause of death in this country is still cardiovascular disease.

SUMMARY

The following summary will help you to identify some of the important concepts covered in this chapter.

- Despite the fact that the death rate from cardiovascular disease has decreased by 25% in the last 10 years, cardiovascular disease is still by far the leading cause of death in the United States.
- This decrease in deaths from cardiovascular disease has been associated with many positive lifestyle changes.

- The three major risk factors associated with cardiovascular disease are cigarette smoking, high blood pressure, and an elevated cholesterol level.
- Cigarette smokers also tend to have poorer health habits than those who do not smoke.
- Reducing your sodium intake and your body weight may significantly reduce your blood pressure.
- With regard to cholesterol, you will be at a very low risk for cardiovascular disease if your cholesterol level is <169 mg/dl, your ratio of cholesterol/HDL is <5.0 (men) or <4.4 (women), and your LDL is <130 mg/dl.
- The more major risk factors that apply to you, the greater your chances of cardiovascular disease.
- Contributing risk factors associated with cardiovascular disease include elevated triglyceride level, high level of stress or tension, obesity or excess weight, diabetes, and inactivity.
- Despite the fact that many of the risk factors associated with cardiovascular disease have decreased significantly in recent years, there are still far too many Americans who place themselves at high risk.

KEY TERMS

angina pectoris   A chest pain caused by insufficient blood supply to the heart.

arteriosclerosis   A hardening of the arteries that causes the arterial walls to thicken and lose elasticity.

atherosclerosis   A narrowing and hardening of the arteries as fatty substances build up on arterial walls.

cardiovascular   Pertaining to the heart and blood vessels.

cerebral thrombosis   Damage to part of the brain caused by an insufficient supply of oxygen.

collateral circulation   A system of small arteries that may carry blood to part of the heart when a coronary artery is blocked.

cholesterol   A fatlike substance that is obtained only from foods of animal origin and that may be manufactured by the body.

cholesterol/HDL ratio   The ratio of total cholesterol to high-density lipoprotein cholesterol (HDL).

coronary arteries   The arteries that supply blood to the heart.

diabetes   A disease characterized by an abnormal level of blood glucose.

high-density lipoprotein (HDL)   A lipoprotein that contains the highest proportion of protein; often referred to as "good" cholesterol.

hypertension   Blood pressure that is consistently higher than normal.

lipoprotein   The combination of lipid with protein so that lipids can be transported in the blood.

low-density lipoprotein (LDL)   A lipoprotein that contains the highest proportion of cholesterol; high levels of LDL have been associated with increased incidence of cardiovascular disease.

myocardial infarction   Damage to the heart when it is deprived of sufficient oxygen.

plaque   A deposit of fatty substances (such as cholesterol) on the inner lining of an artery wall.

thrombus   A blood clot.

triglycerides   Fats consisting of three fatty acids and glycerol.

type I diabetes   A type of diabetes in which the body is unable to produce sufficient insulin.

type II diabetes   A type of diabetes in which insulin is ineffective in controlling the blood sugar level.

REFERENCES

1. Anspaugh DJ, Hamrick MH, and Rosato FD: *Wellness concepts and applications*, St Louis, 1991, Mosby–Year Book.
2. Castelli WP et al: Incidence of coronary heart disease and lipoprotein cholesterol, *Journal of the American Medical Association* 256:2835-2838, 1986.
3. Egan B: Nutritional and lifestyle approaches to the prevention and management of hypertension, *Comprehensive Therapy* 11(8):15-20, 1985.
4. Elias M: Exercise lowers heart risk a third, *USA Today*, p. 1, March 12, 1984.
5. *Facts about blood cholesterol*, Pub. No. 882696, US Department of Health and Human Services, November 1987.
6. Findlay S: Cut cholesterol 25%, reduce heart attacks 50%, *USA Today*, p. 1, Jan 12, 1984.
7. Health Vantage: *Exercise and CHD risk reduction*, Battle Creek, Mich, April 1988, Kellogg.
8. *Heart book: a guide to prevention and treatment of cardiovascular disease*, New York, 1980, American Heart Association.
9. *Heart and stroke facts—1992*, Dallas, 1992, American Heart Association.
10. Hubert HB et al: Life-style correlates of risk factor change in young adults—an eight year study of coronary heart disease risk factors in the Framington offspring, *American Journal of Epidemiology* 125:812-831, 1987.
11. *Interpreting your test results*, Fontana, Wisc, 1985, Fitness Monitoring.
12. Jonas S, Silver N: The last cure-all, *American Health*, pp. 62-64, 69, March 1985.
13. Kannel WG: Meaning of the downward trend in cardiovascular mortality, *Journal of the American Medical Association* 247(6):877-881, 1982.
14. Lamb LL, editor: Cigarettes and women, *The Health Letter* 31:4, 1988.
15. Lechere S et al: High density lipoprotein cholesterol, habitual physical activity and physical fitness, *Atherosclerosis* 57:43-51, 1985.
16. McCunney RJ: Fitness, heart disease, and high density lipoprotein: a look at the relationship, *The Physician and Sports Medicine* 15(2):67-79, 1987.
17. Miller RW: On being too rich, too thin and too cholesterol laden, *FDA Consumer*, pp. 31-34, July/August 1981.
18. Miller RW: Diet, exercise and other keys to a healthy heart, *FDA Consumer*, February 1986.
19. Morgan DW et al: HDL concentrations in weight-trained, endurance-trained and sedentary females, *The Physician and Sports Medicine* 14:3, 1986.
20. Morris JN et al: Vigorous exercise in leisure time: protection against coronary heart disease, *Lancet* 8206:1207-1210, 1980.
21. Nieman DC: *Fitness and Sports Medicine*, Palo Alto, Calif, 1990, Bull.
22. Nieman DC et al: *Nutrition*, Dubuque, Ia, 1990, Wm C Brown.
23. Paffenbarger RS et al: Physical activity, all-causes mortality and longevity of college alumni, *New England Journal of Medicine* 314:605-613, 1986.
24. Perry P: Can this man beat the odds? *American Health*, pp. 44-46, April 1987.
25. Powell KE et al: Physical activity—the incidence of coronary heart disease, *Annual Review of Public Health* 8:254-287, 1987.
26. *Salt, sodium and blood pressure*, Dallas, 1979, American Heart Association.
27. Siscovick DS, LaPorte RE, and Newman JM: The disease-specific benefits and risks of physical activity and exercise, Public Health Reports, *Journal of the US Public Health Service* 100(2): 122-126, 1985.
28. Stamler R et al: Nutrition therapy for high blood pressure, *Journal of the American Medical Association* 257:1484-1491, 1987.
29. Storer TW, Ruhling RO: Essential hypertension and exercise, *The Physician and Sports Medicine* 9(6):59, 1981.
30. US Department of Health and Human Services: *The health consequences of smoking*, Washington, DC, 1988, US Government Printing Office.
31. Wood PD et al: Distribution of plasma lipoproteins in middle age male runners, *Metabolism* 25:1249, 1976.
32. Yulsman T: Beating the big ones, *American Health*, p. 49, April 1987.
33. Yulsman T: Sweet news on the sugar disease, *American Health*, pp. 57-59, April 1987.

Arizona Heart Institute Cardiovascular Risk Factor Analysis

Directions: Indicate the points that you have scored in the column on the right for each of the following risk factors. When you finish, total your points and compare that with the results at the end of the activity.

RISK FACTORS	SCORE		
1. Age	Age 56 or over	1	
	Age 55 or under	0	_____
2. Sex	Male	1	
	Female	0	_____
3. Family history	If you have:		
	Blood relatives who have had a heart attack or stroke at or before age 60	12	
	Blood relatives who have had a heart attack or stroke after age 60	6	
	No blood relatives who have had a heart attack or stroke	0	_____
4. Personal history	50 or under: If you had either a heart attack, a stroke, heart or blood vessel surgery	20	
	51 or over: If you had any of the above	10	
	None of the above	0	_____
5. Diabetes	Diabetes before age 40 and now on insulin	10	
	Diabetes at or after age 40 and now on insulin or pills	5	
	Diabetes controlled by diet, or diabetes after age 55	3	
	No diabetes	0	_____
6. Smoking	Two packs per day	10	
	Between one and two packs per day or quit smoking less than a year ago	6	
	If you smoke six or more cigars a day or inhale a pipe regularly	6	
	Less than one pack per day or quit smoking more than 1 year ago	3	
	Never smoked	0	_____
7. Cholesterol (If cholesterol count is not known answer 8)	Cholesterol level—276 or above	10	
	Cholesterol level—between 225 and 275	5	
	Cholesterol level—224 or below	0	
8. Diet (If you have answered 7, do not answer 8)	Does your normal eating pattern include:		
	One serving of red meat daily, more than seven eggs a week, and daily consumption of butter, whole milk, and cheese	8	
	Red meat 4-6 times a week, 4-7 eggs a week, margarine, low fat dairy products, and some cheese	4	

From Anspaugh DJ, Hamrick MH, and Rosato FD: *Wellness*, St Louis, 1991, Mosby–Year Book.

	Poultry, fish, little or no red meat, three or fewer eggs a week, some margarine, skim milk, and skim milk products	0 _____
9. High blood pressure	If either number is:	
	160 over 100 (160/100) or higher	10
	140 over 90 (140/90) but less than 160 over 100 (160/100)	5
	If both numbers are less than 140 over 90 (140/90)	0 _____
10. Weight	Ideal Weight Formula:	
	Men = 110 lb plus 5 lb for each inch over 5 feet	
	Women = 100 lb plus 5 lb for each inch over 5 feet	
	25 lb overweight	4
	10 to 24 lb overweight	2
	Less than 10 lb overweight	0 _____
11. Exercise	Do you engage in any aerobic exercise (brisk walking, jogging, bicycling, racketball, swimming) for more than 15 minutes:	
	Less than once a week	4
	1 to 2 times a week	2
	3 or more times a week	0 _____
12. Stress	Are you:	
	Frustrated when waiting in line, often in a hurry to complete work or keep appointments, easily angered, irritable	4
	Impatient when waiting, occasionally hurried, or occasionally moody	2
	Comfortable when waiting, seldom rushed, and easygoing	0 _____

TOTAL POINTS _____

Score results

PLEASE NOTE: *A high score does not mean you will develop heart disease. It is merely a guide to make you aware of a potential risk. Since no two people are alike, an exact prediction is impossible without further individualized testing.*

WITH ANSWER TO QUESTION 9		WITHOUT ANSWER TO QUESTION 9	
High risk	40 and above	High risk	36 and above
Medium risk	20-39	Medium risk	19-35
Low risk	19 and below	Low risk	18 and below

Personalizing Your Fitness Program

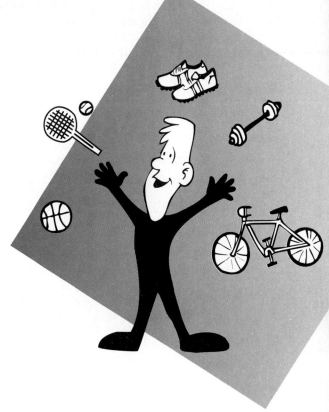

CHAPTER OBJECTIVES

When you understand the material in this chapter, you will be able to:

- Evaluate the importance of regular exercise, and decide whether to make a commitment to exercise regularly
- Discuss why it is important to carefully and systematically plan an exercise program
- Explain why overload and progression are important in a good exercise program
- List appropriate objectives for yourself, and plan an exercise program to achieve these objectives
- Initiate this exercise program, and participate regularly in it

n the preceding chapters, we have done the following:

- Discussed the importance of regular physical activity
- Defined physical fitness and identified each of the health-related components
- Presented the reasons for achieving and maintaining an optimal level of physical fitness
- Included simple tests that allow you to determine your present status in each of the physical fitness components
- Presented norms so that you can evaluate your test results
- Identified the principles and procedures for the development of each of the health-related physical fitness components
- Summarized several existing programs that can be used for developing physical fitness

This information has been presented in the hope that you will recognize the importance of your own physical fitness and that you will do something about it. Knowing about physical fitness and even recognizing its importance are not enough; more than 90% of college students indicate that exercise and fitness are important, but fewer than 40% of these same students exercise on a regular basis.

CHANGING YOUR EXERCISE HABITS

Most people are aware that exercise makes them healthier and more attractive, that it makes them feel better and function more efficiently, and that it helps them deal with stress—in fact, that it is an ideal way to cope with stress. Yet, many of these same people do not exercise on a regular basis, and many who start an exercise program have a hard time sticking with it.

Changing our daily living habits is a difficult task. Even though we realize that we need to make changes, we often lack the necessary motivation or discipline and we often come up with seemingly valid excuses for not exercising. To succeed in changing your daily habits so as to positively influence your health, you must develop a positive way of thinking and believe in your ability to succeed. Without confidence and a positive attitude, you are unlikely to succeed.

The excuses presented in the following box have no place in the minds of persons who wish to be physically fit.

EXCUSES FOR NOT EXERCISING _____

- **"I work hard, and I'm too tired."** This is actually an argument for exercise. It has been shown conclusively that regular exercise increases, not reduces, your level of energy. People who participate regularly in a good exercise program can attest to its value after a stressful day at work.
- **"I don't have the time."** As stated previously, a person will make time for things that are important enough. A recent survey showed that this was true for exercise. People who exercised regularly had the same amount of leisure time available as those who did not exercise regularly. The difference between the two groups was in the priorities that determined how the time was to be used.
- **"I get all the exercise I need each day without doing anything extra."** People who are active each day at work or around the home might burn up calories, but the activity is either not strenuous enough or not continuous enough in most cases to promote cardiovascular fitness.

- **"If I exercise, I will automatically eat more."** This is clearly not true. A person who exercises for 1 hour per day will actually eat less than does a person who does not exercise at all. Exercise tends to suppress your appetite.
- **"When I exercise, I always get sore muscles."** Muscle soreness can be reduced to a minimum by warming up correctly, starting gradually, and progressing slowly. If a person exercises regularly, even if muscle soreness does occur, it does so only at the start of the program and lasts for only a few days.
- **"It is too late to change the way I live."**
- **"I know I should exercise, but . . ."**
- **"I don't like to exercise."**

It's never too late to change your habits, and if exercise is important enough to you, you will take the time to apply the knowledge you now have to designing a program for yourself. Then you must follow this program on a regular basis. Your good intentions must be turned into action.

REVIEW OF THE PRINCIPLES OF EXERCISE

Before you start your program, it might be beneficial to review some of the important principles of exercise. Cardiovascular fitness, or, as it is often called, aerobic fitness, is the most important type of fitness. It involves the efficient functioning of the heart, lungs, and circulatory system, and there are many advantages associated with an optimum level of cardiovascular fitness. Your fitness program should include the following:

A 5- to 10-minute warm-up, as the body gradually moves from a state of minimum activity to a much higher level of activity. Many people drop out of an exercise program during the first few weeks because of muscle soreness. Much of this discomfort can be avoided by taking time to warm up and by starting gradually and progressing slowly in your program.

Twenty to 30 minutes of continuous activity at an intensity that keeps your heart rate in your target zone. Remember that your target zone can be calculated by taking 70% to 85% of your predicted maximum heart rate, which is determined by subtracting your age from 220. Any continuous activity that involves the use of large muscle groups can fulfill this purpose. Suitable activities include walking, jogging, bicycling, swimming, cross-country skiing, aerobic dancing, basketball, and racquetball.

Activities for the development of strength and muscular endurance. Many people prefer some type of weight training for this part of their program.

A 5- to 10-minute cool-down session. It is important to slow down gradually, and depending on the type of activities you have selected, it may be equally important to again stretch the various muscle groups that have been used.

Frequency. For aerobic fitness, you need to exercise a minimum of three times and a maximum of five times each week. If your main objective for exercise is to lose weight and fat, you need to make a commitment to exercise for 45 minutes, 5 days each week.

OTHER CONSIDERATIONS

In planning your program, it is also important to remember the following:
- Exercise sessions must be scheduled regularly three to five times each week.

- **Overload** must be built into the program. Overload involves subjecting the body to a task slightly beyond its normal level, so that enough stress is placed on the body to stimulate the desired response. In the development of strength and cardiovascular and muscular endurance, improvement occurs only if the body is subjected to a workload greater than that to which it is accustomed.
- **Progression** is another important part of every exercise program. The body will adapt to the increased level of resistance as improvement takes place. For this reason, it is necessary to measure progress and to increase the workload frequently. Progress is greatest and most apparent at the start of a program, particularly if you have been inactive. In aerobic activities, progression can be incorporated by carefully checking the heart rate each day and adjusting the intensity to ensure that the heart rate remains in the desired target zone.
- An exercise program will result in **specificity of improvement.** Each exercise program is specific and results in improvement only in the area or areas it is designed to develop. For example, a person who lifts weights regularly develops strength and muscular endurance in those muscle groups for which exercises are included. Similarly, unless you include an aerobic exercise that keeps your heart rate in the target zone for an extended period, you should not expect a significant improvement in cardiovascular endurance. The activities making up the program determine the results attained.

STARTING A SUCCESSFUL EXERCISE PROGRAM

Beginning a successful exercise program involves several steps.

Make a commitment to exercise

We have seen that the first step in beginning an exercise program is to commit yourself to the idea that exercise and fitness are important to you. Having made this commitment, you must now put into practice the principles you have learned and exercise must become a permanent part of your life.

It is important to realize that it will take time and effort to achieve your objectives and experience significant changes. It requires discipline and determination. There are no short cuts or easy methods. This does not mean, however, that exercise cannot be enjoyable. It is very important to select an activity that you enjoy and that will contribute to your objectives. You must then participate at a level that is comfortable but of sufficient intensity to produce the desired changes. If you become bored with an activity, vary your program and include other activities.

Do you need a physical examination before starting your program?

If you are less than 35 years of age and starting a serious exercise program and you have no medical problems, you do not need a physical examination. Just make sure that if you are out of shape that you gradually "ease" into your program and you do not do too much too soon.

If you are over 35 years of age and out of shape and haven't exercised regularly for some time, it is important to find out whether it is safe for you to exercise. This is because the demand placed on your heart while you exercise is much greater than the effort required for most everyday activities.

A good physical examination will include a graded exercise test, which will evaluate your blood pressure, heart rate, and electrocardiogram responses while you are exercising. These data can also be used to evaluate your aerobic fitness level. The examination should also include measurements of strength, muscular endurance, flexibility, and body fat.

By taking such tests, you will not only know if it is safe for you to exercise, you will have baseline figures to use in planning your program. This will allow you to establish realistic objectives, and you will be able to measure your progress. This should increase your motivation.

Define your goals

You can waste much time and energy if you don't establish certain goals for your program. These goals should be based on your individual needs. They should be both challenging and realistic. You must allow yourself a reasonable amount of time to reach them. Do not expect too much too soon.

In determining your goals, you should think about why you want to get fit. For example, your exercise program will be different if your major objective is to lose weight than if it is simply to develop an optimal level of aerobic fitness. Of course, an exercise program can be designed for both of these objectives.

What are realistic objectives? Knowing what are realistic objectives is very important when you start an exercise program. You need to set your objectives so that you can attain some degree of success. Losing 20 lb in a month or running 10 miles in an hour are unrealistic goals for most people. These are not the types of objectives to be set if you follow the procedures outlined in the previous chapters.

A realistic objective for the development of cardiovascular fitness might be to average four exercise sessions for 15 consecutive weeks and accumulate from 12 to 16 miles per week by jogging at an intensity sufficient to maintain your heart rate in the desired target zone. A realistic goal for weight control might be to average 20 miles per week walking and to reduce your caloric intake so that in 12 weeks you will lose 15 lb. Often it is advantageous to write out your objectives in the form of a "contract." In this way, you can periodically evaluate your progress to determine how effective and consistent your exercise program is and whether you need to make any adjustments in your program. Instructions for this are given in Laboratory Experience 11-1.

> You need to determine objectives that are important to you, that are realistic and challenging, and that will require discipline, determination, and effort.

Have a plan of action

Your exercise program must be systematic and carefully planned. All too frequently, exercise is performed irregularly, with little thought given to the objectives or to the reasons for including specific exercises. In designing your program you need to know how much exercise is enough for you, and you must set weekly goals as you move toward your objectives. Remember consistency from week to week will determine your degree of success.

The first few weeks are very important; it is during this time that a large number of people become disheartened and give up. It should be emphasized that you cannot start out at too low a level. It has probably taken you a long time to get out of shape, and it will take you more than a few days to get back into shape. You need patience and determination.

It will take at least 8 weeks for you to experience many of the major changes that take place. However, during the first few weeks you should be able to see definite progress as you become more skilled at adjusting the intensity of the exercise to match your level of fitness. Activities that initially appear difficult become much easier, and you will quickly find out how much work you can do.

The personal checklist in the box below may help you identify your preferences for an exercise program. The decisions you make will help you plan your program.

PERSONAL CHECKLIST

1. I would prefer to exercise
   - ☐ on my own
   - ☐ with a friend
   - ☐ with a group of people
2. In scheduling my program
   - ☐ I have the motivation to exercise regularly on my own or with others
   - ☐ I need to participate in an organized program at a set time and place each day
3. I prefer to exercise
   - ☐ indoors
   - ☐ outdoors
4. I prefer to work out regularly
   - ☐ early in the morning
   - ☐ at noon
   - ☐ immediately after work
   - ☐ later in the evening
5. I feel that I am best suited to
   - ☐ competitive activities
   - ☐ noncompetitive activities
6. As far as expense is concerned
   - ☐ I am willing to spend money and join a health club or YMCA
   - ☐ I am willing to spend money to buy equipment of my own, such as an exercise bike or weight-training set
   - ☐ I want a program with little or no expense
7. I am interested in
   - ☐ the same activity year-round
   - ☐ a variety of activities

From Fitness: the facts, Book 6, *The final ingredient*, Participation, Canada, 1979, Ministry of Culture and Recreation.

Activity selection

You must select activities that you enjoy and that will enable you to achieve your objectives for the program. You may wish to exercise on your own, where you are in complete control of what you do. This way you do not have to worry about or rely on anyone else, and you can get away from everyone and be by yourself. Another advantage is that *you* can decide when and where you exercise. Exercises such as walking, jumping rope, bicycling, jogging, swimming, and skating are examples of activities you can do alone.

If you thrive on competition, you may wish to participate against a person of equal ability in a sport such as racquetball or one-on-one basketball. These activities can be enjoyable and very good for cardiovascular fitness. For those who are competitive and lack the skill or interest to participate in individual sports, team sports may be the answer. They are equally enjoyable and beneficial. Basketball, water polo, ice hockey, soccer, rugby, and field hockey are examples of sports that make a major contribution to the development of cardiovascular fitness.

The objective is to find an activity that is both enjoyable and strenuous enough to contribute to cardiovascular fitness and/or weight loss. If you enjoy what you are doing and it is challenging and satisfying, exercise is much more likely to become a regular part of your daily routine.

Regularity of exercise

Choose a regular time for exercise. To achieve your specific objectives, you must participate on a regular basis. Those who wait until they "find" time to exercise do not exercise very often. If you believe strongly enough in the importance of exercise, you will make time available on a regular basis and exercise will become a habit. A good exercise program requires less than 5 hours per week. This is very little time to spend, considering all the benefits you will receive.

If you are trying to lose weight, exercising in the late afternoon might be advantageous because it will help you decrease your caloric intake. By exercising you may be able to avoid the temptation to stop at a local hotel, restaurant, or bar for "happy hour," where you tend to consume a large number of extra calories. Also, a vigorous workout late in the day will often suppress your appetite.

Be willing to work at it

In any endeavor, people who are successful work hard at it. Nothing comes easy. The familiar phrase "I know I should, but . . ." is not part of a winner's vocabulary. It has been stated that "man is the architect of his own destiny." This is certainly true when it comes to attaining physical fitness.

Many people who do not exercise use the excuse that they just do not have enough energy. You should not let the grind of your daily routine keep you from exercising. Regular exercise will actually increase your energy level and enable you to be more productive in your everyday tasks. You should feel refreshed after a good workout.

Monitor your progress

It is important to monitor your progress on a regular basis, which you can do by keeping a record of your workouts. This enables you to chart your progress and get some immediate feedback on the total time spent each week, number of calories burned, aerobic points earned, and changes in body weight. Many different computer programs are available that can be used on home computers for this purpose.

An exercise logging program is part of the computer software package available for use with this textbook. A sample printout similar to the one from this program appears in Fig. 11-1 on the next page.

Date: 10/31/1983   Height: 72 in   Name: Joe Jock   SSN: 345-67-8901

Sex: Male
Age: 30 yr

Session	Date	Mode	Weight (lb)	Duration (min)	Run/Walk Distance (mi)	Bicycle Distance (mi)	Swim Distance (mi)	Calories Burned	Aerobic Points
1	10/01/1983	Warm-up activities	175	20				115.5	0.5
		Walking/running treadmill	175	45	4.5			630.0	21.5
2	10/02/1983	Walking/running	175	50	5.0			700.0	24.0
3	10/03/1983	Basketball	173	55				428.2	8.3
4	10/05/1983	Racquetball	173	60				685.1	9.0
5	10/06/1983	Stationary bicycle riding	173	40		8.3		379.8	9.5
6	10/09/1983	Bicycle riding	172	30		7.5		361.2	9.8
7	10/10/1983	Swimming	170	20			0.7	530.4	19.5
8	10/12/1983	Aerobic dance	170	55				467.5	5.8
9	10/15/1983	Racquetball	170	45				504.9	6.8
		Walking/running	170	45	4.0			573.8	16.3
10	10/20/1983	Racquetball	169	60				669.2	9.0
11	10/22/1983	Walking/running	169	50	6.0			760.5	33.8
12	10/26/1983	Walking/running treadmill	168	45	4.5			604.8	21.5
13	10/27/1983	Aerobic dance	168	30				252.0	3.1
		TOTALS		650	24.0	15.8	0.7	7662.9	198.4
		AVERAGE (PER EXERCISE DAY)		50	4.8	7.9	0.7	589.5	15.3

Activity	Totals Last Month	Lifetime
Walking/running	21.0 miles	123.6 miles
Bicycle riding	13.0 miles	96.4 miles
Swimming	1.3 miles	12.4 miles
Raquetball	6 hours 30 min.	45 hours 20 minutes
Aerobic dance	22 hours 36 min.	42 hours 10 minutes

Data from the Department of Health, Physical Education, and Athletics, Trinity University—Exercise Physiology Laboratory.

Fig. 11-1 Sample printout of computer program for summary of physical activity.

This example is a monthly printout. It clearly shows the following:
- The number of exercise days for the month
- Changes in body weight from the beginning to the end of the month
- The total miles accumulated in running, bicycling, and swimming
- The total calories burned for the month
- The total number of aerobic points earned for the month
- Corresponding totals for the previous month, which allows you to compare the 2 months to see whether you are making any progress

COMMON SENSE PRECAUTIONS
Get an adequate amount of rest

Your muscles, as well as your entire body, need an adequate amount of rest if you are to get the most out of your exercise program. You can't expect to have a good workout if you stayed up for most of the night with only 2 or 3 hours of sleep.

We also know that most muscle injuries are caused by "overuse"—it is not reasonable to expect to work out vigorously each day, particularly in a weight-bearing activity, and not get injured. If you exercise 5 days each week, make sure that you do not exercise for 5 consecutive days and then take the next 2 days off. This is a poorly planned program. Your body will react much better if you "split up" the days off and take one at the weekend and one in the middle of the week.

Take good care of your feet

Make sure that you have the correct shoes for the activity in which you participate, so that you get adequate support and cushioning. This will help you to avoid injuries such as shin splints and bone bruises. Wearing a thick pair of socks can help to prevent blisters.

Maintain proper muscle balance

Frequently we neglect specific muscle groups at the expense of others, and this creates an imbalance. This often contributes to muscle injuries. An aerobic program combined with a good weight-training program should result in good muscle balance.

Listen to signals from your body

Most people pay close attention to some signals from their body but completely disregard others. If you experience tightness or pain in the chest and you feel faint or light-headed, you will usually stop exercising immediately and seek medical help to find out the extent of the problem.

On the other hand, many people who are constantly fatigued and/or experience nagging muscle injuries will continue exercising and disregard these signals. These signals are your body's way of telling you that something is wrong. You need to also find out what is causing problems such as these.

Vary your workouts

Most muscle injuries are caused by "overuse." If you are prone to muscle injuries, or if you simply want to try to avoid them, you may need to vary your activities when you work out on consecutive days, so that you include nonimpact activities such as swimming and bicycling on alternate days.

STICKING WITH YOUR PROGRAM

Several different studies show that 60% or more of adults who start an exercise program drop out within the first month. You must be patient. It will take some time to develop your fitness level to the point where you function most efficiently. When you have achieved an optimal level of fitness, you should feel so much better that you will need little or no motivation to continue. Achieving this much has involved a lot of hard work and discipline, and you should be proud of your accomplishments. However, it is very important to continue to exercise on a regular basis to maintain this level of fitness. Exercise must become a lifetime commitment. By now you will realize that the benefits far outweigh the effort.

SUMMARY

The following summary will help you to identify some of the important concepts covered in this chapter:

- Knowledge concerning exercise and fitness is important if you are to design an exercise program that best fits your individual needs.
- Your exercise program must be systematic and well-planned, and you must participate in it regularly if you are to be successful.
- Because your body will "adapt," progression and overload must be "built" into your program.

- Specific goals and a plan of action will increase you chances of "sticking" with your program.
- If you have a very busy lifestyle, you will need to "schedule" a time to exercise if you are to develop the consistency that is necessary to be successful.

KEY TERMS

overload   Subjecting the body to a task slightly more difficult than that to which it is accustomed.

progression   Increasing the amount of work from time to time so that the body must work harder.

specificity of improvement   Improvement occurs only in the area or areas that each exercise is designed to develop (applies only to strength, muscular endurance, and flexibility).

REFERENCES

1. Berger BG: In pursuit of fitness, *Shape,* p. 85, July 4, 1986.
2. Findlay S, Shoyer T: Smart ways to shape up, *US News and World Report,* pp. 46-55, July 18, 1988.
3. Fisher GA: *Your heart rate: the key to real fitness,* Provo, Utah, 1976, Brigham Young University Press.
4. Fitness: the facts, Book 4, *The activities,* Participation, Canada, 1979, Ministry of Culture and Recreation.
5. Fitness: the facts, Book 6, *The final ingredient,* Participation, Canada, 1979, Ministry of Culture and Recreation.
6. Kusinitz I, Fine M: *Your guide to getting fit,* ed 2, Mountain View, Calif, 1991, Mayfield.
7. *Nutrition exercise health lifestyle,* 1987, Pritikin Resource Book.
8. Rosenstein AH: The benefits of health maintenance, *Physician and Sports Medicine* 15:4, April 1987.
9. *Wellness Newsletter,* Randall Sports/Medical Products, Kirkland, Wash, 3:1, 1991.

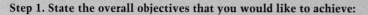

Personal Fitness Contract

By writing a personal fitness contract, you will formulate some specific objectives and you will be more likely to make a lasting commitment to exercise. The example in the box on p. 368 at the end of this section may be of help to you.

Step 1. State the overall objectives that you would like to achieve:

Step 2. State specifically what you will do to achieve these objectives: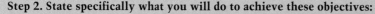

(You need to state which activities you will participate in, and you will need to determine goals for these in terms of frequency, duration, and so on.)

Step 3. State the specific time you will allow yourself to attain these objectives:

CONTRACT:

I, _____ , *am making a contract with myself to regularly follow an exercise program as specified above, as I work toward achieving the specified objectives.*

I will begin my program on _____

I will achieve all my objectives by _____

Signed _____   *Date* _____

Witness _____

Continued.

EXAMPLE: JILL JOCK

Step 1. Overall objectives:

1. To develop consistent exercise habits
2. To improve my aerobic fitness level to where I can jog slowly and complete 3 miles in 30 minutes
3. To reduce my percentage of body fat from 24% to 20%

Step 2. Specific objectives:

1. To develop consistent exercise habits, I need to make a commitment to exercise at least 3 times each week. I will initially exercise for a minimum of 30 minutes on each of the exercise days.
2. To improve my aerobic fitness level, I need to check my intensity level each time I exercise to make sure that my heart rate remains in my target zone.
3. Every 3 weeks I will test myself to see how far I can run in 30 minutes. I will need to see gradual improvement until I can run my 3 miles in 30 minutes.
4. I plan on walking and/or jogging each exercise session, depending on my initial level of fitness.
5. After 4 weeks of exercise, I will increase the duration of each exercise session to 45 minutes and will increase the frequency from 3 to 5 times each week.

Step 3. Time schedule:

1. By the start of the third week, I will have met my first overall objective and each week thereafter, this will continue to be met.
2. I will allow myself 12 additional weeks to meet the other two overall objectives.

CONTRACT

I,   Jill Jock   , am making a contract with myself to regularly follow an exercise program as specified above, as I work toward achieving the specified objectives.

I will begin my program on September 1, 1992

I will achieve all my objectives by December 15, 1992

Signed _____   Date 9/01/92

Witness _____

Food Exchange Lists

MILK

Nonfat

Each serving of milk or milk product on this list contains approximately 12 g of carbohydrate and 8 g of protein (approximately 80 calories).

Skim milk	1 cup
$1/2$% milk	1 cup
1% milk	1 cup
Low-fat buttermilk	1 cup
Evaporated skim milk	$1/2$ cup
Dry nonfat milk	$1/3$ cup dry
Plain nonfat yogurt	1 cup (8 oz)

Low fat

Each serving of milk or milk product on this list contains approximately 12 g of carbohydrates, 8 g of protein, and 5 g of fat (approximately 125 calories).

2% milk	1 cup
Plain low-fat yogurt	1 cup (8 oz)
Low-fat cottage cheese	$1/3$ cup

Whole

Each serving of milk or milk product on this list contains approximately 12 g of carbohydrates, 8 g of protein, and 8 g of fat (approximately 150 calories).

Whole milk	1 cup
Evaporated whole milk	$1/2$ cup
Whole plain yogurt (unflavored)	1 cup (8 oz)

FRUIT

Each item on this list contains approximately 15 g of carbohydrates (approximately 60 calories). Portion sizes for each food are as indicated.

Apple (2-in diam)	1 apple
Apple juice	$1/3$ cup
Banana	$1/2$ banana
Blueberries	$3/4$ cup
Cantaloupe (small)	$1/3$ melon
Cherries (large, raw)	12 cherries

Cherries (canned)	1/2 cup
Cranberry juice cocktail (low-calorie)	3/4 cup
Figs (raw, 2-in)	2 figs
Grapefruit (medium)	1/2 grapefruit
Grapes	15 grapes
Kiwi (large)	1 kiwi
Mango (small)	1/2 mango
Nectarine	1 small
Orange (2 1/2 inch)	1 orange
Orange juice	1/2 cup
Peach (medium)	1 peach
Pear	1/2 large or 1 small
Pineapple (raw)	3/4 cup
Pineapple chunks (unsweetened)	1/2 cup
Plum (2-in)	2 plums
Prunes (dried)	2 medium
Raisins	2 tbsp
Strawberries	1 cup
Watermelon	1 cup

VEGETABLES

Each vegetable serving on this list contains approximately 5 g of carbohydrates and 2 g of protein (approximately 25 calories). Unless otherwise specified, the serving size is 1/2 cup of cooked vegetables, 1 cup of raw vegetables, and 1/2 cup of all vegetable juices. Starchy vegetables such as potatoes and corn are found on the starch/grains list.

Artichoke (1/2 medium)
Asparagus
Bean sprouts
Beans (green)
Beets
Broccoli
Brussels sprouts
Cabbage
Carrots
Cauliflower
Celery
Cucumbers
Eggplant
Green chilies
Greens
Mushrooms
Okra
Onions
Peppers (green and red)
Radishes
Spinach (cooked)
Summer squash
Tomato
Zucchini

STARCH/GRAINS

Each item on this list contains approximately 15 g of carbohydrates and 3 g of protein (approximately 70 calories). The portion for each item is as indicated.

Bread

Bagel	1/2
English muffin	1/2
Pita bread (6-in)	1/2
Tortilla (6-in diam)	1
Bread	1 slice
Bread roll (plain)	1 small or 1/2 large

Hamburger bun	½
Frankfurter roll	½

NOTE: The following also contain 1 fat exchange (5 g of fat and an additional 45 calories).

Pancakes (4-in)	2
Waffles (4 ½-in)	1
Taco shell (6-in)	2
Muffin (small)	1
Corn bread (2-in cube)	1 (2 oz)
Stuffing (bread)	¼ cup

Cereals/grains/pasta

Bran cereals (flaked)	½ cup
Bran cereals (concentrated, e.g., All Bran)	⅓ cup
Cooked cereals	½ cup
Grapenuts	3 tbsp
Other unsweetened cereals	¾ cup
Pasta (cooked)	½ cup
Rice (cooked)	½ cup
Shredded Wheat	½ cup

Starchy vegetables

Baked beans	¼ cup
Beans and peas (cooked)	⅓ cup
Corn	½ cup
Corn on the cob (6 in long)	1 piece
Popcorn (air popped)	3 cups
Potato (baked)	1 small (3 oz)
Potato (mashed)	½ cup
Squash (winter)	¾ cup
Yams	⅓ cup

Crackers/snacks

Many commercial crackers are high in fat. Look at the label and avoid them. The following are usually better choices:

Animal crackers	8
Graham crackers (2 ½-in square)	3
Melba toast	5 slices
Pretzels	¾ oz
Whole-wheat crackers (no fat)	2 to 4 slices (¾ oz)

Miscellaneous

Barbeque sauce	¼ cup
Ketchup	¼ cup
Corn meal	2 tbsp
Cornstarch	2 tbsp
Flour	2½ tbsp
Tomato paste	6 tbsp
Tomato sauce	1 cup

MEAT
Meat (lean)

Each item on this list contains approximately 7 g of protein and 3 g of fat (approximately 55 calories).

Beef: USDA good or choice grades of lean beef (e.g., round, sirloin, flank, tenderloin)	1 oz
Pork: Fresh ham, lean cuts, tenderloin	1 oz
Veal: Chops, roasts	1 oz
Poultry: Chicken, turkey, cornish hen (no skin)	1 oz
Fish: Crab, lobster, scallops, shrimp, clams	2 oz
Fresh, frozen fish	1 oz
Tuna (canned in water)	1/4 cup
Wild game: Venison, rabbit, pheasant, duck, goose (no skin)	1 oz
Other: 95% fat-free luncheon meat	1 oz
Egg whites	3 whites

Meat (medium fat)

Each item on this list contains approximately 7 g of protein and 6 g of fat (approximately 80 calories).

Beef: Ground beef, roast, steak	1 oz
Pork: Most pork products (chops, loin, roast)	1 oz
Lamb: Most lamb products (chops, leg, roast)	1 oz
Veal: Cutlet (unbreaded)	1 oz
Poultry: Chicken with skin, domestic duck, goose, ground turkey	1 oz
Fish: Tuna (canned in oil, drained)	1/4 cup
Salmon (canned in oil, drained)	1/4 cup
Cheese: Skim or part-skim cheeses	
Ricotta	1/4 cup
Mozzarella	1 oz
Diet cheeses (56 to 80 calories/oz)	1 oz
Other: 86% fat-free luncheon meat	1 oz
Tofu	4 oz
Organ meats (high cholesterol)	1 oz
Egg (high in cholesterol)	1

Meat (high fat)

Each item on this list contains approximately 7 g of protein and 8 g of fat (approximately 105 calories). Most foods on this list are high in saturated fat, cholesterol, and calories. They should be limited to three times per week.

Beef: Prime cuts (ribs, corned beef)	1 oz
Pork: Spare ribs, pork sausage	1 oz
Lamb: Patties	1 oz
Fish: Fried fish products	1 oz
Cheese: American, blue, cheddar, swiss, monterey jack	1 oz
Other: Luncheon meat (salami, bologna)	1 oz
Sausage	1 oz

Frankfurter (turkey or chicken)	1
Peanut butter (contains unsaturated fat)	1 tbsp

Many prepared meat/meat substitute dishes are high in fat. Check the percentage of fat in all frozen dinners and canned meals.

FAT

Each serving on this list contains approximately 5 g of fat (approximately 45 calories). Limit your fat intake and, where possible, try to select unsaturated fats.

Unsaturated fats

Safflower oil	1 tsp
Corn oil	1 tsp
Sunflower oil	1 tsp
Sesame oil	1 tsp
Olive oil	1 tsp
Olives	10 small/5 large
Peanut oil	1 tsp
Peanuts	20 small/10 large
Peanut butter	2 tsp
Avocados	1/8 medium
Margarine	1 tsp
Mayonnaise (low-calorie)	1 tbsp
Almonds (dry roasted)	6 whole
Pecans	2 whole
Walnuts	2 whole
Salad dressing (low-calorie)	2 tbsp

Saturated fats

Butter	1 tsp
Bacon	1 slice
Coffee whitener	4 tsp
Sour cream	2 tbsp
Cream cheese	1 tbsp
Salad dressing (mayonnaise type)	2 tsp
French dressing	1 tbsp
Italian dressing	1 tbsp

Nutritional Information for Selected Foods

Food item	Serving size	Grams	Calories	Protein (g)	Carbohydrate (g)	Fat (g)	Cholesterol (mg)	Sodium (mg)
Beverages								
Alcoholic								
Beer								
Regular	12 fl oz	360	150	1	13	0	0	18
Light	12 fl oz	355	95	1	5	0	0	11
Gin, rum, vodka, whiskey								
80-proof	1½ fl oz	42	95	0	Tr	0	0	Tr
86-proof	1½ fl oz	42	105	0	Tr	0	0	Tr
90-proof	1½ fl oz	42	110	0	Tr	0	0	Tr
Wines								
Dessert	3½ fl oz	103	140	Tr	8	0	0	9
Table								
Red	3½ fl oz	102	75	Tr	3	0	0	5
White	3½ fl oz	102	80	Tr	3	0	0	5
Carbonated								
Club soda	12 fl oz	355	0	0	0	0	0	78
Cola type								
Regular	12 fl oz	369	160	0	41	0	0	18
Diet, artificially sweetened	12 fl oz	355	Tr	0	Tr	0	0	32[a]
Ginger ale	12 fl oz	366	125	0	32	0	0	29
Grape	12 fl oz	372	180	0	46	0	0	48
Lemon-lime	12 fl oz	372	155	0	39	0	0	33
Orange	12 fl oz	372	180	0	46	0	0	52
Pepper type	12 fl oz	369	160	0	41	0	0	37
Root beer	12 fl oz	370	165	0	42	0	0	48

Tr, Trace amount.

[a]Blend of aspartame and saccharin; if only saccharin is used, sodium is 75 mg; if only aspartame is used, sodium is 23 mg.
Information summarized from *Nutritive value of foods*, Superintendent of Documents, US Government Printing Office, Washington, DC, Revised 1981.

Food item	Serving size	Grams	Calories	Protein (g)	Carbohydrate (g)	Fat (g)	Cholesterol (mg)	Sodium (mg)
Beverages—cont'd								
Fruit drinks, noncarbonated								
Canned								
Fruit punch drink	6 fl oz	190	85	Tr	22	0	0	15
Grape drink	6 fl oz	187	100	Tr	26	0	0	11
Pineapple–grapefruit juice drink	6 fl oz	187	90	Tr	23	Tr	0	24
Frozen lemonade concentrate, diluted with 4$\frac{1}{3}$ parts water by volume	6 fl oz	185	80	Tr	21	Tr	0	1
Dairy products								
Butter. See Fats and Oils								
Cheese								
Cheddar								
Cut pieces	1 oz	28	115	7	Tr	9	30	176
	1 in	17	70	4	Tr	6	18	105
Shredded	1 cup	113	455	28	1	37	119	701
Creamed (cottage cheese, 4% fat):								
Large curd	1 cup	225	235	28	6	10	34	911
Small curd	1 cup	210	215	26	6	9	31	850
With fruit	1 cup	226	280	22	30	8	25	915
Lowfat (2%)	1 cup	226	205	31	8	4	19	918
Cream	1 oz	28	100	2	1	10	31	84
Feta	1 oz	28	75	4	1	6	25	316
Mozzarella, made with								
Whole milk	1 oz	28	80	6	1	6	22	106
Part skim milk (low moisture)	1 oz	28	80	8	1	5	15	150
Muenster	1 oz	28	105	7	Tr	9	27	178
Parmesan, grated	1 oz	28	130	12	1	9	22	528
Provolone	1 oz	28	100	7	1	8	20	248
Swiss	1 oz	28	105	8	1	8	26	74
Pasteurized process cheese								
American	1 oz	28	105	6	Tr	9	27	406
Swiss	1 oz	28	95	7	1	7	24	388

Tr, Trace amount.

Food item	Serving size	Grams	Calories	Protein (g)	Carbohydrate (g)	Fat (g)	Cholesterol (mg)	Sodium (mg)
Dairy products—cont'd								
Pasteurized process cheese food, American	1 oz	28	95	6	2	7	18	337
Pasteurized process cheese spread, American	1 oz	28	80	5	2	6	16	381
Cream, sweet								
Half-and-half (cream and milk)	1 cup	242	315	7	10	28	89	98
	1 tbsp	15	20	Tr	1	2	6	6
Light, coffee, or table	1 cup	240	470	6	9	46	159	95
	1 tbsp	15	30	Tr	1	3	10	6
Cream, sour	1 cup	230	495	7	10	48	102	123
	1 tbsp	12	25	Tr	1	3	5	6
Ice cream. See Milk desserts, frozen								
Milk								
Whole (3.3% fat)	1 cup	244	150	8	11	8	33	370
Low-fat (2%)	1 cup	244	120	8	12	5	18	377
Low-fat (1%)	1 cup	244	100	8	12	3	10	381
Nonfat (skim)	1 cup	245	85	8	12	Tr	4	406
Chocolate milk (commercial)								
Regular	1 cup	250	210	8	26	8	31	149
Low-fat (2%)	1 cup	250	180	8	26	5	17	151
Low-fat (1%)	1 cup	250	160	8	26	3	7	152
Milk beverages								
Cocoa and chocolate-flavored beverages								
Prepared (8 oz whole milk plus ³/₄ oz powder)	1 serving	265	225	9	30	9	33	176
Eggnog (commercial)	1 cup	254	340	10	34	19	149	138
Malted milk								
Chocolate	³/₄ oz	21	85	1	18	1	1	49
Prepared (8 oz whole milk plus ³/₄ oz powder)	1 serving	265	235	9	29	9	34	168
Shakes, thick								
Chocolate	10-oz container	283	335	9	60	8	30	314
Vanilla	10-oz container	283	315	11	50	9	33	270

Tr, Trace amount.

Food item	Serving size	Grams	Calories	Protein (g)	Carbohydrate (g)	Fat (g)	Cholesterol (mg)	Sodium (mg)
Dairy products—cont'd								
Milk desserts, frozen								
Ice cream, vanilla								
Regular (about 11% fat)	1 cup	133	270	5	32	14	59	116
Yogurt								
Made with low-fat milk								
Fruit-flavored[b]	8-oz container	227	230	10	43	2	10	133
Plain	8-oz container	227	145	12	16	4	14	159
Made with nonfat milk	8-oz container	227	125	13	17	Tr	4	174
Made with whole milk	8-oz container	227	140	8	11	7	29	105
Eggs								
Eggs, large (24 oz per dozen):								
Cooked								
Fried in margarine	1 egg	46	90	6	1	7	211	162
Hard-cooked, shell removed	1 egg	50	75	6	1	5	213	62
Poached	1 egg	50	75	6	1	5	212	140
Scrambled (milk added) in margarine	1 egg	61	100	7	1	7	215	171
Fats and oils								
Butter (4 sticks per lb)								
Stick	1/2 cup	113	810	1	Tr	92	247	933[c]
Tablespoon (1/8 stick)	1 tbsp	14	100	Tr	Tr	11	31	116[c]
Pat (1 in square, 1/3 in high; 90 per lb)	1 pat	5	35	Tr	Tr	4	11	41[c]
Margarine								
Regular (about 80% fat)								
Stick	1/2 cup	113	810	1	1	91	0	1066[d]
Tablespoon (1/8 stick)	1 tbsp	14	100	Tr	Tr	11	0	132

Tr, Trace amount.

[b]Carbohydrate content varies widely because of amount of sugar added and amount of added flavoring. Consult the label if more precise values for carbohydrate and calories are needed.

[c]For salted butter; unsalted butter contains 12 mg sodium per stick, 2 mg per tbsp, or 12 mg per pat.

[d]For salted margarine.

Food item	Serving size	Grams	Calories	Protein (g)	Carbohydrate (g)	Fat (g)	Cholesterol (mg)	Sodium (mg)
Fats and oils—cont'd								
Pat (1 in square, ⅓ in high; 90 per lb)	1 pat	5	35	Tr	Tr	4	0	47[d]
Oils, salad or cooking								
Corn	1 tbsp	14	125	0	0	14	0	0
Olive	1 tbsp	14	125	0	0	14	0	0
Peanut	1 tbsp	14	125	0	0	14	0	0
Safflower	1 tbsp	14	125	0	0	14	0	0
Sunflower	1 tbsp	14	125	0	0	14	0	0
Salad dressings								
Blue cheese	1 tbsp	15	75	1	1	8	3	164
French								
Regular	1 tbsp	16	85	Tr	1	9	0	188
Low-calorie	1 tbsp	16	25	Tr	2	2	0	306
Italian								
Regular	1 tbsp	15	80	Tr	1	9	0	162
Low-calorie	1 tbsp	15	5	Tr	2	Tr	0	136
Mayonnaise								
Regular	1 tbsp	14	100	Tr	Tr	11	8	80
Thousand island								
Regular	1 tbsp	16	60	Tr	2	6	4	112
Low-calorie	1 tbsp	15	25	Tr	2	2	2	150
Fish and shellfish								
Crabmeat, canned	1 cup	135	135	23	1	3	135	1350
Fish sticks, frozen, reheated (stick, 4 by 1 by ½ in)	1 fish stick	28	70	6	4	3	26	53
Flounder or sole, baked, with lemon juice								
With butter	3 oz	85	120	16	Tr	6	68	145
Ocean perch, breaded, fried[e]	1 fillet	85	185	16	7	11	66	138
Salmon								
Baked (red)	3 oz	85	140	21	0	5	60	55
Smoked	3 oz	85	150	18	0	8	51	1700
Scallops, breaded, frozen, reheated	6 scallops	90	195	15	10	10	70	298
Shrimp, French fried (7 medium)[f]	3 oz	85	200	16	11	10	168	384

Tr, Trace amount.

[e]Dipped in egg, milk, and bread crumbs; fried in vegetable shortening.

[f]Dipped in egg, milk, and bread crumbs; fried in vegetable shortening.

Food item	Serving size	Grams	Calories	Protein (g)	Carbohydrate (g)	Fat (g)	Cholesterol (mg)	Sodium (mg)
Fish and shellfish—cont'd								
Trout, broiled, with butter and lemon juice	3 oz	85	175	21	Tr	9	71	122
Tuna, canned, drained solids								
Oil pack, chunk light	3 oz	85	165	24	0	7	55	303
Water pack, solid white	3 oz	85	135	30	0	1	48	468
Tuna salad[g]	1 cup	205	375	33	19	19	80	877
Fruits and fruit juices								
Apples								
Raw								
Unpeeled, without cores 3¼-in diam. (about 2 per lb with cores)	1 apple	212	125	Tr	32	1	0	Tr
Peeled, sliced	1 cup	110	65	Tr	16	Tr	0	Tr
Apple juice, bottled or canned	1 cup	248	115	Tr	29	Tr	0	7
Apricots								
Raw, without pits (about 12 per lb with pits)	3 apricots	106	50	1	12	Tr	0	1
Bananas, raw, without peel								
Whole (about 2½ per lb with peel)	1 banana	114	105	1	27	1	0	1
Sliced	1 cup	150	140	2	35	1	0	2
Blueberries, raw	1 cup	145	80	1	20	1	0	9
Cherries, sweet, raw, without pits and stems	10 cherries	68	50	1	11	1	0	Tr
Grapefruit, raw, without peel, membrane and seeds (3¾-in diam. 1 lb 1 oz, whole, with refuse)	½ grapefruit	120	40	1	10	Tr	0	Tr

Tr, Trace amount.
[g]Made with drained, chunk light tuna, celery, onion, pickle relish, and mayonnaise-type salad dressing.

Food item	Serving size	Grams	Calories	Protein (g)	Carbohydrate (g)	Fat (g)	Cholesterol (mg)	Sodium (mg)
Fruits and fruit juices—cont'd								
Grapes, European type (adherent skin) raw, Thompsn Seedless	10 grape-fruit	50	35	Tr	9	Tr	0	1
Melons, raw, without rind and cavity contents								
Cantaloup, orange-fleshed (5-in diam, 2⅓ lb, whole, with rind and cavity contents)	½ melon	267	95	2	22	1	0	24
Honeydew (6½-in diam, 5¼ lb, whole, with rind and cavity contents)	⅒ melon	129	45	1	12	Tr	0	13
Nectarines, raw, without pits (about 3 per lb with pits)	1 nectarine	136	65	1	16	1	0	Tr
Oranges, raw, whole, without peel and seeds (2⅝-in diam, about 2½ per lb, with peel and seeds)	1 orange	131	60	1	15	Tr	0	Tr
Orange juice								
Raw, all varieties	1 cup	248	110	2	26	Tr	0	2
Canned, unsweetened	1 cup	249	105	1	25	Tr	0	5
Peaches								
Raw								
Whole, 2-½–in diam., peeled, pitted (about 4 per lb with peels and pits)	1 peach	87	35	1	10	Tr	0	Tr
Sliced	1 cup	170	75	1	19	Tr	0	Tr
Pears, raw, with skin, cored, Bartlett, 2-½–in diam (about 2-½ per lb with cores and stems)	1 pear	166	100	1	25	1	0	Tr

Tr, Trace amount.

Food item	Serving size	Grams	Calories	Protein (g)	Carbohydrate (g)	Fat (g)	Cholesterol (mg)	Sodium (mg)
Fruits and fruit juices—cont'd								
Pineapple, raw, diced	1 cup	155	75	1	19	1	0	2
Pineapple juice, un-sweetened, canned	1 cup	250	140	1	34	Tr	0	3
Plums, without pits, raw, 2-^{1}/$_8$–in diam (about 6-^{1}/$_2$ per lb with pits)	1 plum	66	35	1	9	Tr	0	Tr
Raisins, seedless, cup, not pressed down	1 cup	145	435	5	115	1	0	17
Raspberries, raw	1 cup	123	60	1	14	1	0	Tr
Strawberries, raw, capped, whole	1 cup	149	45	1	10	1	0	1
Watermelon, raw, without rind and seeds, piece (4 by 8 in wedge with rind and seeds; ^{1}/$_{16}$ of 32-^{2}/$_3$–lb melon, 10 by 16 in)	1 piece	482	155	3	35	2	0	10
Grain products								
Bagels, plain or water, enriched, 3-^{1}/$_2$–in diam[h]	1 bagel	68	200	7	38	2	0	245
Breads								
French or vienna bread, enriched[i]								
Slice								
French, 5 by 2-^{1}/$_2$ by 1 in	1 slice	35	100	3	18	1	0	203
Vienna, 4-^{3}/$_4$ by 4 by ^{1}/$_2$ in	1 slice	25	70	2	13	1	0	145
Italian bread, enriched								
Slice, 4-^{1}/$_2$ by 3-^{1}/$_4$ by ^{3}/$_4$ in	1 slice	30	85	3	17	Tr	0	176
Mixed grain bread, enriched[i]								
Slice (18 per loaf)	1 slice	25	65	2	12	1	0	106
Pita bread, enriched, white, 6-^{1}/$_2$–in diam	1 pita	60	165	6	33	1	0	339

Tr, Trace amount.

[h]Egg bagels have 44 mg cholesterol and 22 IU or 7 RE vitamin A per bagel.

[i]Made with vegetable shortening.

Food item	Serving size	Grams	Calories	Protein (g)	Carbohydrate (g)	Fat (g)	Cholesterol (mg)	Sodium (mg)
Grain products—cont'd								
Pumpernickel (²/₃ rye flour, ¹/₃ enriched wheat flour)ʲ:								
Slice, 5 by 4 by ³/₈ in	1 slice	32	80	3	16	1	0	177
Rye bread, light (²/₃ enriched wheat flour, ¹/₃ rye flour)ʲ								
Slice, 4-³/₄ by 3-³/₄ by ⁷/₁₆ in	1 slice	25	65	2	12	1	0	175
Wheat bread, enrichedʲ								
Slice (18 per loaf)	1 slice	25	65	2	12	1	0	138
Whole-wheat breadʲ								
Slice (16 per loaf)	1 slice	28	70	3	13	1	0	180
Breakfast cereals								
All-Bran (about ¹/₃ cup)	1 oz	28	70	4	21	1	0	320
Cap'n Crunch (about ³/₄ cup)	1 oz	28	120	1	23	3	0	213
Cheerios (about 1¹/₄ cup)	1 oz	28	110	4	20	2	0	307
Corn Flakes (about 1¹/₄ cup)								
Kellogg's	1 oz	28	110	2	24	Tr	0	351
Toasties	1 oz	28	110	2	24	Tr	0	297
40% Bran Flakes								
Kellogg's (about ³/₄ cup)	1 oz	28	90	4	22	1	0	264
Post (about ²/₃ cup)	1 oz	28	90	3	22	Tr	0	260
Froot Loops (about 1 cup)	1 oz	28	110	2	25	1	0	145
Lucky Charms (about 1 cup)	1 oz	28	110	3	23	1	0	201
100% Natural Cereal (about ¹/₄ cup)	1 oz	28	135	3	18	6	Tr	12
Product 19 (about ³/₄ cup)	1 oz	28	110	3	24	Tr	0	325

Tr, Trace amount.
ʲMade with vegetable shortening.

Food item	Serving size	Grams	Calories	Protein (g)	Carbohydrate (g)	Fat (g)	Cholesterol (mg)	Sodium (mg)
Grain products—cont'd								
Raisin Bran								
Kellogg's (about ³/₄ cup)	1 oz	28	90	3	21	1	0	207
Post (about ½ cup)	1 oz	28	85	3	21	1	0	185
Special K (about 1-¹/₃ cup)	1 oz	28	110	6	21	Tr	Tr	265
Sugar Frosted Flakes, Kellogg's (about ³/₄ cup)	1 oz	28	110	1	26	Tr	0	230
Wheaties (about 1 cup)	1 oz	28	100	3	23	Tr	0	354
Cakes prepared from cake mixes with enriched flour[k]								
Angelfood, piece, ¹/₁₂ of cake	1 piece	53	125	3	29	Tr	0	269
Devil's food with chocolate frosting								
Piece, ¹/₁₆ of cake	1 piece	69	235	3	40	8	37	181
Cupcake, 2-½–in diam	1 cupcake	35	120	2	20	4	19	92
Cakes prepared from home recipes using enriched flour								
Carrot, with cream cheese frosting[l]								
Piece, ¹/₁₆ of cake	1 piece	96	385	4	48	21	74	279
Pound								
Slice, ¹/₁₇ of loaf	1 slice	30	120	2	15	5	32	96
Cheesecake								
Piece, ¹/₁₂ of cake	1 piece	92	280	5	26	18	170	204
Cookies made with enriched flour								
Brownies with nuts, commercial, with frosting, 1-½ by 1-³/₄ by ⁷/₈ in	1 brownie	25	100	1	16	4	14	59
Chocolate chip, commercial, 2-¼–in diam, ³/₈ in thick	4 cookies	42	180	2	28	9	5	140

Tr, Trace amount.

[k]Excepting angel food cake, cakes were made from mixes containing vegetable shortening and frostings were made with margarine.

[l]Made with vegetable oil.

Food item	Serving size	Grams	Calories	Protein (g)	Carbohydrate (g)	Fat (g)	Cholesterol (mg)	Sodium (mg)
Grain products—cont'd								
Oatmeal with raisins, 2-5/8–in diam, 1/4 in thick	4 cookies	52	245	3	36	10	2	148
Peanut butter cookie, from home recipe, 2-5/8–in diam[m]	4 cookies	48	245	4	28	14	22	142
Corn chips	1-oz package	28	155	2	16	9	0	233
Crackers[n]								
Graham, plain, 2-1/2 in square	2 crackers	14	60	1	11	1	0	86
Melba toast, plain	1 piece	5	20	1	4	Tr	0	44
Saltines[o]	4 crackers	12	50	1	9	1	4	165
Wheat, thin	4 crackers	8	35	1	5	1	0	69
Croissants, made with enriched flour, 4-1/2 by 4 by 1-3/4 in	1 croissant	57	235	5	27	12	13	452
Doughnuts, made with enriched flour								
Cake type, plain, 3-1/4–in diam, 1 in high	1 doughnut	50	210	3	24	12	20	192
Yeast-leavened, glazed, 3-3/4–in diam, 1-1/4 in high	1 doughnut	60	235	4	26	13	21	222
English muffins, plain, enriched	1 muffin	57	140	5	27	1	0	378
French toast, from home recipe	1 slice	65	155	6	17	7	112	257
Macaroni, enriched, cooked (cut lengths, elbows, shells), firm stage (hot)	1 cup	130	190	7	39	1	0	1
Muffins made with enriched flour, 2-1/2–in diam, 1-1/2 in high								
From home recipe								
Blueberry[m]	1 muffin	45	135	3	20	5	19	198
Bran	1 muffin	45	125	3	19	6	24	189
Corn	1 muffin	45	145	3	21	5	23	169

Tr, Trace amount.
[m]Made with vegetable shortening.
[n]Crackers made with enriched flour except for rye wafers and whole-wheat wafers
[o]Made with lard.

Food item	Serving size	Grams	Calories	Protein (g)	Carbohydrate (g)	Fat (g)	Cholesterol (mg)	Sodium (mg)
Grain products—cont'd								
Noodles (egg noodles), enriched, cooked	1 cup	160	200	7	37	2	50	3
Noodles, chow mein, canned	1 cup	45	220	6	26	11	5	450
Pancakes, 4-in diam								
Buckwheat, from mix (with buckwheat and enriched flours), egg and milk added	1 pancake	27	55	2	6	2	20	125
Plain								
From home recipe using enriched flour	1 pancake	27	60	2	9	2	16	115
From mix (with enriched flour), egg, milk, and oil added	1 pancake	27	60	2	8	2	16	160
Pies, piecrust made with enriched flour, vegetable shortening, 9-in diam								
Apple, piece, 1/6 of pie	1 piece	158	405	3	60	18	0	476
Blueberry, piece, 1/6 of pie	1 piece	158	380	4	55	17	0	423
Cherry, piece, 1/6 of pie	1 piece	158	410	4	61	18	0	480
Lemon meringue, piece, 1/6 of pie	1 piece	140	355	5	53	14	143	395
Pecan, piece, 1/6 of pie	1 piece	138	575	7	71	32	95	305
Popcorn, popped								
Air-popped, unsalted	1 cup	8	30	1	6	Tr	0	Tr
Popped in vegetable oil, salted	1 cup	11	55	1	6	3	0	86
Sugar syrup coated	1 cup	35	135	2	30	1	0	Tr
Pretzels, made with enriched flour								
Stick, 2-1/4 in long	10 pretzels	3	10	Tr	2	Tr	0	48
Twisted, dutch, 2-3/4 by 2-5/8 in	1 pretzel	16	65	2	13	1	0	258

Tr, Trace amount.

Food item	Serving size	Grams	Calories	Protein (g)	Carbohydrate (g)	Fat (g)	Cholesterol (mg)	Sodium (mg)
Grain products—cont'd								
Rice								
Brown, cooked, served hot	1 cup	195	230	5	50	1	0	0
White, enriched								
Cooked, served hot	1 cup	205	225	4	50	Tr	0	0
Instant, ready-to-serve, hot	1 cup	165	180	4	40	0	0	0
Rolls, enriched								
Commercial								
Dinner, 2-1/2-in diam, 2 in high	1 roll	28	85	2	14	2	Tr	155
Frankfurter and hamburger (8 per 11-1/2-oz pkg.)	1 roll	40	115	3	20	2	Tr	241
Hard, 3-3/4-in diam, 2 in high	1 roll	50	155	5	30	2	Tr	313
Hoagie or submarine, 11-1/2 by 3 by 2-1/2 in	1 roll	135	400	11	72	8	Tr	683
Spaghetti, enriched, cooked								
Firm stage, "al dente," served hot	1 cup	130	190	7	39	1	0	1
Tender stage, served hot	1 cup	140	155	5	32	1	0	1
Tortillas, corn	1 tortilla	30	65	2	13	1	0	1
Waffles, made with enriched flour, 7-in diam								
From home recipe	1 waffle	75	245	7	26	13	102	445
From mix, egg and milk added	1 waffle	75	205	7	27	8	59	515
Legumes, nuts, and seeds								
Almonds, shelled								
Whole	1 oz	28	165	6	6	15	0	3
Beans, dry								
Black	1 cup	171	225	15	41	1	0	1
Lima	1 cup	190	260	16	49	1	0	4
Pea (navy)	1 cup	190	225	15	40	1	0	13
Pinto	1 cup	180	265	15	49	1	0	3

Tr, Trace amount.

Food item	Serving size	Grams	Calories	Protein (g)	Carbohydrate (g)	Fat (g)	Cholesterol (mg)	Sodium (mg)
Legumes, nuts, and seeds—cont'd								
Black-eyed peas, dry, cooked (with residual cooking liquid)	1 cup	250	190	13	35	1	0	20
Brazil nuts, shelled	1 oz	28	185	4	4	19	0	1
Cashew nuts, salted								
Dry roasted	1 oz	28	165	4	9	13	0	181[p]
Roasted in oil	1 oz	28	165	5	8	14	0	177[q]
Lentils, dry, cooked	1 cup	200	215	16	38	1	0	26
Mixed nuts, with peanuts, salted								
Dry roasted	1 oz	28	170	5	7	15	0	190[r]
Roasted in oil	1 oz	28	175	5	6	16	0	185[r]
Peanuts, roasted in oil, salted	1 oz	28	165	8	5	14	0	122[s]
Peanut butter	1 tbsp	16	95	5	3	8	0	75
Peas, split, dry, cooked	1 cup	200	230	16	42	1	0	26
Pistachio nuts, dried, shelled	1 oz	28	165	6	7	14	0	2
Refried beans, canned	1 cup	290	295	18	51	3	0	1228
Sesame seeds, dry, hulled	1 tbsp	8	45	2	1	4	0	3
Sunflower seeds, dry, hulled	1 oz	28	160	6	5	14	0	1
Meat and meat products								
Beef, cooked[t]								
Cuts braised, simmered, or pot roasted								
Relatively fat such as chuck blade								
Lean and fat, piece, 2-1/2 by 2-1/2 by 3/4 in	3 oz	85	325	22	0	26	87	53
Relatively lean, such as bottom round								
Lean and fat, piece, 4-1/8 by 2-1/4 by 1/2 in	3 oz	85	220	25	0	13	81	43

Tr, Trace amount.

[p]Cashews without salt contain 21 mg sodium per cup or 4 mg per oz.

[q]Cashews without salt contain 22 mg sodium per cup or 5 mg per oz.

[r]Mixed nuts without salt contain 3 mg sodium per oz.

[s]Peanuts without salt contain 22 mg sodium per cup or 4 mg per oz.

[t]Outer layer of fat was removed to within approximately 1/2 inch of lean. Deposits of fat within the cut were not removed.

Food item	Serving size	Grams	Calories	Protein (g)	Carbohydrate (g)	Fat (g)	Cholesterol (mg)	Sodium (mg)
Meats and meat products—cont'd								
Ground beef, broiled, patty, 3 by $^5/_8$ in								
Lean	3 oz	85	230	21	0	16	74	65
Regular	3 oz	85	245	20	0	18	76	70
Roast, oven cooked, no liquid added								
Relatively fat, such as rib								
Lean and fat, 2 pieces, 4-$^1/_8$ by 2-$^1/_4$ in	3 oz	85	315	19	0	26	72	54
Relatively lean, such as eye of round								
Lean and fat, 2 pieces, 2-$^1/_2$ by 2-$^1/_2$ by $^3/_8$ in	3 oz	85	205	23	0	12	62	50
Steak								
Sirloin, broiled								
Lean and fat, piece, 2-$^1/_2$ by 2-$^1/_2$ by $^3/_4$ in	3 oz	85	240	23	0	15	77	53
Lamb, cooked								
Chops, (3 per lb with bone)								
Arm, braised								
Lean and fat	2.2 oz	63	220	20	0	15	77	46
Loin, broiled								
Lean and fat	2.8 oz	80	235	20	0	16	78	62
Leg, roasted								
Lean and fat, 2 pieces, 4-$^1/_8$ by 2-$^1/_4$ by $^1/_4$ in	3 oz	85	205	22	0	13	78	57
Rib, roasted								
Lean and fat, 3 pieces, 2-$^1/_2$ by 2-$^1/_2$ by $^1/_4$ in	3 oz	85	315	18	0	26	77	60
Pork, cured, cooked								
Bacon								
Regular	3 medium slices	19	110	6	Tr	9	16	303
Canadian-style	2 slices	46	85	11	1	4	27	711

Tr, Trace amount.

Food item	Serving size	Grams	Calories	Protein (g)	Carbohydrate (g)	Fat (g)	Cholesterol (mg)	Sodium (mg)
Meats and meat products—cont'd								
Ham, light cured, roasted								
Lean and fat, 2 pieces, 4-1/8 by 2-1/4 by 1/4 in	3 oz	85	205	18	0	14	53	1009
Luncheon meat								
Canned, spiced or unspiced, slice, 3 by 2 by 1/2 in	2 slices	42	140	5	1	13	26	541
Chopped ham (8 slices per 6 oz pkg)	2 slices	42	95	7	0	7	21	576
Cooked ham (8 slices per 8-oz pkg)								
Regular	2 slices	57	105	10	2	6	32	751
Extra lean	2 slices	57	75	11	1	3	27	815
Pork, fresh, cooked								
Chop, loin (cut 3 per lb with bone)								
Broiled								
Lean and fat	3.1 oz	87	275	24	0	19	84	61
Ham (leg), roasted								
Lean and fat, piece, 2-1/2 by 2-1/2 by 3/4 in	3 oz	85	250	21	0	18	79	50
Rib, roasted								
Lean and fat, piece, 2-1/2 by 3/4 in	3 oz	85	270	21	0	20	69	37
Shoulder cut, braised								
Lean and fat, 3 pieces, 2-1/2 by 2-1/2 by 1/4 in	3 oz	85	295	23	0	22	93	75
Sausages								
Bologna	2 slices	57	180	7	2	16	31	581
Frankfurter	1 frank	45	145	5	1	13	23	504
Pork link	1 link	13	50	3	Tr	4	11	168
Salami								
Cooked type, slice (8 per 8-oz pkg)	2 slices	57	145	8	1	11	37	607
Veal, medium fat, cooked, bone removed								
Cutlet, 4-1/8 by 2-1/4 by 1/2 in, braised or broiled	3 oz	85	185	23	0	9	109	56

Tr, Trace amount.

Food item	Serving size	Grams	Calories	Protein (g)	Carbohydrate (g)	Fat (g)	Cholesterol (mg)	Sodium (mg)
Meats and meat products—cont'd								
Rib, 2 pieces, 4-1/8 by 2-1/4 by 1/4 in, roasted	3 oz	85	230	23	0	14	109	57
Mixed dishes and fast foods								
Mixed dishes								
Beef and vegetable stew, from home recipe	1 cup	245	220	16	15	11	71	292
Beef potpie, from home recipe, baked, piece, 1/3 of 9-in diam pie	1 piece	210	515	21	39	30	42	596
Chicken a la king, cooked, from home recipe	1 cup	245	470	27	12	34	221	760
Chicken and noodles, cooked, from home recipe	1 cup	240	365	22	26	18	103	600
Chicken chow mein								
Canned	1 cup	250	95	7	18	Tr	8	725
From home recipe	1 cup	250	255	31	10	10	75	718
Chicken potpie, from home recipe, baked, piece, 1/3 of 9-in diam pie	1 piece	232	545	23	42	31	56	594
Chili con carne with beans, canned	1 cup	255	340	19	31	16	28	1354
Chop suey with beef and pork, from home recipe	1 cup	250	300	26	13	17	68	1053
Macaroni (enriched) and cheese								
Canned	1 cup	240	230	9	26	10	24	730
From home recipe[u]	1 cup	200	430	17	40	22	44	1086
Spaghetti (enriched) in tomato sauce with cheese								
Canned	1 cup	250	190	6	39	2	3	955
From home recipe[u]	1 cup	250	260	9	37	9	8	955
Spaghetti (enriched) with meatballs and tomato sauce								
From home recipe	1 cup	248	330	19	39	12	89	1009

Tr, Trace amount.
[u]Made with margarine.

Food item	Serving size	Grams	Calories	Protein (g)	Carbohydrate (g)	Fat (g)	Cholesterol (mg)	Sodium (mg)
Poultry and poultry products								
Chicken								
Fried, flesh, with skin[v]								
Batter dipped								
Breast, ½ breast (5.6 oz with bones)	4.9 oz	140	365	35	13	18	119	385
Drumstick (3.4 oz with bones)	2.5 oz	72	195	16	6	11	62	194
Flour coated								
Breast, ½ breast (4.2 oz with bones)	3.5 oz	98	220	31	2	9	87	74
Drumstick (2.6 oz with bones)	1.7 oz	49	120	13	1	7	44	44
Roasted, flesh only								
Breast, ½ breast (4.2 oz with bones and skin)	3.0 oz	86	140	27	0	3	73	64
Drumstick (2.9 oz with bones and skin)	1.6 oz	44	75	12	0	2	41	42
Turkey, roasted, flesh only								
Dark meat, piece, 2-½ by 1-⅝ by ¼ in	4 pieces	85	160	24	0	6	72	67
Light meat, piece, 4 by 2 by ¼ in	2 pieces	85	135	25	0	3	59	54
Light and dark meat								
Chopped or diced	1 cup	140	240	41	0	7	106	98
Pieces (1 slice white meat, 4 by 2 by ¼ in and 2 slices dark meat, 2-½ by 1-⅝ by ¼ in)	3 pieces	85	145	25	0	4	65	60

Tr, Trace amount.
[v]Fried in vegetable shortening.

Food item	Serving size	Grams	Calories	Protein (g)	Carbohydrate (g)	Fat (g)	Cholesterol (mg)	Sodium (mg)
Soups, sauces, and gravies								
Soups								
Canned, condensed								
Prepared with equal volume of milk								
Clam chowder, New England	1 cup	248	165	9	17	7	22	992
Cream of chicken	1 cup	248	190	7	15	11	27	1047
Cream of mushroom	1 cup	248	205	6	15	14	20	1076
Tomato	1 cup	248	160	6	22	6	17	932
Prepared with equal volume of water								
Bean with bacon	1 cup	253	170	8	23	6	3	951
Beef noodle	1 cup	244	85	5	9	3	5	952
Chicken noodle	1 cup	241	75	4	9	2	7	1106
Chicken rice	1 cup	241	60	4	7	2	7	815
Clam chowder, Manhattan	1 cup	244	80	4	12	2	2	1808
Cream of chicken	1 cup	244	115	3	9	7	10	986
Cream of mushroom	1 cup	244	130	2	9	9	2	1032
Minestrone	1 cup	241	80	4	11	3	2	911
Pea, green	1 cup	250	165	9	27	3	0	988
Tomato	1 cup	244	85	2	17	2	0	871
Vegetable beef	1 cup	244	80	6	10	2	5	956
Sauces								
From dry mix								
Cheese, prepared with milk	1 cup	279	305	16	23	17	53	1565
Hollandaise, prepared with water	1 cup	259	240	5	14	20	52	1564
Gravies								
Canned								
Beef	1 cup	233	125	9	11	5	7	1305
Chicken	1 cup	238	190	5	13	14	5	1373
Mushroom	1 cup	238	120	3	13	6	0	1357

Tr, Trace amount.

Food item	Serving size	Grams	Calories	Protein (g)	Carbohydrate (g)	Fat (g)	Cholesterol (mg)	Sodium (mg)
Sugars and sweets								
Candy								
Caramels, plain or chocolate	1 oz	28	115	1	22	3	1	64
Chocolate								
Milk, plain	1 oz	28	145	2	16	9	6	23
Milk, with almonds	1 oz	28	150	3	15	10	5	23
Milk, with peanuts	1 oz	28	155	4	13	11	5	19
Milk, with rice cereal	1 oz	28	140	2	18	7	6	46
Fudge, chocolate, plain	1 oz	28	115	1	21	3	1	54
Gum drops	1 oz	28	100	Tr	25	Tr	0	10
Hard candy	1 oz	28	110	0	28	0	0	7
Jelly beans	1 oz	28	105	Tr	26	Tr	0	7
Marshmallows	1 oz	28	90	1	23	0	0	25
Custard, baked	1 cup	265	305	14	29	15	278	209
Honey, strained or extracted	1 cup	339	1030	1	279	0	0	17
	1 tbsp	21	65	Tr	17	0	0	1
Jams and preserves	1 tbsp	20	55	Tr	14	Tr	0	2
	1 packet	14	40	Tr	10	Tr	0	2
Jellies	1 tbsp	18	50	Tr	13	Tr	0	5
	1 packet	14	40	Tr	10	Tr	0	4
Popsicle, 3-fl-oz size	1 popsicle	95	70	0	18	0	0	11
Puddings								
Canned								
Chocolate	5-oz can	142	205	3	30	11	1	285
Tapioca	5-oz can	142	160	3	28	5	Tr	252
Vanilla	5-oz can	142	220	2	33	10	1	305
Dry mix, prepared with whole milk								
Chocolate								
Instant	½ cup	130	155	4	27	4	14	440
Regular (cooked)	½ cup	130	150	4	25	4	15	167
Rice	½ cup	132	155	4	27	4	15	140
Tapioca	½ cup	130	145	4	25	4	15	152
Vanilla								
Instant	½ cup	130	150	4	27	4	15	375
Regular (cooked)	½ cup	130	145	4	25	4	15	178
Sugars								
Brown, pressed down	1 cup	220	820	0	212	0	0	97

Tr, Trace amount.

Food item	Serving size	Grams	Calories	Protein (g)	Carbohydrate (g)	Fat (g)	Cholesterol (mg)	Sodium (mg)
Sugars and sweets—cont'd								
White								
Granulated	1 cup	200	770	0	199	0	0	5
	1 tbsp	12	45	0	12	0	0	Tr
	1 packet	6	25	0	6	0	0	Tr
Syrups								
Chocolate-flavored syrup or topping								
Thin type	2 tbsp	38	85	1	22	Tr	0	36
Fudge type	2 tbsp	38	125	2	21	5	0	42
Vegetables and vegetable products								
Asparagus, green								
Cooked, drained								
From raw								
Cuts and tips	1 cup	180	45	5	8	1	0	7
From frozen								
Cuts and tips	1 cup	180	50	5	9	1	0	7
Beans								
Lima, immature seeds, frozen, cooked, drained Thick-seeded types (Ford hooks)	1 cup	170	170	10	32	1	0	90
Beets								
Cooked, drained								
Diced or sliced	1 cup	170	55	2	11	Tr	0	83
Black-eyed peas, immature seeds, cooked and drained								
From raw	1 cup	165	180	13	30	1	0	7
Broccoli								
Raw	1 spear	151	40	4	8	1	0	41
Spears, cut into $^{1}/_{2}$-in pieces	1 cup	155	45	5	9	Tr	0	17
Brussels sprouts, cooked, drained From raw, 7-8 sprouts, 1-$^{1}/_{4}$ to 1-$^{1}/_{2}$–in diam	1 cup	155	60	4	13	1	0	33
Cabbage, common varieties								
Raw, coarsely shredded or sliced	1 cup	70	15	1	4	Tr	0	13

Tr, Trace amount.

Food item	Serving size	Grams	Calories	Protein (g)	Carbohydrate (g)	Fat (g)	Cholesterol (mg)	Sodium (mg)
Vegetables and vegetable products—cont'd								
Carrots								
Raw, without crowns and tips, scraped								
Whole, 7-¹/₂ by 1-¹/₈ in, or strips, 2-¹/₂ to 3 in long	1 carrot or 18 strips	72	30	1	7	Tr	0	25
Cooked, sliced, drained								
From raw	1 cup	156	70	2	16	Tr	0	103
Cauliflower								
Raw (flowerets)	1 cup	100	25	2	5	Tr	0	15
Cooked, drained From raw (flowerets)	1 cup	125	30	2	6	Tr	0	8
Celery, pascal type, raw								
Stalk, large outer, 8 by 1-¹/₂ in (at root end)	1 stalk	40	5	Tr	1	Tr	0	35
Corn, sweet								
Cooked, drained From raw, ear 5 by 1-³/₄ in	1 ear	77	85	3	19	1	0	13
From frozen	1 ear	63	60	2	14	Tr	0	3
Cucumber, with peel, slices, ¹/₈ in thick (large, 2-¹/₈-in diam; small, 1-³/₄-in diam)	6 large or 8 small slices	28	5	Tr	1	Tr	0	1
Eggplant, cooked, steamed	1 cup	96	25	1	6	Tr	0	3
Lettuce, raw								
Butterhead, as Boston types:								
Head, 5-in diam	1 head	163	20	2	4	Tr	0	8
Leaves	1 outer or 2 inner leaves	15	Tr	Tr	Tr	Tr	0	1

Tr, Trace amount.

Food item	Serving size	Grams	Calories	Protein (g)	Carbohydrate (g)	Fat (g)	Cholesterol (mg)	Sodium (mg)
Vegetables and vegetable products—cont'd								
Crisphead, as iceberg								
Pieces, chopped or shredded	1 cup	55	5	1	1	Tr	0	5
Looseleaf (bunching varieties including romaine or cos), chopped or shredded pieces	1 cup	56	10	1	2	Tr	0	5
Mushrooms								
Raw, sliced or chopped	1 cup	70	20	1	3	Tr	0	
Cooked, drained	1 cup	156	40	3	8	1	0	3
Onions								
Raw								
Chopped	1 cup	160	55	2	12	Tr	0	3
Cooked (whole or sliced), drained	1 cup	210	60	2	13	Tr	0	17
Peas, edible pod, cooked, drained	1 cup	160	65	5	11	Tr	0	6
Peas, green								
Canned, drained solids	1 cup	170	115	8	21	1	0	372[w]
Frozen, cooked, drained	1 cup	160	125	8	23	Tr	0	139
Potatoes, cooked								
Baked (about 2 per lb, raw)								
With skin	1 potato	202	220	5	51	Tr	0	16
Flesh only	1 potato	156	145	3	34	Tr	0	8
Broiled (about 3 per lb, raw)								
Peeled after boiling	1 potato	136	120	3	27	Tr	0	5
Peeled before boiling	1 potato	135	115	2	27	Tr	0	7
French fried, strip, 2 to 3-1/2 in long, frozen								
Oven heated	10 strips	50	110	2	17	4	0	16
Fried in vegetable oil	10 strips	50	160	2	20	8	0	108
Potato products, prepared								

Tr, Trace amount.

[w]For regular pack; special dietary pack contains 3 mg sodium.

Food item	Serving size	Grams	Calories	Protein (g)	Carbohydrate (g)	Fat (g)	Cholesterol (mg)	Sodium (mg)
Vegetables and vegetable products—cont'd								
Au gratin								
From dry mix	1 cup	245	230	6	31	10	12	1076
From home recipe	1 cup	245	325	12	28	19	56	1061
Hashed brown, from frozen	1 cup	156	340	5	44	18	0	53
Mashed								
From home recipe								
Milk added	1 cup	210	160	4	37	1	4	636
Milk and margarine added	1 cup	210	225	4	35	9	4	620
Potato salad, made with mayonnaise	1 cup	250	360	7	28	21	170	1323
Scalloped								
From dry mix	1 cup	245	230	5	31	11	27	835
From home recipe	1 cup	245	210	7	26	9	29	821
Potato chips	10 chips	20	105	1	10	7	0	94
Pumpkin								
Cooked from raw, mashed	1 cup	245	50	2	12	Tr	0	2
Radishes, raw, stem ends, rootlets cut off	4 radishes	18	5	Tr	1	Tr	0	4
Sauerkraut, canned, solids and liquid	1 cup	236	45	2	10	Tr	0	1560
Spinach								
Raw, chopped	1 cup	55	10	2	2	Tr	0	43
Cooked, drained								
From raw	1 cup	180	40	5	7	Tr	0	126
From frozen (leaf)	1 cup	190	55	6	10	Tr	0	163
Sweetpotatoes								
Cooked (raw, 5 by 2 in; about 2-1/2 per lb)								
Baked in skin, peeled	1 potato	114	115	2	28	Tr	0	11
Boiled, without skin	1 potato	151	160	2	37	Tr	0	20
Tomatoes								
Raw, 2-3/5–in diam (3 per 12 oz pkg)	1 tomato	123	25	1	5	Tr	0	10
Tomato juice, canned	1 cup	244	40	2	10	Tr	0	881[x]
Tomato products, canned								
Paste	1 cup	262	220	10	49	2	0	170[y]
Sauce	1 cup	245	75	3	18	Tr	0	1482[z]

Tr, Trace amount.

[x]For added salt; if none is added, sodium content is 24 mg.

[y]With no added salt; if salt is added, sodium content is 2070 mg.

[z]With no added salt; if salt is added, sodium content is 998 mg.

Food item	Serving size	Grams	Calories	Protein (g)	Carbohydrate (g)	Fat (g)	Cholesterol (mg)	Sodium (mg)
Vegetables and vegetable products—cont'd								
Vegetable juice cocktail, canned	1 cup	242	45	2	11	Tr	0	883
Miscellaneous items								
Catsup	1 cup	273	290	5	69	1	0	2845
	1 tbsp	15	15	Tr	4	Tr	0	156
Chili powder	1 tsp	2.6	10	Tr	1	Tr	0	26
Mustard, prepared, yellow	1 tsp or individual packet	5	5	Tr	Tr	Tr	0	63
Olives, canned								
Green	4 medium or 3 extra large	13	15	Tr	Tr	2	0	312
Ripe, Mission, pitted	3 small or 2 large	9	15	Tr	Tr	2	0	68
Pickles, cucumber								
Dill	1 pickle	65	5	Tr	1	Tr	0	928
Sweet	1 pickle	15	20	Tr	5	Tr	0	107
Salt	1 tsp	5.5	0	0	0	0	0	2132

Nutritional Information for Selected Fast-Food Restaurants

Item	Serving (oz)	(g)	Calories	Protein (g)	Carbohydrate (g)	Total fat (g)	Dietary fiber (g)	Cholesterol (mg)	Sodium (mg)
Restaurant: Arby's									
Regular Roast Beef	5	147	353	22.2	31.6	14.8	1	39	588
Beef 'N Cheddar	7	197	455	25.7	27.7	26.8	1	63	955
Chicken Breast Sandwich	7	184	493	23.0	47.9	25.0	1	91	1019
Roast Chicken Club	8	234	610	31.0	40.0	33.0	1	80	1500
Turkey Deluxe	7	197	375	23.8	32.5	16.6	2	39	1047
Ham 'N Cheese	6	156	292	22.9	19.2	13.7	1	45	1350
Super Roast Beef	8	234	501	25.1	50.4	22.1	1	40	798
French Fries	3	71	246	2.1	29.8	13.2	2	0	114
Restaurant: Burger King									
Whopper/Everything	10	270	628	27.0	46.0	36.0	2	90	880
Whopper/Cheese	10	294	706	32.0	47.0	43.0	2	113	1164
Hamburger	4	108	272	15.0	29.0	12.0	1	37	509
Cheeseburger	4	121	318	17.0	30.0	15.0	1	48	651
Bacon Double Cheeseburger	6	160	515	33.0	27.0	31.0	1	104	728
Hamburger Deluxe	5	138	344	15.0	30.0	17.0	1	41	486
Cheeseburger Deluxe	5	151	390	17.0	31.0	20.0	2	52	628
Ocean Catch Filet	7	194	488	19.0	45.0	25.0	2	77	592
Chicken Specialty Sandwich	8	229	685	26.0	56.0	40.0	2	82	1423
Chicken Tenders™	3	90	236	20.0	10.0	10.0	1	47	636
French Fries	4	111	341	3.0	24.0	13.0	3	14	160
Onion Rings	3	86	302	4.0	28.0	16.0	2	0	665
Breakfast Croissan'wich/ Bacon	4	118	355	14.0	20.0	24.0	1	249	762
Breakfast Croissan'wich/ Sausage	6	159	538	20.0	20.0	40.0	1	293	1042

Information for all restaurants, except Jack In The Box, from Ross Laboratories, Columbus, Ohio, 43216, from *Dietetic Currents*, 18:4, 1991. Information for Jack in the Box from Boyle MA, Zyla G: *Personal Nutrition*, ed 2, St Paul, Minn, 1992, West Publishing.

Item	Serving (oz)	(g)	Calories	Protein (g)	Carbohydrate (g)	Total fat (g)	Dietary fiber (g)	Cholesterol (mg)	Sodium (mg)
Restaurant: Burger King—cont'd									
Breakfast Croissan'wich/ Ham/Egg/Cheese	5	144	346	19.0	19.0	21.0	1	241	962
Breakfast Bagel Sandwich/ Bacon	6	169	438	20.0	46.0	20.0	2	274	905
Breakfast Bagel Sandwich/ Sausage/Egg/Cheese	7	210	626	27.0	49.0	36.0	2	318	1137
Breakfast Bagel Sandwich/ Ham/Egg/Cheese	7	196	418	23.0	46.0	15.0	2	287	1130
Scrambled Egg Platter	7	211	549	17.0	44.0	30.0	3	370	808
Scrambled Egg Platter/ Sausage	9	260	768	26.0	47.0	53.0	3	412	1271
Scrambled Egg Platter/ Bacon	8	221	610	21.0	44.0	39.0	3	373	1043
French Toast Sticks	5	141	538	10.0	53.0	32.0	2	80	537
Great Danish	3	71	500	5.0	40.0	36.0	3	6	288
Vanilla Shake	10	284	334	9.0	51.0	10.0	0	39	205
Chocolate Shake	10	284	326	9.0	49.0	10.0	1	33	202
Apple Pie	4	125	311	3.0	44.0	14.0	2	4	412
Chicken Salad	9	258	142	20.0	8.0	4.0	2	50	440
Chef Salad	10	273	178	17.0	7.0	9.0	2	120	570
Garden Salad	8	223	95	6.0	8.0	5.0	2	15	125
Side Salad	5	135	25	1.0	5.0	0.0	2	0	20
Thousand Island Dressing	2	63	290	1.0	15.0	26.0	0	36	470
Bleu Cheese Dressing	2	59	300	3.0	2.0	32.0	0	40	600
Reduced Calorie Italian	2	59	170	0.0	3.0	18.0	0	3	762
French Dressing	2	64	290	0.0	23.0	22.0	1	2	400
Bacon Bits	0.1	3	16	1.0	0.0	1.0	0	5	1
Croutons	0.3	7	31	1.0	5.0	1.0	0	0	90
Restaurant: Dairy Queen									
Cone, Small	3	85	140	3.0	22.0	4.0	0	10	45
Cone, Regular	5	142	240	6.0	38.0	7.0	0	15	80
Cone, Large	8	213	340	9.0	57.0	10.0	0	25	115
Cone, Small, Chocolate-Dipped	3	92	190	3.0	25.0	9.0	2	10	55
Cone, Regular, Chocolate-Dipped	6	156	340	6.0	42.0	16.0	3	20	100
Cone, Large, Chocolate-Dipped	8	234	510	9.0	64.0	24.0	4	30	145
Chocolate Sundae, Small	4	106	190	3.0	33.0	4.0	1	10	75
Chocolate Sundae, Regular	6	177	310	5.0	56.0	8.0	1	20	120
Chocolate Sundae, Large	9	248	440	8.0	78.0	10.0	2	30	165
Chocolate Shake, Small	9	241	409	8.0	69.0	11.0	1	30	150
Chocolate Shake, Regular	15	418	710	14.0	120.0	19.0	2	50	260
Chocolate Shake, Large	17	489	831	16.0	140.0	22.0	2	60	304

Item	Serving (oz)	(g)	Calories	Protein (g)	Carbohydrate (g)	Total fat (g)	Dietary fiber (g)	Cholesterol (mg)	Sodium (mg)
Restaurant: Dairy Queen—cont'd									
Chocolate Malt, Small	9	241	438	8.0	77.0	10.0	2	30	150
Chocolate Malt, Regular	15	418	760	14.0	134.0	18.0	3	50	260
Chocolate Malt, Large	17	489	889	16.0	157.0	21.0	3	60	304
Float	14	397	410	5.0	82.0	7.0	0	20	85
Peanut Buster Parfait	11	305	740	16.0	94.0	34.0	6	30	250
Parfait	10	283	430	8.0	76.0	8.0	1	30	140
Freeze	14	397	500	9.0	89.0	12.0	0	30	180
Mr Misty, Small	9	248	190	0.0	48.0	0.0	0	0	10
Mr Misty, Regular	12	330	250	0.0	63.0	0.0	0	0	10
Mr Misty, Large	16	439	340	0.0	84.0	0.0	0	0	10
Mr Misty Kiss	3	89	70	0.0	17.0	0.0	0	0	10
Mr Misty Freeze	15	411	500	9.0	91.0	12.0	0	30	140
Mr Misty Float	15	411	390	5.0	74.0	7.0	0	20	95
Buster Bar	5	149	448	10.0	41.0	29.0	6	10	175
Fudge Nut Bar	5	142	406	8.0	40.0	25.0	2	10	167
Dilly Bar	3	85	210	3.0	21.0	13.0	1	10	50
DQ Sandwich	2	60	140	3.0	24.0	4.0	0	5	40
Chipper Sandwich	4	113	318	5.0	56.0	7.0	0	13	170
Heath Blizzard, Regular	14	404	800	15.0	125.0	24.0	3	65	325
Single Hamburger	5	148	360	21.0	33.0	16.0	1	45	630
Double Hamburger	7	210	530	36.0	33.0	28.0	1	85	660
Triple Hamburger	10	272	710	51.0	33.0	45.0	1	135	690
Single Hamburger/Cheese	6	162	410	24.0	33.0	20.0	1	50	790
Double Hamburger/Cheese	8	239	650	43.0	34.0	37.0	1	95	980
Triple Hamburger/Cheese	11	301	820	58.0	34.0	50.0	1	145	1010
Hot Dog	4	100	280	11.0	21.0	16.0	1	45	830
Hot Dog/Chili	5	128	320	13.0	23.0	20.0	1	55	985
Hot Dog/Cheese	4	114	330	15.0	21.0	21.0	1	55	990
Super Hot Dog	6	175	520	17.0	44.0	27.0	1	80	1365
Super Hot Dog/Chili	8	218	570	21.0	47.0	32.0	2	100	1595
Super Hot Dog/Cheese	7	196	580	22.0	45.0	34.0	1	100	1605
Fish Filet	6	177	430	20.0	45.0	18.0	1	40	674
Fish Filet/Cheese	7	191	483	23.0	46.0	22.0	1	49	870
Chicken Breast Filet	7	202	608	27.0	46.0	34.0	2	78	725
Chicken Breast Filet/Cheese	8	216	661	30.0	47.0	38.0	2	87	921
All White Chicken Nuggets	4	99	276	16.0	13.0	18.0	1	39	505
BBQ Nugget Sauce	1	28	41	0.0	9.0	0.7	0	0	130
French Fries, Small	3	71	200	2.0	25.0	10.0	2	10	115
French Fries, Large	4	113	320	3.0	40.0	16.0	3	15	185
Onion Rings	3	85	280	4.0	31.0	16.0	3	15	140
Restaurant: Domino's Pizza (2 slices of each pizza)									
Cheese Pizza	6	168	376	21.6	56.3	10.0	6	19	483
Pepperoni Pizza	7	187	460	24.1	55.6	17.5	5	28	825
Sausage/Mushroom Pizza	7	200	430	24.2	55.3	15.8	8	28	552

Item	Serving (oz)	(g)	Calories	Protein (g)	Carbohydrate (g)	Total fat (g)	Dietary fiber (g)	Cholesterol (mg)	Sodium (mg)
Restaurant: Domino's Pizza (2 slices of each pizza)—cont'd									
Veggie Pizza	9	261	498	31.0	60.0	18.5	8	36	1035
Deluxe Pizza	8	234	498	26.7	59.2	20.4	7	40	954
Double Cheese/Pepperoni Pizza	8	227	545	32.1	55.2	25.3	8	48	1042
Ham Pizza	7	186	417	23.2	58.0	11.0	2	26	805
Restaurant: Jack in the Box									
Breakfast Jack Sandwich	4	126	307	18	30	13	<1	203	871
Canadian Crescent	5	134	472	19	25	31	<1	226	851
Sausage Crescent	6	156	584	22	28	43	<1	187	1012
Supreme Crescent	5	146	547	20	27	40	<1	178	1053
Pancakes Breakfast Platter	8	231	612	15	87	22	<1	99	888
Scrambled Egg Breakfast Platter	9	249	662	24	52	40	<1	354	1188
Hamburger	3	98	276	13	30	12	<1	29	521
Cheeseburger	4	113	323	16	32	15	<1	42	749
Jumbo Jack	7	205	485	26	38	26	<1	64	905
Jumbo Jack w/Cheese	9	246	630	32	45	35	<1	110	1665
Bacon Cheeseburger Supreme	8	231	724	34	44	46	<1	70	1307
Swiss and Baconburger	8	231	643	33	31	43	<1	99	1354
Ham and Swiss Burger	7	203	638	36	37	39	<1	117	1330
Chicken Supreme	8	228	601	31	39	36	<1	60	1582
Double Cheeseburger	5	149	467	21	33	27	—	72	842
Tacos									
Regular	3	81	191	8	16	11	<1	21	460
Super	5	135	288	12	21	17	<1	—	—
French Fries	2	68	221	2	27	12	<1	8	164
Hash Brown Potatoes	2	62	116	2	11	7	<1	3	211
Onion Rings	4	108	382	5	39	23	<1	27	407
Milkshakes									
Chocolate	11	322	330	11	55	7	0	25	270
Strawberry	12	328	320	10	55	7	0	25	240
Vanilla	11	317	320	10	57	6	0	25	230
Apple Turnover	4	119	410	4	45	24	<1	15	350
Restaurant: Kentucky Fried Chicken									
Nuggets	1	16	46	2.8	2.2	2.9	0	12	140
Barbeque Sauce	1	28	35	0.3	7.1	0.6	0	0	450
Sweet and Sour Sauce	1	28	58	0.1	13.0	0.6	0	0	148
Chicken Littles Sandwich	2	47	169	5.7	13.8	10.1	0	18	331
Buttermilk Biscuit	2	65	235	4.5	28.0	11.9	1	1	655
Mashed Potatoes/Gravy	4	98	71	2.4	11.9	1.6	1	0	339
French Fries, Regular	3	77	244	3.2	31.1	11.9	2	2	139
Corn-on-the-cob	5	143	176	5.1	31.9	3.1	7	0	21

Item	Serving (oz)	(g)	Calories	Protein (g)	Carbohydrate (g)	Total fat (g)	Dietary fiber (g)	Cholesterol (mg)	Sodium (mg)
Restaurant: Kentucky Fried Chicken—cont'd									
Coleslaw	3	91	119	1.5	13.3	6.6	1	5	197
Original Recipe Chicken									
Wing	2	55	178	12.2	6.0	11.7	0	64	372
Breast	4	115	283	27.5	8.8	15.3	0	93	672
Drumstick	2	57	146	13.1	4.2	8.5	0	67	275
Thigh	4	104	294	17.9	11.1	19.7	1	123	619
Extra Crispy Chicken									
Wing	2	65	254	12.4	9.3	18.6	0	67	422
Breast	5	135	342	33.0	11.7	19.7	1	114	790
Drumstick	2	69	204	13.6	6.1	13.9	0	71	324
Thigh	4	119	406	20.0	14.4	29.8	1	129	688
Restaurant: Long John Silver's Seafood Shoppe									
Three-piece Fish Light/ Paprika (Baked)	5	134	120	28.0	1.0	1.0	0	110	120
Three-piece Fish/Lemon Crumb (Baked)	5	141	150	29.0	4.0	1.0	0	110	370
Three-piece Fish/Scampi Sauce (Baked)	5	148	170	28.0	2.0	5.0	0	110	270
Shrimp/Scampi Sauce (Baked)	5	148	120	15.0	2.0	5.0	0	205	610
Chicken Light/Herbs (Baked)	4	117	140	25.0	1.0	4.0	0	70	670
Rice Pilaf	5	142	210	5.0	43.0	2.0	1	0	570
Green Beans	4	113	30	1.0	6.0	1.0	3	5	540
Garden Vegetables	4	113	120	4.0	16.0	6.0	5	5	95
Coleslaw	3	98	140	1.0	20.0	6.0	1	15	260
Breadstick	1	34	110	3.0	18.0	3.0	1	0	120
Small Salad	2	54	8	1.0	2.0	0.0	1	0	0
Restaurant: McDonald's									
Egg McMuffin	5	138	290	18.2	28.1	11.2	1	226	740
Hotcakes/Butter/Syrup	6	176	410	8.2	74.4	9.2	2	21	640
Scrambled Eggs	4	100	140	12.4	1.2	9.8	0	399	290
Pork Sausage	2	48	180	8.4	0.0	16.3	0	48	350
English Muffin/Butter	2	59	170	5.4	26.7	4.6	1	9	270
Hashbrown Potatoes	2	53	130	1.4	14.9	7.3	2	9	330
Biscuit/Biscuit Spread	3	75	260	4.6	31.9	12.7	1	1	730
Biscuit/Sausage	4	123	440	13.0	31.9	29.0	1	49	1080
Biscuit/Sausage/Egg	6	180	520	19.9	32.6	34.5	1	275	1250
Biscuit/Bacon/Egg/Cheese	6	156	440	17.5	33.3	26.4	1	253	1230
Sausage McMuffin	4	117	370	16.5	27.3	21.9	1	64	830
Sausage McMuffin/Cheese	6	167	440	22.6	27.9	26.8	1	263	980
Apple Danish	4	115	390	5.8	51.2	17.9	2	25	370
Iced Cheese Danish	4	110	390	7.4	42.3	21.8	1	47	420

Item	Serving (oz)	(g)	Calories	Protein (g)	Carbohydrate (g)	Total fat (g)	Dietary fiber (g)	Cholesterol (mg)	Sodium (mg)
Restaurant: McDonald's—cont'd									
Cinnamon Raisin Danish	4	110	440	6.4	57.5	21.0	2	34	430
Raspberry Danish	4	117	410	6.1	61.5	15.9	2	26	310
Apple Bran Muffin	3	85	190	5.0	46.0	0.0	2	0	230
Blueberry Muffin	3	85	170	3.0	40.0	0.0	1	0	220
Chicken McNuggets	4	113	290	19.0	16.5	16.3	1	65	520
Hot Mustard Sauce	1	30	70	0.5	8.2	3.6	0	5	250
Barbeque Sauce	1	32	50	0.3	12.1	0.5	0	0	340
Sweet and Sour Sauce	1	32	60	0.2	13.8	0.2	0	0	190
Hamburger	4	102	260	12.3	30.6	9.5	1	37	500
Cheeseburger	4	116	310	15.0	31.2	13.8	1	53	750
McLean Deluxe	7	203	310	20.0	34.0	10.0	2	37	650
Quarter Pounder	6	166	410	23.1	34.0	20.7	1	86	660
Quarter Pounder/Cheese	7	194	520	28.5	35.1	29.2	1	118	1150
Big Mac	8	215	560	25.2	42.5	32.4	1	103	950
Filet-O-Fish	5	142	440	13.8	37.9	26.1	1	50	1030
McD.L.T.	8	234	580	26.3	36.0	36.8	2	109	990
McChicken	7	190	490	19.2	39.8	28.6	1	43	780
Chef Salad	10	283	230	20.5	7.5	13.3	2	128	490
Garden Salad	8	213	110	7.1	6.2	6.6	2	83	160
Chicken Salad Oriental	9	244	140	23.1	5.0	3.4	2	78	230
Side Salad	4	115	60	3.7	3.3	3.3	1	41	85
Bleu Cheese Dressing	1	14	70	0.5	1.2	6.9	0	6	150
French Dressing	1	14	58	0.1	2.7	5.2	0	0	180
Ranch Dressing	1	14	83	0.2	1.3	8.6	0	5	130
1000 Island Dressing	1	14	78	0.2	2.4	7.5	0	8	100
Lite Vinaigrette Dressing	1	14	15	0.2	2.0	0.5	0	0	75
Oriental Dressing	1	14	24	0.2	5.8	0.1	0	0	180
Red French Reduced Calorie Dressing	1	14	40	0.1	5.2	1.9	0	0	110
Caesar Dressing	1	14	60	0.4	0.6	6.1	0	7	170
Peppercorn Dressing	1	14	80	0.2	0.5	8.7	0	7	85
French Fries, Small	2	68	220	3.1	25.6	12.0	2	9	110
French Fries, Medium	3	97	320	4.4	36.3	17.1	3	12	150
French Fries, Large	4	122	400	5.6	45.9	21.6	3	16	200
Apple Pie	3	83	260	2.2	30.0	14.8	2	6	240
Vanilla Low-fat Milk Shake	11	293	290	10.8	60.0	1.3	0	10	170
Chocolate Low-fat Milk Shake	11	293	320	11.0	66.0	1.7	1	10	240
Strawberry Low-fat Milk Shake	11	293	320	10.7	67.0	1.3	0	10	170
Soft Serve Cone	3	86	140	3.9	21.9	4.5	0	16	70
Strawberry Sundae	6	171	210	5.7	49.2	1.1	1	5	95
Hot Fudge Sundae	6	169	240	7.3	50.5	3.2	1	6	170
Hot Caramel Sundae	6	174	270	6.6	59.3	2.8	0	13	180
McDonaldland Cookies	2	56	290	4.2	47.1	9.2	1	0	300

Item	Serving (oz)	(g)	Calories	Protein (g)	Carbohydrate (g)	Total fat (g)	Dietary fiber (g)	Cholesterol (mg)	Sodium (mg)
Restaurant: McDonald's—cont'd									
Chocolaty Chip Cookies	2	56	330	4.2	41.9	15.6	0	4	280
Restaurant: Pizza Hut									
Pan Pizza, 2 slices									
Cheese	7	205	492	30.0	57.0	18.0	5	34	940
Pepperoni	8	211	540	29.0	62.0	22.0	5	42	1127
Supreme	9	255	589	32.0	53.0	30.0	7	48	1363
Super Supreme	9	257	563	33.0	53.0	26.0	6	55	1447
Thin 'n Crispy Pizza, 2 slices									
Cheese	5	148	398	28.0	37.0	17.0	4	33	867
Pepperoni	5	146	413	26.0	20.0	20.0	4	46	986
Supreme	7	200	459	28.0	41.0	22.0	5	42	1328
Super Supreme	7	203	463	29.0	44.0	21.0	5	56	1336
Hand-Tossed Pizza, 2 slices									
Cheese	8	220	518	34.0	55.0	20.0	7	55	1276
Pepperoni	7	197	500	28.0	50.0	23.0	6	50	1267
Supreme	8	239	540	32.0	50.0	26.0	7	55	1470
Super Supreme	9	243	556	33.0	54.0	25.0	7	54	1648
Personal Pan Pizza, 1 pizza									
Pepperoni	9	256	675	37.0	76.0	29.0	8	53	1335
Supreme	9	264	647	33.0	76.0	28.0	9	49	1313
Restaurant: Taco Bell									
Bean Burrito/Red Sauce	7	191	356	13.1	54.4	10.2	5	9	888
Beef Burrito/Red Sauce	7	191	403	22.5	39.1	17.3	3	57	1051
Burrito Supreme/Red Sauce	9	241	413	18.0	46.6	17.6	4	33	921
Double Beef Burrito									
Supreme/Red Sauce	9	255	457	23.7	41.7	21.8		57	1053
Tostada/Red Sauce	6	156	243	9.5	26.6	11.1	6	16	596
Enchirito/Red Sauce	8	213	382	19.8	30.9	19.7	4	54	1243
Pintos and Cheese/Red Sauce	5	128	191	9.0	19.0	8.7	4	16	642
Nachos	4	106	346	7.5	37.5	18.5	4	9	399
Nachos Bellgrande	10	287	649	21.6	60.6	35.3	7	36	997
Taco	28	778	183	10.3	11.0	10.8	1	32	276
Taco Bellgrande	6	163	355	18.3	17.7	23.1	2	56	472
Taco Light	6	170	410	19.0	18.1	28.8	2	56	594
Soft Taco	3	92	228	11.8	17.9	11.9	1	32	516
Soft Taco Supreme	4	124	275	12.6	19.1	16.3	1	32	516
Taco Salad/Salsa	21	595	941	36.0	63.1	61.3	10	80	1662
Taco Salad/Salsa Without									
Shell	19	530	520	30.6	30.0	31.4	6	80	1431
Taco Salad Without Shell	19	530	520	29.5	26.3	31.3	6	80	1056
Mexican Pizza	8	223	575	21.3	39.7	36.8	6	52	1031
Taco Sauce	<1	<1	2	0.1	0.4	0.0	0	0	126
Hot Taco Sauce	<1	<1	3	0.1	0.3	0.1	0	0	82

Item	Serving (oz)	(g)	Calories	Protein (g)	Carbohydrate (g)	Total fat (g)	Dietary fiber (g)	Cholesterol (mg)	Sodium (mg)
Restaurant: Taco Bell—cont'd									
Jalapeno Peppers	5	100	20	1.0	4.0	0.2	1	0	1370
Steak Fajita	5	135	234	14.6	19.5	10.9	1	14	485
Chicken Fajita	5	135	226	13.6	19.8	10.2	1	44	619
Sour Cream	1	21	46	0.6	0.9	4.4	0	16	10
Pico De Gallo	1	28	8	0.3	1.1	0.2	0	1	88
Guacamole	1	21	34	0.4	3.0	2.3	1	0	113
Meximelt	4	106	266	12.9	18.7	15.4	1	38	689
Restaurant: Wendy's									
Junior Hamburger	3	104	260	15.0	32.0	9.0	1	35	570
Junior Cheeseburger	3	116	300	18.0	33.0	13.0	1	35	770
Small Hamburger	4	111	260	15.0	33.0	9.0	1	34	570
Small Cheeseburger	4	125	310	18.0	33.0	13.0	1	34	770
Chicken Sandwich	8	219	430	26.0	41.0	19.0	2	60	725
Big Classic/Cheese	10	295	640	30.0	46.0	38.0	4	100	1370
Plain Single	4	126	340	24.0	30.0	15.0	1	65	500
Single/Everything	8	210	420	25.0	35.0	21.0	1	70	890
Plain Single/Cheese	5	137	410	25.0	29.0	22.0	1	80	710
Garden Salad (Take-Out)	10	227	102	7.0	9.0	5.0	4	0	110
Chef Salad (Take-Out)	12	331	180	15.0	10.0	9.0	4	120	140
New Chili	9	256	220	21.0	23.0	7.0	7	45	750
Taco Salad	28	791	660	40.0	46.0	37.0	9	35	1110
French Fries, Small	3	91	240	3.0	33.0	12.0	2	15	145
Baked Potatoes									
Plain	9	250	250	6	52	<1	5	0	60
W/bacon and cheese	12	350	570	19	57	30	5	22	1180
W/broccoli and cheese	13	365	500	13	54	25	5	22	430
W/cheese	12	350	590	17	55	34	5	22	450
W/chili and cheese	14	400	510	22	63	20	8	22	610
W/sour cream and chives	11	310	460	7	53	24	5	15	230

Glossary

aerobic activity   Any organized activity that is rhythmic in nature and involves continuous movement in which large muscle groups are involved. Examples include walking, jogging, aerobic dance, swimming, cross-country skiing, and a variety of other activities.

aerobic capacity   The maximal rate at which work can be performed with the body supplying energy aerobically.

aerobic dance   A series of exercises or dance routines performed to music. Also referred to as "aerobics to music" or simply "aerobics."

aerobic fitness   See cardiovascular endurance.

aerobic work   Activities using large muscle groups at an intensity that can be sustained for a long period during which the body is able to provide sufficient energy aerobically.

amino acids   The constituents of protein. An adequate amount of each of these is necessary for the body to make protein.

anaerobic work   A high-intensity activity that can be sustained for only a short period, because energy demands are greater than the capacity of the heart and circulatory system to supply the energy.

angina pectoris   A chest pain caused by insufficient blood supply to the heart.

arteriosclerosis   A hardening of the arteries that causes the arterial walls to thicken and lose elasticity.

artery   A blood vessel that transports blood away from the heart.

atherosclerosis   A narrowing and hardening of the arteries as fatty substances build up on arterial walls.

atrium   An upper chamber of the heart (blood being returned to the heart first enters the right or left atrium).

ball-and-socket joint   A joint where the rounded head of one bone fits into the hollow cavity of another.

ballistic stretching   A series of bouncing and jerking movements, where force generated by the moving segment provides the force necessary to stretch the muscle.

bench aerobics   A sequence of exercises performed to music where participants step up to and down from a bench using a variety of step combinations.

blood pressure   The force exerted by blood against the walls of blood vessels.

body composition   A comparison of the relative amounts of lean body weight and fat tissue in the body.

caloric expenditure   The total calories for all activities performed over a given period.

caloric intake   The caloric content of all food that is ingested.

calorie   A unit for measuring energy—calories in food represent the energy value of foods.

capillary   The smallest blood vessel in which exchange of gases takes place between blood and tissues.

carbohydrate   An organic nutrient derived from a plant source that provides the major source of energy in the body.

cardiac output   The amount of blood circulated by the heart each minute.

cardiovascular   Pertaining to the heart and blood vessels.

cardiovascular disease   All disease pertaining to the heart and blood vessels—includes hypertension, coronary heart disease, rheumatic heart disease, and stroke.

cardiovascular endurance   An extremely high efficiency in the functioning of the heart, lungs, and blood vessels that results in increased efficiency in the performance of continuous work involving large muscle groups. Also referred to as aerobic fitness.

cholesterol   A fatlike substance that is obtained only from foods of animal origin and that may be manufactured by the body.

cholesterol/HDL ratio   The ratio of total cholesterol to high-density lipoprotein cholesterol (HDL).

circuit   A given number of exercises arranged and numbered consecutively.

circuit training   A series of exercises arranged in a specific sequence so that participants can complete a predetermined number of repetitions as quickly as possible at each exercise "station."

circuit weight training   A combination of circuit training and weight training to develop an aerobic fitness routine.

collateral circulation   A system of small arteries that may carry blood to part of the heart when a coronary artery is blocked.

complete protein   Any food containing all nine of the essential amino acids—includes meats, fish, poultry, eggs, and dairy products.

complex carbohydrate   A compound consisting of many sugar molecules linked together—includes starches and fiber.

concentric contraction   An isotonic contraction where the muscle shortens and works against gravity.

contract-relaxation stretching technique   A stretching technique to increase the ability of muscles to relax.

cool down   A process whereby you gradually slow down after a workout or exercise session, rather than stopping abruptly. Walking until your heart returns to near your resting value is an example of a cool-down activity.

critical or threshold heart rate   The minimal heart rate necessary for the development of cardiovascular endurance.

desirable weight   The weight at which a person looks good, feels good, and functions efficiently.

diabetes   A disease characterized by an abnormal level of blood glucose.

diastole   The relaxation phase of the cardiac cycle when the heart is not contracting.

distress   A high level of stress associated with negative responses such as anxiety, tension, and frustration.

duration   The time that an activity must be continued with the heart rate at a specified level to result in improvement of cardiovascular fitness.

eccentric contraction   An isotonic contraction in which the muscle lengthens while it performs work as it returns to its original position.

elasticity (muscle)   The ability of a muscle to regain its original shape after being stretched.

energy nutrient   A nutrient that provides energy in the form of calories—carbohydrates, fat, and protein.

essential nutrient   A necessary nutrient that cannot be manufactured by the body and therefore must be obtained from the food you eat.

eustress   A positive reaction to stress, resulting in responses such as joy and happiness.

fat   A nutrient that is a secondary source of energy in the body and that can be stored in the body (also referred to as lipids or oils).

fiber   Any part of a food plant that cannot be broken down and digested by the human body—usually found in the stems, leaves, and seeds of plants.

flexibility   The range of motion that is possible at a joint or joints.

frequency   The number of times you must exercise each week to result in improvement in cardiovascular endurance.

hamstring   The large muscle group located at the back of the thigh that crosses both the hip and knee joint.

health   A state of complete physical, mental, and emotional well-being.

heart   The muscular pump responsible for circulation of blood through the circulatory system.

heart rate   The number of times the heart contracts per minute.

hemoglobin   An iron-containing protein found in blood that is responsible for transportation of oxygen.

high-density lipoprotein (HDL)   A lipoprotein that contains the highest proportion of protein; often referred to as "good" cholesterol.

hinge joint   A joint that allows movement to take place in one direction and where the only movements possible are flexion and extension.

hypertension   Blood pressure that is consistently higher than normal.

hypokinetic disease   A disease related to or resulting from lack of sufficient activity—includes such diseases as cardiovascular disease, osteoporosis, low back pain, hypertension, and type II diabetes.

incomplete protein   Any food containing protein that does not contain all nine of the essential amino acids—includes grain products, green leafy vegetables, nuts and seeds, and legumes.

insoluble fiber   The type of fiber that does not dissolve in water—it is found in the cell walls of many grains, vegetables, and fruits.

intensity   Stress placed on the body by an activity. It can usually be measured by the heart rate response to the work involved.

intensity of exercise   The stress placed on the body by the activity. With aerobic activities it can be adequately determined by the heart rate response to the work involved.

isokinetic contraction   An isotonic contraction where the speed of motion is controlled so that the maximal force is applied by the muscle through a full range of motion.

isometric contraction   A contraction where the force exerted by the muscle is equal to or less than the resistance. No movement takes place at the joint, and there is no change in the length of the muscles. Also called static contradiction.

isotonic contraction   A contraction where movement occurs at the joint and there is a shortening and lengthening of muscles involved. Also called dynamic contraction.

jogging   A slow form of running.

joint   A junction of two or more bones.

lean body weight   The total amount of body weight that is not attributable to fat—includes muscles, ligaments, tendons, bones, and fluids.

ligament   A tough band of tissue that holds bones together.

lipoprotein   The combination of lipid with protein so that lipids can be transported in the blood.

low-density lipoprotein (LDL)   A lipoprotein that contains the highest proportion of cholesterol; high levels of LDL have been associated with increased incidence of cardiovascular disease.

maximal heart rate   The maximal heart rate the body is capable of attaining. It can be estimated by subtracting your age from 220.

maximal oxygen consumption   The maximal level of oxygen the body is capable of processing and using. It is considered to be the best measure of cardiovascular endurance. It is also referred to as maximal oxygen uptake, aerobic capacity, and physical work capacity.

migraine headache   Intense pain in the head, usually confined to one side of the head. May be preceded by changes in vision.

minerals   Inorganic substances needed by the body for specific functions.

muscular endurance   The ability of a muscle or muscle group to apply force repeatedly or to sustain a contraction for a period.

negative energy balance   Occurs when the number of calories consumed is less than the number of calories used and results in a loss of body weight or body fat.

neutral energy balance   When the caloric intake and caloric expenditure are approximately equal, and body weight remains relatively constant.

nutrients   Basic substances needed by the body for a variety of functions.

obesity   An excessive accumulation of body fat.

one-repetition maximum (1 RM)   The maximum force that can be exerted only once by a muscle or muscle group.

organic   A nutrient containing carbon that can usually be oxidized or burned to produce energy.

overload   Subjecting a muscle to a workload greater than that to which it is accustomed.

overweight   When a person weighs 10% or more than his or her desirable weight.

percent body fat   The percentage of the total body weight that is attributable to fat.

physical fitness   An optimum level of efficiency in the functioning of the body.

plaque   A deposit of fatty substances (such as cholesterol) on the inner lining of an artery wall.

positive energy balance   Occurs when the caloric intake is greater than the caloric expenditure and results in an increase in body weight.

progression   Increasing the amount of work from time to time so that the body must work harder.

protein   Primary food substance formed from amino acids—used by the body primarily to build, repair, regulate, and replace the cells of the body.

quadriceps   The large muscle group at the front of the thigh responsible for extension at the knee joint.

rebound running   Stepping or bouncing on a mini-trampoline.

Recommended Dietary Allowance (RDA)   The amounts of essential nutrients considered adequate to meet the known nutritional needs of most healthy persons.

refined sugar   A term used to describe sweeteners, such as table sugar, that are created by processing and added to other foods as sweeteners.

repetition   Completion of a designated movement through a full range of motion.

resting heart rate   The number of times your heart contracts each minute while the body is at rest.

saturated fat   Fat found mainly in animal products that carries the maximum number of hydrogen atoms.

set   A specified number of repetitions attempted consecutively.

shin splints   A "catch-all" term that refers to a painful condition that occurs on the anterior portion of the lower leg. This condition often results from exercise performed on hard surfaces.

skinfold measurement The measurement of fat at a particular site using skinfold calipers.

soluble fiber Fiber that dissolves in water to form a gel—it is the nonstructural material in plant cells such as pectins and gums.

specificity of improvement Improvement occurring only in the area or areas that each exercise is designed to develop (applies only to strength, muscular endurance, and flexibility).

starch The most familiar form of carbohydrates found in plants, in seeds, and in the grain from which bread, cereal, spaghetti, and pasta are made.

static stretching Movement of a joint that occurs slowly and gradually through the maximal range of motion.

sticking point The point in the range of motion in an isotonic contraction where force applied by a muscle is weakest.

strength The amount of force a muscle or muscle group can exert against a resistance.

stressor Any change that causes a person to react in a stressful manner.

stretch reflex A mechanism that prevents overstretching of a muscle by forcing the muscle to contract.

stroke volume The amount of blood pumped from the left ventricle each time the heart contracts.

submaximal task A task performed aerobically at an intensity where the body can supply the necessary energy aerobically.

systole The contraction phase of the cardiac cycle when the ventricles contract and force blood out of the heart.

target-zone heart rate The heart rate necessary for maximal development of cardiovascular endurance. It is 70% to 85% of the maximal heart rate.

tendon Fibrous tissue that connects muscle to bone.

thrombus A blood clot.

triglycerides Fats consisting of three fatty acids and glycerol.

Type I diabetes A type of diabetes in which the body is unable to produce sufficient insulin.

Type II diabetes A type of diabetes in which insulin is ineffective in controlling the blood sugar level.

Type A personality A person who is aggressive, anxious, and impatient and who works excessively.

Type B personality A person who is relaxed, not rushed, and not affected by deadlines or demands.

unsaturated fat A fat found mainly in plant products that is usually liquid at room temperature. It contains less than the maximum number of hydrogen atoms.

vein A blood vessel that returns blood to the heart.

ventricle The lower chamber of the heart; responsible for pumping blood from the heart.

vitamins Organic compounds needed in small quantities by the body to perform specific functions.

warm-up The initial phase of the workout where you exercise at a low level of intensity and increase your body temperature and the temperature of the muscles involved in the exercise in preparation for a more strenuous level of activity.

wellness Accepting responsibility for one's lifestyle and making decisions that will result in a high level of physical well-being.

Index